TAKING SIDES

Clashing Views on

Bioethical Issues

TWELFTH EDITION

TAKING SIDES

Clashing Views on

Bioethical Issues

TWELFTH EDITION

Selected, Edited, and with Introductions by

Carol Levine
United Hospital Fund

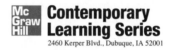
Contemporary Learning Series
2460 Kerper Blvd., Dubuque, IA 52001

Visit us on the Internet
http://www.mhcls.com

For Hannah, Amy, Asher, Maddy, and Max

Photo Acknowledgment
Cover image: Digital Vision/Getty Images

Cover Acknowledgment
Maggie Lytle

Compositor: ICC Macmillan Inc.

Manufactured in the United States of America

Twelfth Edition

123456789DOCDOC987

Library of Congress Cataloging-in-Publication Data
Main entry under title:
Taking sides: clashing views on controversial bioethical issues/selected, edited, and with
introductions by Carol Levine.—12th ed.
Includes bibliographical references and index.
1. Bioethics. I. Levine, Carol, *comp.*
174.957'4

MHID: 0-07-339718-0
ISBN: 978-0-07-339718-4
1091-8809

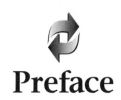

Preface

T his is a book about choices—hard and tragic choices. The choices are hard not only because they often involve life and death but also because there are convincing arguments on both sides of the issues. An ethical dilemma, by definition, is one that poses a conflict not between good and evil but between one good principle and another that is equally good. The choices are hard because the decisions that are made—by individuals, groups, and public policy-makers—will influence the kind of society we have today and the one we will have in the future.

Although the views expressed in the selections in this volume are strong—even passionate—they are also subtle, concerned with the nuances of the particular debate. *How* one argues matters in bioethics; you will see and have to weigh the significance of varying rhetorical styles and appeals throughout this volume.

Although there are no easy answers to any of the issues in the book, the questions will be answered in some fashion—partly by individual choices and partly by decisions that are made by professionals and government. We must make them the best answers possible, and that can only be done by informed and thoughtful consideration. This book, then, can serve as a beginning for what ideally will become an ongoing process of examination and reflection.

Changes to this edition   Many popular issues and the basic structure of the book remain from the previous edition. There are seven units: Medical Decision Making; Death and Dying; Choices in Reproduction; Children and Bioethics; Genetics; Human and Animal Experimentation; and Bioethics and Public Policy. There are four completely new issues: "Do Standard Medical Ethics Apply in Disaster Conditions?" (Issue 5), "Is Genetic Enhancement an Unacceptable Use of Technology?" (Issue 13), "Should Prisoners Be Allowed to Participate in Research?" (Issue 15), and "Should Federally Funded Health Care Be Tied to Following Doctors' Orders?" (Issue 16). In addition, two issues have been retitled and new articles substituted. Issue 12 is now titled "Is the Ban on Federal Funding of Stem Cell Research Justifiable?" and both the YES and NO selections are new. In all, there are 11 new selections. Unit introductions, issue introductions, and postscripts have been revised as necessary. Also, the *Internet References* page that begins each unit offers relevant Internet site addresses (URLs) that should prove useful as starting points for further research.

A word to the instructor   An *Instructor's Manual With Test Questions* (multiple-choice and essay) is available through the publisher, and a general guidebook, *Using Taking Sides in the Classroom*, which discusses methods and techniques for using the pro-con approach in any classroom setting, is also available. An online version of *Using Taking Sides in the Classroom* and a correspondence service for *Taking Sides* adopters can be found at http://www.mhcls.com/usingts/.

Taking Sides: Clashing Views on Bioethical Issues is only one title in the Taking Sides series. If you are interested in seeing the table of contents for any of the other titles, please visit the Taking Sides Web site at http://www.mhcls.com/takingsides/.

For this edition, Martha Hogan prepared the *Instructor's Manual*. Many people have helped on previous editions, chief among them Alexis Kuerbis, Dillan Siegler, Ben Munisteri, and Lauri Posner. Paul Homer, Eric Feldman, and Arthur Caplan were generously helpful at earlier stages of the series. Daniel Callahan and Willard Gaylin, co-founders of The Hastings Center, were instrumental in encouraging me to take on this project.

Carol Levine
United Hospital Fund

Contents In Brief

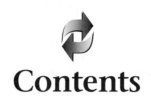

Contents

Physician Marcia Angell asserts that a physician's main duties are to respect patient autonomy and to relieve suffering, even if that sometimes means assisting in a patient's death. Physician Kathleen M. Foley counters that if physician-assisted suicide becomes legal, it will begin to substitute for interventions that otherwise might enhance the quality of life for dying patients.

Physician Steven H. Miles maintains that physicians' duty to follow patients' wishes ends when the requests are inconsistent with what medical care can reasonably be expected to achieve, when they violate community standards of care, and when they consume an unfair share of collective resources. Philosopher Felicia Ackerman contends that it is ethically inappropriate for physicians to decide what kind of life is worth prolonging and that decisions involving personal values should be made by the patient or family.

Philosopher Patrick Lee and professor of jurisprudence Robert P. George assert that human embryos and fetuses are complete (though immature) human beings and that intentional abortion is unjust and objectively immoral. Philosopher Margaret Olivia Little believes that the moral status of the fetus is only one aspect of the morality of abortion. She points to gestation as an intimacy, motherhood as a relationship, and creation as a process to advance a more nuanced approach.

In a case involving a pregnant woman's use of crack cocaine, a majority of the supreme court of South Carolina ruled that a state legislature may impose additional criminal penalties on pregnant drug-using women without violating their constitutional right of privacy. Attorney Lynn M. Paltrow argues that treating drug-using pregnant women as criminals targets poor, African American women while ignoring other drug usage and fails to provide the resources to assist them in recovery.

Ethicist Robert F. Weir and pediatrician Charles Peters assert that adolescents with normal cognitive and developmental skills have the capacity to make decisions about their own health care. Advance directives, if used appropriately, can give older pediatric patients a voice in their care. Pediatrician Lainie Friedman Ross counters that parents should be responsible for making their child's health care decisions. Children need to develop virtues, such as self-control, that will enhance their long-term, not just immediate, autonomy.

Massachusetts Citizens for Children, an advocacy organization, asserts that laws exempting parents from responsibility to provide medical care for their seriously ill children, on the basis of religious beliefs, result in needless deaths and mislead parents about their legal responsibilities. Professor of philosophy Mark Sheldon assesses the case of Jehovah's Witness parents who refuse to allow their children to undergo blood transfusions and concludes that they cannot be said to be truly harming or neglecting their children. Rather, they are placing their children's spiritual interests above worldly ones.

The President's Council on Bioethics supports the current ban on federal funding of embryonic stem call research based on the law and its underlying principle, and the significance of federal funding. Jerome Groopman, professor of medicine at Harvard, says that the policy fails on scientific and moral accounts and is essentially a political choice.

Political philosopher Michael J. Sandel believes that using genetic technology to enhance performance, design children, and perfect human nature is a flawed attempt at human mastery, and banishes appreciation of life as a gift. Physician Howard Trachtman says that the medical community should embrace enhancement as a never-ending quest for health that recognizes that perfection can never be achieved.

Jerod M. Loeb and his colleagues, representing the American Medical Association's Group on Science and Technology, assert that concern for animals, admirable in itself, cannot impede the development of methods to improve the welfare of humans. Philosopher Tom Regan argues that conducting research on animals exacts the grave moral price of failing to show proper respect for animals' inherent value, whatever the benefits of the research.

The Institute of Medicine Committee believes that the current protections for prisoners rely too much on their vulnerability as a category and should be revised to consider the potential risks and benefits of each study, thus allowing prisoners to participate in some kinds of research. Silja J. A. Talvi, an investigative journalist, believes that all prison research should end because prison medical care is so poor and there is such a high potential for abuse.

Philosopher J. Radcliffe-Richards and colleagues of the International Forum for Transplant Ethics contend that bans on selling organs remove the only hope of the destitute and dying. Arguments against selling organs are weak attempts to justify the repugnance felt by people who are rich or healthy. The Institute of Medicine Committee argues that a free market in organs is problematic because in live organ donation both buyers and sellers may not have complete or accurate information, and selling organs of dead people raises concerns about commodification of human bodies.

Law student Donald W. Herbe asserts that pharmacists' moral beliefs concerning abortion and emergency contraception are genuinely fundamental and deserve respect. He proposes that professional pharmaceutical organizations lead the way to recognizing a true right of conscience, which would eventually result in universal legislation protecting against all potential ramifications of choosing conscience. Julie Cantor, a lawyer, and Ken Baum, a physician and lawyer, reject an absolute right to object, as well as no right to object, to these prescriptions but assert that pharmacists who cannot or will not dispense a drug have a professional obligation to meet the needs of their customers by referring them elsewhere.

Law and public health professor Lawrence O. Gostin states that the threat of bioterrorism makes it imperative to reframe the balance between individual interests and society's need to protect itself so that the common good prevails. Law professor George J. Annas contends that taking human rights seriously is our best defense against terrorism and fosters public health on both a federal and global scale.

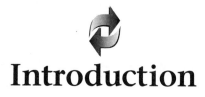

Introduction

Medicine and Moral Arguments

Carol Levine

In the fall of 1975 a 21-year-old woman lay in a New Jersey hospital—as she had for months—in a coma, the victim of a toxic combination of barbiturates and alcohol. Doctors agreed that her brain was irreversibly damaged and that she would never recover. Her parents, after anguished consultation with their priest, asked the doctors and hospital to disconnect the respirator that was artificially maintaining their daughter's life. When the doctors and hospital refused, the parents petitioned the court to be made her legal guardian so that they could authorize the withdrawal of treatment. After hearing all the arguments, the court sided with the parents, and the respirator was removed. Contrary to everyone's expectations, however, the young woman did not die but began to breathe on her own (perhaps because, in anticipation of the court order, the nursing staff had gradually weaned her from total dependence on the respirator). She lived for 10 years until her death in June 1985—comatose, lying in a fetal position, and fed with tubes—in a New Jersey nursing home.

The young woman's name was Karen Ann Quinlan, and her case brought national attention to the thorny ethical questions raised by modern medical technology: When, if ever, should life-sustaining technology be withdrawn? Is the sanctity of life an absolute value? What kinds of treatment are really beneficial to a patient in a "chronic vegetative state" like Karen's? And, perhaps the most troubling question, who shall decide? These and similar questions are at the heart of the growing field of biomedical ethics, or (as it is usually called) *bioethics*.

Ethical dilemmas in medicine are, of course, nothing new. They have been recognized and discussed in Western medicine since a small group of physicians—led by Hippocrates—on the Isle of Cos in Greece, around the fourth century B.C., subscribed to a code of practice that newly graduated physicians still swear to uphold today. But unlike earlier times, when physicians and scientists had only limited abilities to change the course of disease, today they can intervene in profound ways in the most fundamental processes of life and death. Moreover, ethical dilemmas in medicine are no longer considered the sole province of professionals. Professional codes of ethics, to be sure, offer some guidance, but they are usually unclear and ambiguous about what to do in specific situations. More important, these codes assume that whatever decision is to be made is up to the professional, not the patient. Today, to an ever-greater degree, laypeople—patients, families, lawyers, clergy, and others—want to and have become involved in ethical decision making not only in individual cases, such as the Quinlan case, but also in large societal decisions, such as how to allocate scarce medical resources, including high-technology machinery, newborn intensive care units, and the expertise of physicians. While questions about the physician-patient relationship and individual cases are still prominent in bioethics (see, for example, the issues on truth telling and assisting dying patients in suicide), today the field covers a broad range of other decisions as well, such as the use of reproductive technology, the harvesting and transplantation of organs, equity in access to health care, and the future of animal experimentation.

This involvement is part of broader social trends: a general disenchantment with the authority of all professionals and, hence, a greater readiness to challenge the traditional belief that "doctor knows best"; the growth of various civil rights movements among women, the aged, and minorities—of which the patients' rights movement is a spin-off; the enormous size and complexity of the health care delivery system, in which patients and families often feel alienated from the professional; the increasing cost of medical care, much of it at public expense; and the growth of the "medical model," in which conditions that used to be considered outside the scope of physicians' control, such as alcoholism and behavioral problems, have come to be considered diseases.

Bioethics began in the 1950s as an intellectual movement among a small group of physicians and theologians who started to examine the questions raised by the new medical technologies that were starting to emerge as the result of the heavy expenditure of public funds in medical research after World War II. They were soon joined by a number of philosophers who had become disillusioned with what they saw as the arid abstractions of much analytic philosophy at the time and by lawyers who sought to find principles in the law that would guide ethical decision making or, if such principles were not there, to develop them by case law and legislation or regulation. Although these four disciplines—medicine, theology, philosophy, and law—still dominate the field, today bioethics is an interdisciplinary effort, with political scientists, economists, sociologists, anthropologists, nurses, allied health professionals, policymakers, psychologists, and others contributing their special perspectives to the ongoing debates.

The issues discussed in this volume attest to the wide range of bioethical dilemmas, their complexity, and the passion they arouse. But if bioethics today is at the frontiers of scientific knowledge, it is also a field with ancient roots. It goes back to the most basic questions of human life: What is right? What is wrong? How should people act toward others? And why?

While the *bio* part of *bioethics* gives the field its urgency and immediacy, we should not forget that the root word is *ethics*.

Applying Ethics to Medical Dilemmas

To see where bioethics fits into the larger framework of academic inquiry, some definitions are in order. First, *morality* is the general term for an individual's or a society's standards of conduct, both actual and ideal, and of the character traits that determine whether people are considered "good" or "bad." The scientific study of morality is called *descriptive ethics*; a scientist—generally an anthropologist, sociologist, or historian—can describe in empirical terms what the moral beliefs, judgments, or actions of individuals or societies are and what reasons are given for the way they act or what they believe. The philosophical study of morality, on the other hand, approaches the subject of morality in one of two different ways: either as an analysis of the concepts, terms, and methods of reasoning (*metaethics*) or as an analysis of what those standards or moral judgments ought to be (*normative ethics*). Metaethics deals with meanings of moral terms and logic; normative ethics, with which the issues in this volume are concerned, reflects on the kinds of actions and principles that will promote moral behavior.

Because normative ethics accepts the idea that some acts and character traits are more moral than others (and that some are immoral), it rejects the rather popular idea that ethics is relative. Because different societies have different moral codes and values, ethical relativists have argued that there can be no universal moral judgments: What is right or wrong depends on who does it and where, and whether or not society approves. Although it is certainly true that moral values are embedded in a social, cultural, and political context, it is also true that certain moral judgments are universal. We think it is wrong, for example, to sell people into slavery—whether or not a certain society approved or even whether or not a person wanted to be a slave. People may not agree about what these universal moral values are or ought to be, but it is hard to deny that some such values exist.

The other relativistic view rejected by normative ethics is the notion that whatever feels good *is* good. In this view, ethics is a matter of personal preference, weightier than one's choice of which automobile to buy, but not much different in kind. Different people, having different feelings, can arrive at equally valid moral judgments, according to the relativistic view. Just as we should not disregard cultural factors, we should not overlook the role of emotion and personal experience in arriving at moral judgments. But to give emotion ultimate authority would be to consign reason and rationality—the bases of moral argument—to the ethical trash heap. At the very least, it would be impossible to develop a just policy concerning the care of vulnerable persons, like the mentally retarded or newborns, who depend solely on the vagaries of individual caretakers.

Thus, if normative ethics is one branch of philosophy, bioethics is one branch of normative ethics; it is normative ethics applied to the practice of medicine and science. There are other branches—business ethics, legal ethics, journalism ethics, and military ethics, for example. One common term for the entire grouping is *applied and professional ethics*, because these ethics deal with the ethical standards of the members of a particular profession and how they are applied in the professionals' dealings with each other and the rest of society. Bioethics is based on the belief that some solutions to the dilemmas that arise in medicine and science are more moral than others and that these solutions can be determined by moral reasoning and reflection.

Ethical Theories

If the practitioners of bioethics do not rely solely on cultural norms and emotions, what are their sources of determining what is right or wrong? The most comprehensive source is a theory of ethics—a broad set of moral principles (or perhaps just one overriding principle) that is used in measuring human conduct. Divine law is one such source, of course, but even in the Western religious traditions of bioethics (both the Jewish and Catholic religions have rich and comprehensive commentaries on ethical issues, and the Protestant religion has a less cohesive but still important tradition) the law of God is interpreted in terms of human moral principles. Recently, bioethicists have paid more attention to analyzing the teachings of other religious traditions, such as Islam, Buddhism, Confucianism, and other Eastern religions. A theory of ethics must be acceptable to many groups, not just the followers of one religious tradition. Most writers outside the religious traditions (and some within them) have looked to one of three major traditions in ethics: teleological theories, deontological theories, and natural law theories.

Teleological Theories

Teleological theories are based on the idea that the end or purpose (from the Greek *telos,* or end) of the action determines its rightness or wrongness. The most prominent teleological theory is *utilitarianism*. In its simplest formulation, an act is moral if it brings more good consequences than bad ones. Utilitarian theories are derived from the works of two English philosophers: Jeremy Bentham (1748–1832) and John Stuart Mill (1806–1873). Rejecting the absolutist religious morality of his time, Bentham proposed that "utility"—the greatest good for the greatest number—should guide the actions of human beings. Invoking the hedonistic philosophy of Epicurean Greeks, Bentham said that pleasure (*hedon* in Greek) is good and pain is bad. Therefore, actions are right if they promote more pleasure than pain and wrong if they promote more pain than pleasure. Mill found the highest utility in "happiness," rather than pleasure. (Mill's philosophy is echoed in the Declaration of Independence's espousal of "life, liberty, and the pursuit of happiness.") Other utilitarians have looked to a range of utilities, or goods (including friendship, love, devotion, and the like) that they believe ought to be weighed in the balance—the utilitarian calculus.

Utilitarianism has a pragmatic appeal. It is flexible, and it seems impartial. However, its critics point out that utilitarianism can be used to justify suppression of individual rights for the good of society ("the ends justify the means") and that it is difficult to quantify and compare "utilities," however they are defined.

Utilitarianism, in its many forms, has had a powerful influence on bioethical discussion, partly because it is the closest to the case-by-case risk/benefit ratio that physicians use in clinical decision making. Joseph Fletcher, a Protestant theologian who was one of the pioneers in bioethics in the 1950s, developed utilitarian theories that he called *situation ethics*. He argued that a true Christian morality does not blindly follow moral rules but acts from love and sensitivity to the particular situation and the needs of those involved. He has enthusiastically supported most modern technologies on the grounds that they lead to good ends.

Writers in this volume who use utilitarian theories to arrive at their moral judgments include Lawrence O. Gostin, who defends giving public health agencies sweeping powers in a bioterrorist threat; and Jerod M. Loeb and his colleagues, who defend animal experimentation.

Deontological Theories

The second major type of ethical theory is *deontological* (from the Greek *deon,* or duty). The rightness or wrongness of an act, these theories hold, should be judged on whether or not it conforms to a moral principle or rule, not on whether it leads to good or bad consequences. The primary exponent of a deontological theory was Immanuel Kant (1724–1804), a German philosopher. Kant declared that there is an ultimate norm, or supreme duty, which he called the "Moral Law." He held that an act is moral only if it springs from a "good will," the only thing that is good without qualification.

We must do good things, said Kant, because we have a duty to do them, not because they result in good consequences or because they give us pleasure (although that can happen as well). Kant constructed a formal "Categorical Imperative," the ultimate test of morality: "I ought never to act except in such a way that I can also will that my maxim should become universal law." Recognizing that this formulation was far from clear, Kant said the same thing in three other ways. He explained that a moral rule must be one that can serve as a guide for everyone's conduct; it must be one that permits people to treat each other as ends in themselves, not solely as means to another's ends; and it must be one that each person can impose on himself by his own will, not one that is solely imposed by the state, one's parents, or God. Kant's Categorical Imperative, in the simplest terms, says that all persons have equal moral worth and that no rule can be moral unless all people can apply it autonomously to all other human beings. Although on its own Kant's Categorical Imperative is merely a formal statement with no moral content at all, he gave some examples of what he meant: "Do not commit suicide," and "Help others in distress."

Kantian ethics is criticized by many who note that Kant gives little guidance on what to do when ethical principles conflict, as they often do. Moreover, they say, his emphasis on autonomous decision making and individual will neglects the social and communal context in which people live and make decisions. It leads to isolation and unreality. These criticisms notwithstanding, Kantian ethics has stimulated much current thinking in bioethics. In this volume, the idea that certain actions are in and of themselves right or wrong underlies, for example, Patrick Lee and Robert P. George's argument against abortion because it involves killing a human being; Tom Regan's opposition to animal research; and President's Council on Bioethics' opposition to federal funding of human stem cell research.

Two modern deontological theorists are philosophers John Rawls and Robert M. Veatch. In *A Theory of Justice* (1971), Rawls places the highest value on equitable distribution of society's resources. He believes that society has a fundamental obligation to correct the inequalities of historical circumstance and natural endowment of its least well off members. According to this theory, some action is good only if it benefits the least well off. (It can also benefit others, but that is secondary.) His social justice theory has influenced bioethical writings concerning the allocation of scarce resources.

Veatch has applied Rawlsian principles to medical ethics. In his book, *A Theory of Medical Ethics* (1981), he offers a model of social contract among professionals, patients, and society that emphasizes mutual respect and responsibilities. This contract model will, he hopes, avoid the narrowness of professional codes of ethics and the generalities and ambiguities of more broadly based ethical theories.

Natural Law Theory

The third strain of ethical theory that is prominent in bioethics is *natural law theory*, first developed by St. Thomas Aquinas (1223–1274). According to this theory, actions are morally right if they accord with our nature as human beings. The attribute that is distinctively human is the ability to reason and to exercise intelligence. Thus, argues this theory, we can know the good, which is objective and can be learned through reason. References to natural law theory are prominent in the works of Catholic theologians and writers; they see natural law as ultimately derived from God but knowable through the efforts of human beings. The influence of natural law theory can be seen in the issues on human stem cell research and genetic enhancement.

Theory of Virtue

The *theory of virtue*, another ethical theory with deep roots in the Aristotelian tradition, has recently been revived in bioethics. This theory stresses not the morality of any particular actions or rules but the disposition of individuals to act morally, to be virtuous. In its modern version, its primary exponent is Alasdair MacIntyre, whose book *After Virtue* (1980) urges a return to the Aristotelian model. Gregory Pence has applied the theory of virtue directly to medicine in *Ethical Options in Medicine* (1980); he lists temperance in personal life, compassion for the suffering patient, professional competence, justice, honesty, courage, and practical judgment as the virtues that are most desirable in physicians. Although this theory has not yet been as fully developed in bioethics as the utilitarian or deontological theories, it is likely to have particular appeal for physicians—many of whom have resisted formal ethics education on the grounds that moral character is the critical factor and that one can best learn to be a moral physician by emulating one's mentors. Although not explicit, assumptions about the qualities of a virtuous physician underlie the discussion in Issue 5 on disaster conditions and Issue 6 on physician-assisted suicide.

Although various authors, in this volume and elsewhere, appeal in rather direct ways to either utilitarian or deontological theories, often the various types are combined. One may argue both that a particular action is immoral in and of itself and that it will have bad consequences (some commentators say even Kant used this argument). In fact, probably no single ethical theory is adequate to deal with all the ramifications of the issues. In that case we can turn to a middle level of ethical discussion. Between the abstractions of ethical theories (Kant's Categorical Imperative) and the specifics of moral judgments (always obtain informed consent from a patient) is a range of concepts—ethical principles—that can be applied to particular cases.

Ethical Principles

In its four years of deliberation in the 1970s, the National Commission for the Protection of Human Subjects of Biomedical and Behavioral Research grappled with some of the most difficult issues facing researchers and society: When, if ever, is it ethical to do research on fetuses, on children, or on people in mental institutions? This commission—which was composed of people from various religious backgrounds, professions, and social strata—was finally able to agree on specific recommendations on these questions, but only after they had finished their work did the commissioners try to determine what ethical principles they had used in reaching a consensus. In their Belmont Report (1978), named after the conference center where they met to discuss this question, the commissioners outlined what they considered to be the three most important ethical principles (respect for persons, beneficence, and justice) that should govern the conduct of research with human beings. These three principles, they believed, are generally accepted in our cultural tradition and can serve as basic justifications for the many particular ethical prescriptions and evaluations of human action. Because of the principles' general acceptance and widespread applicability, they are at the basis of most bioethical discussion. Although philosophers argue about whether other principles—preventing harm to others or loyalty, for example—ought to be accorded equal weight with these three or should be included under another umbrella, they agree that these principles are fundamental.

Respect for Persons

Respect for persons incorporates at least two basic ethical convictions, according to the Belmont Report. Individuals should be treated as autonomous agents, and persons with diminished autonomy are entitled to protection. The derivation from Kant is clear. Because human beings have the capacity for rational action and moral choice, they have a value independent of anything that they can do or provide to others. Therefore, they should be treated in a way that respects their independent choices and judgments. Respecting autonomy means giving weight to autonomous persons' considered opinions and choices, and refraining from interfering with their choices unless those choices are clearly detrimental to others. However, since the capacity for autonomy varies with age, mental disability, or other circumstances, those people whose autonomy is diminished must be protected—but only in ways that serve their interests and do not interfere with the level of autonomy that they do possess. This subject is discussed in Issue 10 on adolescent life-and-death decision making.

Two important moral rules are derived from the ethical principle of respect for persons: informed consent and truth telling. Persons can exercise autonomy only when they have been fully informed about the range of options open to them, and the process of informed consent is generally considered to include the elements of information, comprehension, and voluntariness. Thus, a person can give informed consent to some medical procedure only if he or she has full information about the risks and benefits, understands them, and agrees voluntarily—that is, without being coerced or pressured into agreement. Although the principle of informed consent has become an accepted moral rule (and a legal one as well), it is difficult—some say impossible—to achieve in a real-world setting. It can easily be turned into a legalistic parody or avoided altogether. But as a moral ideal it serves to balance the unequal power of the physician and patient.

Another important moral ideal derived from the principle of respect for persons is truth telling. It held a high place in Kant's theory. In his essay "The Supposed Right to Tell Lies From Benevolent Motives," he wrote: "If, then, we define a lie merely as an intentionally false declaration towards another man, we need not add that it must injure another . . . ; for it always injures another; if not another individual, yet mankind generally. . . . To be truthful in all declarations is therefore a sacred and conditional command of reasons, and not to be limited by any other expediency."

Other important moral rules that are derived from the principle of respect for persons are confidentiality and privacy.

Beneficence

Most physicians would probably consider beneficence (from the Latin *bene,* or good) the most basic ethical principle. In the Hippocratic Oath it is used this way: "I will apply dietetic measures for the benefit of the sick according to my ability and judgment; I will keep them from harm and injustice." And further on, "Whatever houses I may visit, I will comfort and benefit the sick, remaining free of all intentional injustice." The phrase *Primum non nocere* (First, do no harm) is another well-known version of this idea, but it appears to be a much later, Latinized version—not from the Hippocratic period.

Philosopher William Frankena has outlined four elements included in the principle of beneficence: (1) One ought not to inflict evil or harm; (2) one ought to prevent evil or harm; (3) one ought to remove evil or harm; and (4) one ought to do or promote good. Frankena arranged these elements in hierarchical order, so that the first takes precedence over the second, and so on. In this scheme, it is more important to avoid doing evil or harm than to do good. But in the Belmont Report, beneficence is understood as an obligation—first, to do no harm, and second, to maximize possible benefits and minimize possible harms.

The principle of beneficence is at the basis of Marcia Angell's support of allowing physicians to assist some patients in suicide and of Christopher James Ryan's concerns that some advance directives are too risky for patients.

Justice

The third ethical principle that is generally accepted is justice, which means "what is fair" or "what is deserved." An injustice occurs when some benefit to which a person is entitled is denied without good reason or when some burden is imposed unduly, according to the Belmont Report. Another way of interpreting the principle is to say that equals should be treated equally. However, some distinctions—such as age, experience, competence, physical condition, and the like—can justify unequal treatment. Those who appeal to the principle of justice are most concerned about which distinctions can be made legitimately and which ones cannot (see Issue 20 on pharmacists' refusals on conscience grounds).

One important derivative of the principle of justice is the recent emphasis on "rights" in bioethics. Given the successes in the 1960s and 1970s of civil rights movements in the courts and political arena, it is easy to understand the appeal of "rights talk." An emphasis on individual rights is part of the American tradition, in a way that emphasis on the "common good" is not. The language of rights has been prominent in the abortion debate, for instance, where the "right to life" has been pitted against the "right to privacy" or the "right to control one's body." The "right to health care" is a potent rallying cry, though it is one that is difficult to enforce legally. Although claims to rights may be effective in marshaling political support and in emphasizing moral ideals, those rights may not be the most effective way to solve ethical dilemmas. Our society, as philosopher Ruth Macklin has pointed out, has not yet agreed on a theory of justice in health care that will determine who has what kinds of rights and—the other side of the coin—who has the obligation to fulfill them.

When Principles Conflict

These three fundamental ethical principles—respect for persons, beneficence, and justice—all carry weight in ethical decision making. But what happens when they conflict? That is what this book is all about.

On each side of the issues included in this volume are writers who appeal, explicitly or implicitly, to one or more of these principles. For example, in Issue 9, Jean Toal sees beneficence as paramount, and she would criminalize drug-using behavior by pregnant women in order to prevent harm to their fetuses. Lynn M. Paltrow finds such a policy unjust because it singles out certain risks and certain women for state intervention.

Some of the issues are concerned with how to interpret a particular principle: Whether, for example, it is more or less beneficent to allow a physician to assist in suicide, or whether society's interest in obtaining transplantable organs for those who need them and allowing payment for them.

Will it ever be possible to resolve such fundamental divisions—those that are not merely matters of procedure or interpretation but of fundamental differences in principle? Lest the situation seem hopeless, consider that some consensus does seem to have been reached on questions that seemed equally tangled a few decades ago. The idea that government should play a role in regulating human subjects research was hotly debated, but it is now generally accepted (at least if the research is medical, not social or behavioral in nature, and is federally funded). And the appropriateness of using the criterion of brain death for determining the death of a person (and the possibility of subsequent removal of their organs for transplantation) has largely been accepted and written into state laws. The idea that a hopelessly ill patient has the legal and moral right to refuse treatment that will only postpone dying is also well established (though it is often hard to exercise because hospitals and physicians continue to resist it). Finally, nearly everyone now agrees that health care is distributed unjustly in the United States—a radical idea only a few years ago. There is, of course, sharp disagreement about whose responsibility it is to rectify the situation—the government's or the private sector's.

In the 20 years since the first edition of this book was published, the dominance of principles as the foundation of bioethics has been challenged. Several philosophers have pointed out, as already noted, that the "mid-level" principles are not grounded in a unified moral theory. Other writers have described the philosophical mode of argument as too arid and abstract, and they have called for the inclusion of other forms of discourse, such as public policy, emotionbased reasoning, and narrative, or "storytelling."

Besides the virtue theory, already described, two other candidates have their defenders. The ethics of caring has been presented as an alternative to traditional bioethics reasoning. Women, it is claimed, embody an ethic of caring, which is itself a prime aim of healing relationships. An ethic of caring would focus on relationships rather than autonomy, on reconciliation rather than winning an argument, and on nurturing rather than imposing dominance. While the absence of caring relationships is clearly a problem in modern health care, this view has been severely criticized by many, including women, as failing to provide a sufficient basis for replacing ethical principles.

Another mode of analysis that is being revived is casuistry. Although associated with the Middle Ages and religious thinking, casuistry is simply a way of reaching consensus on principles by focusing on concrete cases—the clearest ones first, and then the harder ones. The casuist reaches principles from the bottom up, rather than deciding cases from the top (principles first) down.

A final form of analysis is clinical ethics. Its practitioners focus on the clinical realities of moral choices as they emerge in ordinary health care. It is not antithetical to principles but brings abstractions back to reality by measuring proposed solutions against the real world in which doctors and patients live and work. Issue 7 on the refusal of treatment on the grounds of "futility" builds on clinical ethics and real cases.

Edmund Pellegrino, a distinguished physician and ethicist, has seen many changes in the more than 50 years he has been involved in medicine. Looking toward the future, he does not see the death of principles, but he does foresee some changes. "Physicians and other health workers must become familiar with shifts in contemporary moral philosophy," he says, "if they are to maintain a hand in restructuring the ethics of their profession." But clinicians, too, must change, to "provide a reality check on the nihilism and skepticism of contemporary philosophy. Medical ethics is too ancient and too essential . . . to be left entirely to the fortuitous currents of philosophical fashion or the unsupported assertion of clinicians."

Although there is consensus in some areas, in others there is only controversy. This book will introduce you to some of the ongoing debates. Whether or not we will be able to move beyond opposing views to a realm of moral consensus will depend on society's willingness to struggle with these issues and to make the hard choices that are required.

Internet References . . .

Agency for Healthcare Research and Quality (AHRQ)

The AHRQ Web site provides research-based information to increase the scientific knowledge needed to enhance consumer and clinical decision making, improve health care quality, and promote efficiency in the organization of public and private systems of health care delivery.

http://www.ahrq.gov

Biomedical Ethics: Readings on the Internet

This site provides an article that outlines the history of patient autonomy and how it has transformed American medicine. Other articles concerning topics in bioethics are also included.

http://www.fdl.uwc.edu/faculty/rrigteri/biomed.htm

Bioethics Resources on the Web

Created by the National Institutes of Health Office of Science Policy, this is an excellent starting point and has links to other resources.

http://bioethics.od.nih.gov/

The National Reference Center for Bioethics Literature

Located at the Kennedy Institute of Ethics, Georgetown University, this site has extensive resources on physician-patient relationships and other topics and will perform data researches on request.

http://www.georgetown.edu/research/nrcbl/nrc/index.htm

Bioethics: Web Resources

Professor Tom May at Southern Methodist University has created a comprehensive and detailed guide that lists resources by topic, as well as sections on theology and bioethics, institutional links, and journals and newsletters.

http://faculty.smu.edu/tmayo/bioweb.htm

The Alden March Bioethics Institute

This institute maintains a Web site with information, news, and links to a bioethics blog.

http://www.bioethics.net/

Medical Decision Making

In earlier times medical decision making was of concern only to physicians. With their presumed greater knowledge and with patients' best interests at heart, they were entrusted with making life-and-death, as well as ordinary decisions. Ironically, although physicians had greater authority in those times than they do today, they also had less ability to treat. As medicine has grown more technologically and scientifically sophisticated, the range of people who have an interest in making decisions—and in some cases, a right to do so—among the medical options has grown. Law and ethics have reaffirmed the status of the patient as the primary decision maker. Nevertheless, many ambiguous and troubling situations remain in implementing patients' wishes. It is not even clear that patients have the moral right to make arbitrary decisions about aspects of their care, especially when their preferences impinge on the rights of others, such as family members, physicians, and other patients. Many cultural traditions find Western values, such as truth-telling, harmful to patients. Moreover, as marketplace values have entered medicine in dramatic ways, individuals are now seen more often as "consumers" rather than "patients." Prescription drug advertising that appeals directly to consumers raises questions about the balance between individual autonomy and physician beneficence. This section explores some of the issues that arise when making medical decisions.

- Is Informed Consent Still Central to Medical Ethics?

- Should Truth-Telling Depend on the Patient's Culture?

- Does Direct-to-Consumer Drug Advertising Enhance Patient Choice?

ISSUE 1

Is Informed Consent Still Central to Medical Ethics?

YES: Robert M. Arnold and Charles W. Lidz, from "Informed Consent: Clinical Aspects of Consent in Health Care," in Stephen G. Post, ed., *Encyclopedia of Bioethics*, vol. 3, 3rd ed. (Macmillan, 2003)

NO: Onora O'Neill, from *Autonomy and Trust in Bioethics* (Cambridge University Press, 2002)

ISSUE SUMMARY

YES: Physician Robert M. Arnold and professor of psychiatry and sociology Charles W. Lidz assert that informed consent in clinical care is an essential process that promotes good communication and patient autonomy despite the obstacles of implementation.

NO: Philosopher Onora O'Neill argues that the most evident change in medical practice in recent decades may be a loss of trust in physicians rather than any growth of patient autonomy. Informed consent in practice, she says, often amounts simply to a right to choose or refuse treatments, not a deeper and more meaningful expression of self-mastery.

Informed consent is undoubtedly one of the best-known and, arguably, one of the least-implemented concepts in modern medicine. Although much of modern medical ethics has ancient roots, the idea of informed consent is relatively recent. Until the mid-twentieth century most medical ethics were firmly based on the obligations of physicians to act for the benefit of their patients. Information was supposed to be managed carefully in order to protect patients from bad news and to keep them hopeful.

The first "Code of Medical Ethics" of the American Medical Association relied heavily on the work of Thomas Percival, a British physician whose book *Medical Ethics* (1803) played a crucial role in the field for more than a century. Percival believed that the patient's right to the truth was less important than the physician's obligation to benefit the patient. Deception, in the interest of doing good, was thus justified. The patient's consent to treatment, informed or otherwise, is not mentioned in early codes of medical ethics, although on a practical level doctors had to have a patient's permission to perform most procedures.

The modern concept of informed consent came to medical ethics through the courts. The earliest influential decision was *Schloendorff v. New York Hospital* (1914), in which the court ruled that a patient's right to "self-determination" obligated a physician to obtain consent. This case laid the basis for further litigation. The most influential series of decisions occurred in the 1950s and 1960s, when rulings went beyond the obligation to obtain consent to include an explicit duty to disclose information relevant to the patient who is making a decision about consent.

While the earlier cases had been based on the patient's right to be free from unwanted bodily intrusion (legally, "battery"), the court in *Natanson v. Kline* (1960) held that physicians who withheld information while obtaining consent were guilty of negligence. Imposing a legal duty on physicians to inform their patients of the risks, benefits, and alternatives to treatment exposed them to the risk of malpractice suits. Another factor that influenced the ascendance of informed consent in medical treatment were parallel discussions about the ethics of research involving human subjects. Voluntary consent to participate in research was a cornerstone of the Nuremberg Code of 1947, which was issued after the trials of Nazi physicians who had performed lethal experiments on nonconsenting prisoners.

Nevertheless, traditions die hard, and little change was seen in actual practice until the resurgence of interest in medical ethics in the 1970s. In 1972 the case of *Canterbury v. Spence* established a far-reaching patient-centered disclosure standard. The ruling stated, "The patient's right of self-decision can be effectively exercised only if the patient possesses enough information to enable an intelligent choice. . . . Social policy does not accept the paternalistic view that the physician may remain silent because divulgence might prompt the patient to forego needed therapy." In the 1980s and 1990s court cases have focused on individuals who lack the competence to provide informed consent, such as comatose patients, children, and mentally ill persons.

Although the physician's duty to obtain informed consent and the patient's right to information are now firmly established in law and grounded in the ethical principle of respect for persons, medical practice varies considerably. In Stephen G. Post, ed., *Encyclopedia of Bioethics* (2003), Tom L. Beauchamp and Ruth R. Faden, philosophers who have studied informed consent extensively, assert, "The overwhelming impression from the empirical literature and from reported clinical experience is that the actual process of soliciting informed consent often falls short of a serious show of respect for the decisional authority of patients."

The following selections illustrate two views of the future of informed consent. Robert M. Arnold and Charles W. Lidz reassert the importance of informed consent and offer ways in which the process can be improved in the clinical setting, despite the many obstacles. Onora O'Neill argues that informed consent has not enhanced patient autonomy but has had the opposite effect of lessening patient trust.

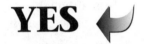

YES

**Robert M. Arnold and
Charles W. Lidz**

Informed Consent: Clinical Aspects
of Consent in Health Care

Clinical Aspects of Consent in Healthcare

Decision making is an everyday event in healthcare, not only for doctors and patients, but also for nurses, psychologists, social workers, emergency medical technicians, dentists, and other health professionals. Since the 1960s, however, the cultural ideal of how these decisions should be made has changed considerably. The concept that medical decision making should rely exclusively on the physician's expertise has been replaced by a model in which healthcare professionals share information and discuss alternatives with patients who then make the ultimate decisions about treatment.

The concept of informed consent gained its initial support as part of the general societal trend toward broadening access to decision making during the 1960s. Thus, the initial support for informed consent came from legal and philosophic circles rather than healthcare professionals. In the legal arena, informed consent has been used to develop minimal standards for doctor–patient interactions and clinical decision making (Berg et al.). Although there are some differences by jurisdiction, widely accepted legal standards require that healthcare professionals inform patients of the risks, benefits, and alternatives of all proposed treatments, and then allow the patient to choose among acceptable therapeutic alternatives.

In academia, informed consent has served as a cornerstone for the development of the discipline of bioethics. Based on the importance of autonomy in moral discourse, philosophers have argued that healthcare professionals are obligated to engage patients in discussions regarding the goals of therapy and the alternatives for reaching those goals, and that patients are the final decision makers regarding all therapeutic decisions.

While many physicians would express some support to the concept of shared decision making, this support is largely theoretical and does not seem to have made its way into routine medical practice. Physicians typically think of informed consent as a legal requirement for a signed piece of paper that is at best a waste of time, and at worst a bureaucratic, legalistic interference with their care for patients. Rather than seeing informed consent as a process that promotes good communication and patient autonomy, many healthcare professionals view it as a complex, legally prescribed recitation of risks and benefits that only frightens or confuses patients.

Objections to Informed Consent

There are various objections to informed consent that clinicians often make, and it will be useful to review those objections here.

Consent cannot be truly "informed"   Many practicing clinicians report that their patients are unable to understand the complex medical information necessary for a fully rational weighing of alternative treatments. There is considerable research support for this view. A variety of studies document that patients recall only a small percentage of the information that professionals present to them (Meisel and Roth); that they are not as good decision makers when they are sick as at other times (Sherlock; Cassell, 2001); and that they often make decisions based on medically trivial factors. Informed consent thus appears either to promote uninformed—and thus suboptimal—decisions, or to encourage patients to blindly accept healthcare professionals' recommendations. In either case informed consent appears to be a charade, and a dangerous one at that.

However, the fact that patients often do have difficulty understanding important aspects of medical decisions does not mean that healthcare professionals are the best decision makers about the patient's treatment. Knowledge about medical facts is not enough. Wise house buyers will have a structural engineer check over an old house, but few would be willing to allow the engineer to choose their house for them. Just as structural engineers cannot decide which house a family should buy—because they lack knowledge about the family's pattern of living, personal tastes, and potential family growth—healthcare professionals cannot scientifically deduce the best treatment for a specific patient simply from the medical facts. What matters to individuals about their health depends on their lifestyles, past experiences, and values, so choosing the *optimal therapy* is not a purely objective matter (U.S. President's Commission). Thus, patients and healthcare professionals both contribute essential knowledge to the decision-making process: patients bring their knowledge of their personal situation, goals, and values; and healthcare professionals bring their expertise on the nature of the problem and the technology that may be used to meet the patient's goals (see Brock).

Informed-consent disclosures, even if they are well done, may not lead to what clinicians might consider optimal decisions. Most people make major life decisions, such as whom to marry and which occupation to take up, based on faulty or incomplete information. Patients' lack of understanding of medical information in choosing treatment is probably no worse than their lack of information in choosing a spouse, nor are medical decisions more important than spousal choice. Respecting patient autonomy means allowing individuals to make their own decisions, even if the healthcare professional disagrees with them. The informed-consent process can improve patient decisions, but it cannot be expected to lead to perfect decisions.

Moreover, although sick persons have defects in their rational abilities, so do healthcare professionals. In fact, some of the most famous research on the difficulties individuals have with the rational use of probabilistic data involves physicians (Dawson and Ackes). Health professionals must be careful not to be too pessimistic about patients' ability to become informed decision makers. Patients may not be able to become as technically well-informed as professionals, but they clearly can understand and make decisions based on relevant information. One study, for example, showed that patients' decisions regarding life-sustaining treatment changed when they were given accurate information about the therapy's chance of success and that patients, when given increased information about screening tests for prostate cancer, were less likely to have the test change their decision on having the test (Murphy et al.). Moreover, what seems to be an irrational decision may turn out to be, from the patient's point of view, rational. Thus, a patient may turn down a recommended treatment because of personal experience with surgery or because the long-term benefit is not seen as being worth the short-term risk.

Most important, the difficulty of educating sick persons does not justify unilateral decision making. Rather, it places a special obligation on healthcare professionals to communicate clearly with patients. Using technical jargon, trying to give all of the available information in one visit, and not asking what the patient wants to know is a recipe for confusing even the most intelligent patient. A growing literature deals with informational aides—ranging from question prompt-sheets to giving patients audiotapes of the interaction and formal decision aides—that can be used to promote patient understanding and shared decision-making. New technologies like interactive DVD offer patients the opportunity to participate more fully in shared decision making at their own rate. A limitation of many of these aides is that they are limited helping with specific decisions and need to be updated frequently (Barry). Healthcare professionals also need to become more familiar with different cultural patterns of communication in order to talk with patients from different cultural backgrounds. For example, although a simple, factual discussion of depression and its treatment may be acceptable to most middle-class Americans, it would be seen as inappropriate by a first-generation Vietnamese male, whose culture discourages viewing depression as a disease (Hahn). There is no reason, in principle, why a person who makes decisions at home and work cannot, with help, understand the medical data sufficiently to become involved in medical decisions. Healthcare professionals must learn how best to present that help and involve patients in the decision-making process.

Patients do not wish to be involved in decision making   Many healthcare professionals believe that it is unfair to force patients to make decisions regarding their medical care. After all, they argue, patients pay their healthcare professionals to make medical decisions. The empirical literature partially supports the view that patients want professionals to make treatment decisions for them (Steel et al.). For example, in a study of male patients' preferences about medical decision making regarding hypertension, only 53 percent wanted to participate at all in the decision-making process (Strull et al.).

More recent data suggest that sicker patients are less interested in information about their disease and more willing to have doctors make decisions (Butow 1997; 2002).

There is no reason to force patients to be involved in decisions if they do not want to be. However, unless the health professional asks, he or she cannot know how involved a patient wants to be. Studies suggest that doctors' ability to predict their patients' interest in information, or their desire to be involved in decision making, is no better than flipping a coin (Butow 1997, 2002). In addition, roughly two-thirds of patients want to be involved in decision making, either by being the primary decision maker (the minority) or in shared decision making with the physician.

Patients may not always want to be involved in decision making, since many have been socialized into believing that "the doctor knows best." This is particularly true for poorer patients. Studies have shown that physicians wrongly assume that because patients with fewer socioeconomic resources ask fewer questions, they do not want as much information. These patients may in fact want just as much information, but they have been socialized into a different way of interacting with healthcare professionals (Waitzkin, 1984).

Patients may choose to allow someone else to make the decision for them. However, when a patient asks, "What would you do if you were me?" the underlying question may be, "As an expert in biomedicine, what alternative do you think will best maximize my values or interest?" If this is the case, the healthcare professional should respond by making a recommendation and justifying it in terms of the patient's values or interests. More frequently, the patient is asking, "If you had this disease, what therapy would you choose?" This question presumes that the professional and patient have the same values, needs, and problems, which is often not the case. Healthcare professionals should respond by pointing this out and emphasizing the importance of the patients' values in the decision-making process.

Although many patients do not want to be actively involved in decision making, they almost always want more information concerning their illness than the healthcare professional gives them. Healthcare professionals should not assume that just because patients do not wish to choose their therapy, they do not want information. Patients may desire information so as to increase compliance or make modifications in other areas of their lives, as well as to make medical decisions.

There are harmful effects of informing patients   Healthcare   professionals often justify withholding information from patients because of their belief that informing patients would be psychologically damaging and therefore contrary to the principle of nonmaleficence. Many healthcare professionals, however, overestimate potential psychological harm and neglect the positive effects of full disclosure (Faden et al.). Some discussions that physicians assume are stressful, such as advance care-planning, have been shown to decrease patient anxiety and increase the patient's sense of control. Moreover, bad news can often be communicated in a way that ameliorates the psychological effects of the disclosure (Quill and Townsend). Truth-telling must be distinguished from "truth dumping." Explanation of the care that can be provided, and empathic attention to the patient's fears and uncertainties can often prevent or mitigate otherwise more painful news. Finally, sometimes the harm associated with bad news is unavoidable. It is normal to be sad after finding out that one has an incurable cancer, for example. That does not mean that one should not convey the information, only that it should be done in as sensitively and supportively as possible.

Informed consent takes too much time   Respecting autonomy and promoting patient well-being—the values served through informed consent—are fundamental to good medicine. However, adhering to the ideals of medical practice takes time—time to help patients understand their illness and work through their emotional reactions to stressful information, to discuss each party's preconceptions and to clarify the therapeutic goals, to decide on a treatment plan, and to elicit questions about diagnosis and treatment.

In U.S. healthcare, time is money. As many commentators have noted, physicians are less well reimbursed for talking to patients than for performing invasive tests. This may discourage doctors from spending enough time discussing treatment options with patients. This, along with the pressures of managed care has decreased the average outpatient encounter, allowing even less time for doctor–patient communication. The ultimate justification for spending time to facilitate patient decisions is the same as that for spending any time in medical care: that patients will be better cared for. Moreover, some of the new decision aides, such as question prompts, may in fact decrease the time spent in the patient visit, while simultaneously increasing patient understanding.

Clinical Approaches to Informed Consent

Many of the problems in implementing informed consent result, at least in part, from the way informed consent has been implemented in clinical practice. Informed consent has become synonymous with the *consent form,* a legal invention with a legitimate role in documenting that informed consent has taken place, but hardly a substitute for the discussion process leading to informed consent (Andrews).

A pro forma approach: an event model of informed consent   In many clinical settings, consent begins when *it is time to get consent,* typically just prior to the administration of treatment. The process of getting the patients' consent consists of the recitation by a physician or nurse of the list of material risks and benefits and a request that the patient sign for the proposed treatment. This "conversation" is a very limited one that emphasizes the transfer of information from the physician or nurse to the patient. While it does meet the minimal legal requirements for informed consent efficiently, it does not meet the higher ethical goal of informed consent, which is to empower patients by educating and involving them in their treatment plans. Instead, it imposes an almost empty ritual on an unchanged relationship between provider and patient (Katz).

The procedure just described assumes that care involves a series of discrete, circumscribed decisions. In fact, much of clinical medicine consists of a series of frequent, interwoven decisions that must be repeatedly reconsidered as more information becomes available. When "it is time to get consent," there may be nothing left to decide. Consider the operative consent form obtained the evening prior to an operation. After patients have discussed with their families whether to be admitted to the hospital, rearranged their work and child-care schedules, and undergone a long and painful diagnostic workup, the decision to have surgery seems preordained. The evening before the operation, patients do not seriously evaluate the operation's risks and benefits, so consent is pro forma. No wonder some healthcare professionals feel that *consent* is a waste of time and energy.

The event model for gathering informed consent falls far short of meeting the ethical goal of ensuring patient participation in the decision-making process. Rather than engaging the patient as an active participant in the decision-making process, the patient's role is to agree to or veto the healthcare professionals' recommendations. Little attempt is made to elicit patient preferences and consider how treatment might address them.

A dialogical approach: the process model of informed consent   Fortuately, it is possible to fulfill legal requirements for informed consent while maximizing active patient participation in the clinical setting. An alternative to the event model described above, which sees informed consent as an aberration from clinical practice, the process model attempts to integrate informed consent into all aspects of clinical care (Berg et al). The process model of informed consent assumes that each party has something to contribute to the decision-making process. The physician brings technical knowledge and experience in treating patients with similar problems, while patients bring knowledge about their life circumstances and the ability to assess the effect that treatment may have on them. Open discussion makes it possible for the patient and the physician to examine critically their views and to determine what might be optimal treatment.

The process model also recognizes that medical care rarely involves only one decision made at a single point in time. Decisions about care frequently begin with the suspicion that something is wrong and that treatment may be necessary, and they end only when the patient leaves follow-up care. Decisions involve diagnostic as well as therapeutic interventions. Some decisions are made in one visit, while others occur over a prolonged period of time. Although some interactions between provider and patient involve explicit decisions, decisions are made at each interaction, even if the decision is only to continue treatment. The process model also recognizes that various healthcare professionals may play a role in making sure that the patients' consent is informed. For example, a woman deciding on various breast cancer treatments may talk with an oncologist and a surgeon about the risks of various treatments, with a nurse about the side effects of medication, with a social worker about financial issues in treatment, and with a patient-support group about her husband's reaction to a possible mastectomy.

Ideally, then, informed consent involves shared decision making over a period of time; in a dialogue throughout the course of the patient's relationship with various healthcare professionals. Such a dialogue aims to facilitate patient participation and to strengthen the therapeutic alliance.

Tasks Involved in Informed Consent

Consent is a series of interrelated tasks. First, the patient and professional must agree on the problem that will be the focus of their work together (Eisenthal and Lazare). Most nonemergency consultations involve complex negotiations between healthcare professional and patient regarding the definition of the patient's problem. The patient may see the problem as a routine physical examination for a work release, the need for advice, or the investigation of a physical symptom. If professionals are to respond effectively to the patients' goals, they must find out the reason for the visit. Whereas physicians typically focus on biomedical information and its implications, patients typically view the problem in the context of their social situation (Fisher and Todd). The differences between the patient's perceptions of the problem and the professional's perceptions must be explicitly worked through, since agreement regarding the focus of the interactions will lead to increased patient satisfaction and compliance with further treatment plans (Meichenbaum and Turk).

Even when the professional and patient have agreed on what the problem is, substantial misunderstandings may arise regarding the treatment goals. Patients may expect the medically impossible, or they may expect outcomes based on knowledge of life circumstances about which the physician is unaware. Since assessing the risks and benefits of any treatment option depends on therapeutic goals, the professional and patient must agree on the goals the therapy aims to accomplish.

Finding out what the patient wants is more complicated than merely inquiring, "What do you want?" A patient typically does not come to the professional with well-developed preferences regarding medical therapy except "to get better," with little understanding of what this may involve (Cassell, 1985). As a patient's knowledge and perspective change over the course of an illness, so too may the patient's views regarding the therapeutic goals.

Because clinicians provide much of the medical information needed to ensure that the patient's preferences are grounded in medical possibility, healthcare professionals play a significant role in how a patient's preferences evolve. It is important that they understand that patients may reasonably hold different goals from those their practitioners hold. This is particularly true when they come from different economic strata. For example, a physician's emphasis on the most medically sophisticated care may pale in the light of the patient's financial problems. Therapeutic goals, like the definition of the problem, require ongoing clarification and negotiation.

After agreeing upon the problem and the therapeutic goals, the healthcare professional and the patient must choose the best way to achieve them. If patients have been involved in the prior two steps, the decision about a treatment plan will more likely reflect their values than if they are merely asked to assent to the clinician's strategy.

Healthcare professionals often ask how much information they must supply to ensure that the patient is an informed participant in the decision-making process

(Mazur). There is, however, a more important question: Has the information been provided in a manner that the patient can understand? While the law only requires that healthcare professionals inform patients, morally valid consent requires that patients understand the information conveyed. Ensuring patient understanding requires attention to the quality as well as the quantity of information presented (Faden).

A great deal of empirical data has been collected concerning problems with consent forms. These forms have been criticized, for example, as being unintelligible because of their length and use of technical language (Berg et al.) Healthcare professionals thus need to be aware of, and facile in using, a variety of methods to increase patients' comprehension of information, including verbal techniques, written information, and interactive videodiscs (Stanley et al.).

Still, the question of how much information to present remains. The legal standards regarding information disclosure—what a reasonable patient would find essential to making a decision or what a reasonably prudent physician would disclose—are not particularly helpful. Howard Brody has suggested two important features: (1) the physician must disclose the basis on which the proposed treatment or the alternative possible treatments have been chosen; and (2) the patient must be encouraged to ask questions suggested by the the physician's reasoning—and the questions need to be answered to the patient's satisfaction (Brody). Healthcare professionals must also inform patients when controversy exists about the various therapeutic options. Similarly, patients should also be told the degree to which the recommendation is based on established scientific evidence rather than personal experience or educated guesses.

Two other factors will influence the amount of information that should be given: the importance of the decision (given the patient's situation and goals) and the amount of consensus within the healthcare professions regarding the agreed-upon therapy. For example, a low-risk intervention, such as giving influenza vaccines to elderly patients, offers a clear-cut benefit with minimal risk. In this case, the professional should describe the intervention and recommend it because of its benefits. A detailed description of the infrequent risks is not needed unless the patient asks or is known to be skeptical of medical interventions. Interventions that present greater risks or a less clear-cut risk-benefit ratio require a longer description—for example, the decision to administer AZT to an HIV (human immunodeficiency virus)-positive, asymptomatic woman with a CD4 cell count of 350. In this situation, the data regarding starting medications are unclear and a patient's preference is critical. In this situation, one would need to talk about the major side effects of the medicines, the burden of taking medicines daily, the immunological benefit of anti-virals, etc. In neither case is a discussion of pathophysiology or biochemistry necessary. It must be emphasized that there is no formula for deciding how much a patient needs to be told or the length of time this will take. The amount of information necessary will depend on the patient's individual situation, values, and goals.

Finally, an adequate decision-making process requires continual updating of information, monitoring of expectations, and evaluation of the patient's progress in reaching the chosen or revised goals. Thus, the final step in informed consent is follow-up. This step is particularly important for patients with chronic diseases for which modifications of the treatment plan are often necessary.

The process model of informed consent has many advantages. Because it assumes many short conversations over time rather than one long interaction, it can be more easily integrated into the professional's ambulatory practice than the event model. It also allows patients to be much more involved in decision making and ensures that treatment is more consistent with their values. Furthermore, the continual monitoring of patients' understanding of their disease, the treatment, and its progress is likely to reduce misunderstandings and increase their investment in, and adherence to, the treatment plan. Thus, the process model of informed consent is likely to promote both patient autonomy and well-being.

Unfortunately, there are situations in which this approach is not very helpful. Some healthcare professionals, anesthesiologists, or emergency medical technicians, for example, are not likely to have ongoing relationships with patients. In emergencies, there is not time for a decision to develop through a series of short conversations. In these cases, informed consent may more closely approximate the event model. However, since most medical care is delivered by primary-care practitioners in an ambulatory setting, the process model of informed consent is more helpful.

Bibliography

Andrews, Lori B. 1984. "Informed Consent Status and the Decision-making Process." *Journal of Legal Medicine* 5(2): 163–217.

Barry, M. 2000. "Involving Patients in Medical Decisions: How Can Physicians Do Better?" *Journal of the American Medical Association* 282(24): 2356–2357.

Berg, Jessica; Appelbaum, Paul S.; Lidz, Charles W.; et al. 2001. *Informed Consent: Legal Theory and Clinical Practice*, 2nd edition. New York: Oxford University Press.

Brock, Dan W. 1991. "The Ideal of Shared Decision Making Between Physicians and Patients." *Kennedy Institute of Ethics Journal* 1(1): 28–47.

Braddock, C. H.; Fihn, S. D.; Levinson, W., et al. 1997. "How Doctors and Patients Discuss Routine Clinical Decisions: Informed Decision Making in the Outpatient Setting." *Journal of General Internal Medicine* 12(6): 339–345.

Brody, Howard. 1989. "Transparency: Informed Consent in Primary Care." *Hastings Center Report* 19(5): 5–9.

Butow, P. N.; Dowsett, S.; Hagerty, R.; et al. 2002. "Communicating Prognosis to Patients with Metastatic Disease: What Do They Really Want to Know?" *Supportive Care in Cancer* 10(2):161–168.

Butow, P. N.; Maclean, M.; Dunn, S. M.; et al. 1997. "The Dynamics of Change: Cancer Patients' Preferences for Information, Involvement, and Support." *Annals of Oncology* 8: 857–863.

Cassell, Eric J. 1985. *Talking with Patients*. 2 vols. Cambridge, MA: MIT Press.

Cassell, Eric J. 2001. "Preliminary Evidence of Impaired Thinking in Sick Patients." *Annals of Internal Medicine* 134(12): 1120–1123.

Dawson, Neal V., and Arkes, Hal R. 1987. "Systematic Errors in Medical Decision Making: Judgment Limitations." *Journal of General Internal Medicine* 2(3): 183–187.

Eisenthal, Sherman, and Lazare, Aaron. 1976. "Evaluation of the Initial Interview in a Walk-In Clinic." *Journal of Nervous and Mental Disease* 162(3): 169–176.

Faden, Ruth R. 1977. "Disclosure and Informed Consent: Does It Matter How We Tell It?" *Health Education Monographs* 5(3): 198–214.

Faden, Ruth R.; Beauchamp, Tom L.; and King, Nancy M. P. 1986. *A History and Theory of Informed Consent.* New York: Oxford University Press.

Fisher, Sue, and Todd, Alexandra D., eds. 1983. *The Social Organization of Doctor–Patient Communication.* Washington, D.C.: Center for Applied Linguistics.

Gadow, Sally. 1980. "Existential Advocacy: Philosophic Foundation of Nursing." In *Nursing: Images and Ideals: Opening Dialogue with the Humanities,* ed. Stuart F. Spicker and Sally Gadow. New York: Springer.

Hahn, Robert A. 1982. "Culture and Informed Consent: An Anthropological Perspective." In *Making Health Care Decisions: The Ethical and Legal Implications of Informed Consent in the Patient–Practitioner Relationship,* vol. 2. Washington, D.C.: U.S. President's Commission for the Study of Ethical Problems in Medicine and Biomedical and Behavioral Research.

Katz, Jay. 1984. *The Silent World of Doctor and Patient.* New York: Free Press.

Lidz, Charles W.; Meisel, Alan; Zerubavel, Eviatar; et al., eds. 1984. *Informed Consent: A study of Decision-Making in Psychiatry.* New York: Guilford.

Mazur, Dennis J. 1986. "What Should Patients Be Told Prior to a Medical Procedure? Ethical and Legal Perspectives on Medical Informed Consent." *American Journal of Medicine* 81(6): 1051–1054.

Meichenbaum, Donald, and Turk, Dennis. 1987. *Facilitating Treatment Adherence: A Practitioner's Guidebook.* New York: Plenum Press.

Meisel, Alan, and Roth, Loren H. 1981. "What We Do and Do Not Know About Informed Consent." *Journal of the American Medical Association* 246(21): 2473–2477.

Murphy, Donald J.; Burrows, David; Santilli, Sara; et al. 1994. "The Influence of the Probability of Survival on Patients' Preferences Regarding Cardiopulmonary Resuscitation." *New England Journal of Medicine* 330(8): 545–549.

Quill, Timothy E., and Townsend. Penelope. 1991. "Bad News: Delivery, Dialogue, and Dilemmas." *Archives of Internal Medicine* 151: 463–468.

Sherlock, Richard. 1986. "Reasonable Men and Sick Human Beings." *American Journal of Medicine* 80(1): 2–4.

Stanley, Barbara; Guido, Jeannine; Stanley, Michael; et al. 1984. "The Elderly Patient and Informed Consent: Empirical Findings." *Journal of the American Medical Association* 252(10): 1302–1306.

Steel, David J.; Blackwell, Barry; Gutmann, Mary C.; et al. 1987. "The Activated Patient: Dogma, Dream, or Desideratum." *Patient Education and Counseling* 10(1): 3–23.

Strull, William M.; Lo, Bernard; and Charles, Gerard. 1984. "Do Patients Want to Participate in Medical Decision-Making?" *Journal of the American Medical Association* 252(21): 2990–2994.

U.S. President's Commission for the Study of Ethical Problems in Medicine and Biomedical and Behavioral Research. 1982. *Making Health Care Decisions: A Report on the Ethical and Legal Implications of Informed Consent in the Patient–Practitioner Relationship.* Washington, D.C.: Author.

Waitzkin, Howard. 1984. "Doctor–Patient Communication: Clinical Implications of Social Scientific Research." *Journal of the American Medical Association* 252(17): 2441–2446.

Waitzkin, Howard. 1991. *The Politics of Medical Encounters: How Patients and Doctors Deal with Social Problems.* New Haven, CT: Yale University Press.

West, Candace. 1984. Routine Complications: *Troubles with Talk between Doctors and Patients.* Bloomington: Indiana University Press.

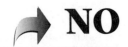 **NO**

Gaining Autonomy and Losing Trust?

Contemporary Bioethics

Bioethics is not a discipline, nor even a new discipline; I doubt whether it will ever be a discipline. It has become a meeting ground for a number of disciplines, discourses and organisations concerned with ethical, legal and social questions raised by advances in medicine, science and biotechnology. The protagonists who debate and dispute on this ground include patients and environmentalists, scientists and journalists, politicians and campaigners and representatives of an array of civic and business interests, professions and academic disciplines. Much of the debate is new and contentious in content and flavour; some of it is alarming and some misleading.

The first occasion on which I can remember a discussion of bioethics—we did not then use the word, although it had been coined[1]—was in the mid-1970s at a meeting of philosophers, scientists and doctors in New York City. We were discussing genetically modified (GM) organisms: a topic of breathtaking novelty that was already hitting the headlines. Towards the end of the evening an elderly doctor remarked, with mild nostalgia, that when he had studied medical ethics as a student, things had been easier: the curriculum had covered referrals, confidentiality—and billing. Those simpler days are now very remote. . . .

During [recent] years no themes have become more central in large parts of bioethics, and especially in medical ethics, than the importance of respecting individual rights and individual autonomy. These are now the dominant ethical ideas in many discussions of topics ranging from genetic testing to geriatric medicine, from psychiatry to *in vitro* fertilisation, from beginning to end of life problems, from medical innovation to medical futility, from heroic medicine to hospices. In writing on these and many other topics, much time and effort has gone into articulating and advancing various conceptions of respect for persons, and hence for patients, that centre on ensuring that their rights and their autonomy are respected. Respect for autonomy and for rights are often closely identified with medical practice that seeks individuals' informed consent to all medical treatment, medical research or disclosure of personal information, and so with major changes in the acceptable relationships between professionals and patients. Medical practice has moved away from paternalistic traditions, in which professionals were seen as the proper judges of patients' best interests. Increased recognition and respect of patients' rights and

From *The Gifford Lectures*, University of Edinburgh, 2002, excerpted from I, 14–15, 17–21, 37–39.
Copyright © 2002 by Onora O'Neill.

insistence on the ethical importance of securing their consent are now viewed as standard and obligatory ways of securing respect for patients' autonomy.[2] . . .

We might expect the increasing attention paid to individual rights and to autonomy to have increased public trust in the ways in which medicine, science and biotechnology are practised and regulated. Greater rights and autonomy give individuals greater control over the ways they live and increase their capacities to resist others' demands and institutional pressures. Yet amid widespred and energetic efforts to respect persons and their autonomy and to improve regulatory structures, public trust in medicine, science and biotechnology has seemingly faltered. The loss of trust is a constant refrain in the claims of campaigning groups and in the press. . . .

Trust and Autonomy in Medical Ethics

[The] traditional model of the trusting doctor–patient relationship has been subject to multiple criticisms for many years. Traditional doctor–patient relationships, it has been said on countless occasions, have in fact nearly always been based on asymmetric knowledge and power. They institutionalise opportunities for abuse of trust. Doctor–patient relationships were viewed as relationships of trust only because a paternalistic view of medicine was assumed, in which the dependence of patients on professionals was generally accepted. The traditional doctor–patient relationship, so its critics claim, may have been one of trust, but not of reasonable trust. Rather, they claimed, patients who placed trust in their doctors were like children who initially must trust their parents blindly. Such trust was based largely on the lack of any alternative, and on inability to discriminate between well-placed and misplaced trust.

If there was one point of agreement about necessary change in the early years of contemporary medical ethics, it was that this traditional, paternalistic conception of the doctor–patient relationship was defective, and could not provide an adequate context for reasonable trust. A more adequate basis for trust required patients who were on a more equal footing with professionals, and this meant that they would have to be better informed and less dependent. The older assumption that relations of trust are in themselves enough to safeguard a weaker, dependent party was increasingly dismissed as naive. The only trust that is well placed is given by those who understand what is proposed, and who are in a position to refuse or choose in the light of that understanding. We can look at the same image with a less innocent eye, and see it as raising all these questions about the traditional doctor–patient relationship. In this second way of seeing the picture the doctor dominates: the white coat and intimidating office are symbols of her professional authority; the patient's anxious and discontented expression reveals how little this is a relationship of trust.

These considerations lie behind many discussions of supposedly better models of the doctor–patient relationship, in which patients are thought of as equal partners in their treatment, in which treatment is given only with the informed consent of patients, in which patient satisfaction is an important indicator of professional adequacy, in which patients are variously seen as consumers, as informed adults and are not infantilised or treated paternalistically and in which the power of doctors is curbed.[3] In this more sophisticated approach to trust, autonomy is seen as a precondition of genuine trust. Here, as one writer puts it, 'informed consent is the modern clinical ritual of trust',[4] a ritual of trust that embeds it in properly institutionalised respect for patient autonomy. So we can also read the image in the frontispiece in a third, more optimistic, way as combining patient autonomy with mutual trust in the new, recommended, respecting way. What we now see is a relationship between equals: the patient too is a professional, dressed in a suit and sitting like an equal at the desk; the patient has heard a full explanation and is being offered a consent form; he is deciding whether to give his fully informed consent. Trust is properly combined with patient autonomy.

This revised model of doctor–patient interaction demands more than a simple change of attitude on the part of doctors, or of patients. It also requires huge changes in the terms and conditions of medical practice and ways of ensuring that treatment is given only where patients have consented. Informed consent has not always been so central to doctor–patient relationships, which were traditionally grounded in doctors' duties not to harm and to benefit. Informed consent came to be seen as increasingly important in part because of legal developments, especially in the USA, and in part because of its significance for research on human subjects, and the dire abuse of research subjects by Nazi doctors. The first principle of the Nuremberg Doctors' Code of 1947 states emphatically that subjects' consent must be 'voluntary, competent, informed and comprehensive'.[5] Only later did the thought emerge clearly that consent was also central to clinical practice, and that patient autonomy or self-determination should not be subordinated to doctors' commitments to act for their patients' benefit or best interest. Yet despite the enormous stress laid on individual autonomy and patient rights in recent years, this heightened concern for patient autonomy does not extend throughout medicine: public health, and the treatment of those unable to consent are major domains of medical practice that cannot easily be subjected to requirements of respecting autonomy and securing informed consent.

From the patient's point of view, however, the most evident change in medical practice of recent decades may be loss of a context of trust rather than any growth of autonomy. He or she now faces not a known and trusted face, but teams of professionals who are neither names nor faces, but as the title of one book aptly put it, *strangers at the bedside*.[6] These strangers have access to large amounts of information that patients give them in confidence. Yet to their patients they remain strangers—powerful strangers. They are the functionaries of medical institutions whose structures are opaque to most patients, although supposedly designed to secure their best interest, to preserve confidentiality and to respect privacy. Seen 'from the patient's point of view every development in the post World War II period distanced the physician and the hospital from the patient, disrupting social connection and serving the bonds of trust'.[7]

From the practitioner's point of view, too, the situation has losses as well as gains. The simplicities of the Hippocratic oath and of other older professional codes have been replaced by far more complex professional codes, by more formal certification of competence to perform specific medical interventions, by enormous increases in requirements for keeping records and by many exacting forms of professional accountability.[8] In medicine, as in most other forms of professional life and public service, and 'audit society' has emerged.[9] The doctor now faces the patient knowing that he or she must comply with explicit standards and codes, that many aspects of medical practice are regulated, that compliance is monitored and that patients who are not properly treated may complain—or even sue.

These new relationships may live up to their billing by replacing traditional forms of trust with a new and better basis for trust. The new structures may provide reasons for patients to trust even if they do not know their doctors personally, and do not understand the details of the rules and codes that constrain doctors' action. Supposedly they can feel reassured that the power of doctors is now duly regulated and constrained, that doctors will act with due respect and that they can seek redress where doctors fail. Although traditional trust has vanished with the contexts in which it arose, a more acceptable basis for reasonable trust has been secured, which anchors it in professional respect for patients' rights. Supposedly the ideals of trust and autonomy have been reshaped and are now compatible. . . .

The Triumph of Informed Consent

Yet what does the supposed triumph of autonomy in medical ethics amount to? . . .

By insisting on the importance of informed consent we *make* it *possible* for individuals to choose autonomously, however that it is to be construed. But we in no way guarantee or require that they do so. Those who insist on the importance of informed consent in medical practice typically say nothing about individuality or character, about self-mastery, or reflective endorsement, or self-control, or rational reflection, or second-order desires, or about any of the other specific ways in which autonomous choices supposedly are to be distinguished from other, mere choices.

In short, the focus of bioethical discussions of autonomy is not on patient autonomy or individual autonomy of any distinctive sort. What is rather grandly called 'patient autonomy' often amounts simply to a right to choose or refuse treatments on offer, and the corresponding obligations of practitioners not to proceed without patients' consent. Of course, some patients may use this liberty to accept or refuse treatment with a high degree of reflection and individuality, hence (on some accounts) with a high degree of individual or personal autonomy. But this need not generally be the case. Requirements for informed consent are relevant to specifically autonomous choice only because they are relevant to choice of all sorts. What passes for patient autonomy in medical practice is operationalised by practices of informed consent: the much-discussed triumph of autonomy is mostly a triumph of informed consent requirements.

This minimalist interpretation of individual or personal autonomy in medical ethics in fact fits rather well with medical practice. When we are ill or injured we often find it hard to achieve any demanding version of individual autonomy. We are all too aware of our need and ignorance, and specifically that we need help from others whose expertise, control of resources and willingness to assist is not guaranteed. A person who is ill or injured is highly vulnerable to others, and highly dependent on their action and competence. Robust conceptions of autonomy may seem a burden and even unachievable for patients; mere choosing may be hard enough. And, in fact, the choices that patients are required to make typically quite limited. It is not as if doctors offer patients a smorgasbord of possible treatments and interventions, a variegated menu of care and cure. Typically a diagnosis is followed with an indication of prognosis and suggestions for treatment to be undertaken. Patients are typically asked to choose from a smallish menu—often a menu of one item—that others have composed and described in simplified terms. This may suit us well when ill, but it is a far cry from any demanding exercise of individual autonomy.

It is probably a considerable relief to many patients that they are not asked to muster much in the way of individual autonomy. When we are ill or injured we often lack the skills or energy for demanding cognitive tasks. Our highest priority is to get help from others and in particular from others with relevant skills and knowledge. The traditional construction of doctor–patient relations as relations of trust, as quasi-personal, as guided by professional concern for the patient's best interests makes sense to many patients because (if achievable) it would secure what they most need. The point and the context of the older, trust-centred model of doctor–patient relationships are not at all obscure.

However, at a time at which the real relations between doctors and patients are no longer personal relationships, nor even one-to-one relationships, but rather relationships between patients and complex organisations staffed by many professionals, the older personal, trust-based model of doctor–patient relationships seems increasingly obsolete. Contemporary relations between professionals and patients are constrained, formalised and regulated in many ways, and may erode patients' reasons for trusting. The very requirements to record and file medical information, for example, while intended to control information and protect patients, can inhibit doctors' abilities to communicate freely. Doctors, like many other professionals, find themselves pressed to be accountable rather than to be communicative, to conform to regulations rather than to enter relations of trust. As layers of regulation and control are added with the aim of protecting dependent, ignorant and vulnerable patients, as professionals are disciplined by multiple systems of accountability backed by threats of litigation on grounds of professional negligence in case of failure to meet these requirements, relations between patients and professionals are inevitably reshaped. Much is demanded of informed consent requirements if they are to substitute for forms of trust that are no longer achievable (or perhaps were never widely achieved, and still less widely warranted), and safeguard the interests of patients who find strangers at their bedsides. . . .

Notes

1.   The Kennedy Institute in Washington DC was founded in 1971 with the full name 'The Joseph and Rose Kennedy Institute for the Study of Human Reproduction and Bioethics'. See W.T. Reich, 'The Word 'Bioethics': Its Birth and

the Legacies of Those Who 'Shaped It', *Kennedy Institute of Ethics Journal,* 4, 1994, 319–35.

2. For a highly informative account of these changes, . . . see Ruth Faden and Tom Beauchamp, *A History and Theory of Informed Consent,* Oxford University Press, 1986; for a sociological perspective see Paul Root Wolpe, 'The Triumph of Autonomy in American Bioethics: A Sociological View', in Raymond DeVries and Janardan Subedi, eds., *Bioethics and Society: Constructing the Ethical Enterprise,* Prentice-Hall, 1998, 38–59.

3. R.A. Hope and K.W.M. Fulford, 'Medical Education: Patients, Principles, Practice Skills', in R. Gillon, ed., *Principles of Health Care Ethics,* John Wiley & Sons, 1993.

4. Wolpe, 'The Triumph of Autonomy', 48.

5. See Faden and Beauchamp, *A History and Theory of Informed Consent;* Ulrich Tröhler and Stella Reiter-Theil, *Ethics Codes in Medicine: Foundations and Achievements of Codification Since 1947,* Ashgate; Lori B. Andrews, 'Informed Consent Statutes and the Decision-Making Process', *Journal of Legal Medicine,* 30, 163–217; World Medical Association, Declaration of Helsinki, 2000; see institutional bibliography.

6. David J. Rothman, *Strangers at the Bedside: A History of How Law and Ethics Transformed Medical Decision-Making,* Basic Books, 1991. Rosamond Rhodes and James J. Strain, 'Trust and Transforming Healthcare Institutions', *Cambridge Journal of Healthcare Ethics,* 9, 2000, 205–17.

7. Rothman, *Strangers at the Bedside.*

8. Nigel G.E. Harris 'Professional Codes and Kantian Duties', in Ruth Chadwick, ed., *Ethics and the Professions,* Amesbury, 1994, 104–15.

9. Michael Power, *The Audit Explosion,* Demos, 1994 and *The Audit Society: Rituals of Verification,* Oxford University Press, 1994.

POSTSCRIPT

Is Informed Consent Still Central to Medical Ethics?

The Patient Self-Determination Act, a federal law that went into effect in 1991, requires health care institutions to advise patients about their right to accept or refuse medical care and to offer them an opportunity to create an advance directive indicating their medical choices should they become incompetent. Nevertheless, there is considerable evidence that patients and their designated health care proxies are not brought into decision making at the end of life in a timely and effective way. There are also some limits on what kinds of information must be provided to patients. In the 1993 case of *Arato v. Avedon,* the California Supreme Court supported information sharing and patient-centered decision making but ruled that doctors need not supply explicit statistical information about life expectancy to patients. See George J. Annas, "Informed Consent, Cancer, and Truth in Prognosis," *The New England Journal of Medicine* (January 20, 1994).

Nonetheless, the concept of informed consent, from Western political and ethical theories that place a high value on individual self-determination, remains a central principle in the United States. Cultural groups who have different traditions may not share this value. Two articles in the *Journal of the American Medical Association* (September 13, 1995)—"Western Bioethics on the Navajo Reservation," by Joseph A. Carrese and Lorna A. Rhodes, and "Ethnicity and Attitudes Toward Patient Autonomy," by Leslie J. Blackhall—suggest that disclosing negative information and involving patients in decision making may be contrary to the beliefs of certain ethnic populations. For more on this subject, see Issue 2, *Should Truth-Telling Depend on the Patient's Culture?*

The most comprehensive account of informed consent is *A History and Theory of Informed Consent* by Ruth L. Faden, Tom L. Beauchamp, and Nancy M. P. King (Oxford University Press, 1986). Another useful volume, particularly in terms of psychiatric treatment, is *Informed Consent: Legal Theory and Clinical Practice* by Paul S. Appelbaum, Charles W. Lidz, and Alan Meisel (Oxford University Press, 1987). Jay Katz's *The Silent World of Doctor and Patient* (Free Press, 1984; paper edition 2002, Johns Hopkins University Press) is an insightful discussion of the reasons physicians may be reluctant to disclose information to their patients. See also, Jessica W. Berg, Paul S. Appelbaum, Charles W. Lidz, and Lisa S. Parker, *Informed Consent: Legal Theory and Clinical Practice,* 2d ed. (Oxford University Press, 2001), and Terrance C. McConnell, *Inalienable Rights: The Limits of Consent in Medicine and the Law* (Oxford University Press, 2000).

ISSUE 2

Should Truth-Telling Depend on the Patient's Culture?

YES: Leslie J. Blackhall, Gelya Frank, Sheila Murphy, and Vicki Michel, from "Bioethics in a Different Tongue: The Case of Truth-Telling," *Journal of Urban Health* (March 2001)

NO: Mark Kuczewski and Patrick J. McCruden, from "Informed Consent: Does It Take a Village? The Problem of Culture and Truth Telling," *Cambridge Quarterly of Healthcare Ethics* (2001)

ISSUE SUMMARY

YES: Leslie J. Blackhall, Gelya Frank, and Sheila Murphy, from the University of Southern California, and Vicki Michel, from the Loyola Law School, advise clinical and bioethics professionals facing truth-telling dilemmas to make room for the diverse ethical views of the populations they serve.

NO: Philosopher Mark Kuczewski and bioethicist Patrick J. McCruden argue that by insisting on informed consent or an appropriate waiver process, the health care system respects cultural differences rather than stereotyping them.

In his powerful short story "The Death of Ivan Ilych," Leo Tolstoy graphically portrays the physical agony and the social isolation of a dying man. However, "What tormented Ivan Ilych most was the deception, the lie, which for some reason they all accepted, that he was not dying but was simply ill, and that he only need keep quiet and undergo a treatment and then something very good would result." Instrumental in setting up the deception is Ivan's doctor, who reassures him to the very end that all will be well. Hearing the banal news from his doctor once again, "Ivan Ilych looks at him as much as to say: 'Are you really never ashamed of lying?' But the doctor does not wish to understand this question."

Unlike many of the ethical issues discussed in this volume, which have arisen as a result of modern scientific knowledge and technology, the question of whether or not to tell dying patients the truth is an old and persistent one. But this debate has been given a new urgency in two ways. First, medical practices today are so complex that it is often difficult to know just what the "truth" really is. A dying patient's life can often be prolonged, although at great financial and personal cost, and many people differ even over the definition of a terminal illness. Second, the American population now includes many people from different cultures whose beliefs about truth-telling differ from those of conventional Western medicine.

At a basic level what must be balanced in this decision are two significant principles of ethical conduct: the obligation to tell the truth and the obligation not to harm others, in this case, not just the patient but the patient's family members who seek to withhold the truth from their dying relative. Moral philosophers, beginning with Aristotle, have regarded truth as an absolute value or one that, at the very least, is preferable to deception. The great nineteenth-century German philosopher Immanuel Kant argued that there is no justification for lying (although some later commentators feel that his absolutist position has been overstated). Other philosophers have argued that deception is sometimes justified. For example, Henry Sidgwick, an early-twentieth-century British philosopher, believed that it was entirely acceptable to lie to invalids and children to protect them from the shock of the truth. Although the question has been debated for centuries, no clear-cut answer has been reached. In fact, the case of a benevolent lie to a dying patient is often given as the prime example of an excusable deception.

While the philosophical debate continued, American medical practice underwent a pronounced shift beginning in the 1960s. Influenced by the growing attention to the principle of patient autonomy, doctors began involving patients in their health care decisions and telling them the facts of their diagnosis and prognosis. In recent years, however, greater attention to cultural sensitivity has led to a new debate: whether or not to withhold the truth from dying patients because family members demand it in the name of their cultural belief that truth-telling would harm the patient.

In the following selections, Leslie J. Blackhall and her colleagues present data from their study of cultural beliefs about truth-telling to argue that it is important to respect the ways in which people differ as to how the truth should be told. They question even what "truth" and "telling" really mean. Mark Kuczewski and Patrick J. McCruden rebut this emphasis on cultural relativism and reinforce the significance of informed consent.

YES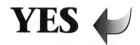

Leslie J. Blackhall et al.

Bioethics in a Different Tongue: The Case of Truth-Telling

Introduction

The study discussed in this [selection] began with the concern that much of bioethics was a top-down affair. The ethical problems surrounding end-of-life care and the solutions to these problems have been defined by professionals (like the authors) who are mainly white, middle-class people with advanced educational degrees and good (or at least decent) health insurance. When we looked at care at the end of life, we were concerned about excessive, burdensome, and futile medical technology and with the right to choose and, especially, to refuse treatments. Advance care directives were invented to address these problems, to ensure that patients' rights to refuse excessive care were preserved when they were so demented or comatose that they were unable to communicate, or even know, what those wishes were. Having decided what the problem was (too much futile care at the end of life) and the solution (advance care directives), much space then was devoted in the literature on bioethics to promoting these documents. However, most studies that look at the use of advance directives, even those studies with interventions designed to increase accessibility, show that relatively few people actually have completed a directive.[1-6]

The reasons why people do not complete advance directives are many and complex, but one reason may be that the concerns of bioethics professionals about care at the end of life are not necessarily those most important to all segments of the population. For example, it is questionable whether patients, many of whom have no health insurance, who receive care at major urban hospitals are worried about getting too much medical care at the end of life. At these hospitals, their experience is more likely to be a fight for every bit of medical attention they receive, not fending off excessive care. Also, in the clinical experience of one of us (L.J.B.), it is not uncommon for patients and their families, particularly recent immigrants, to seem puzzled by, if not downright hostile to, attempts to involve them in end-of-life decisions.

Observations and reflections such as these led us to undertake a study to look at attitudes concerning end-of-life care among elderly people of different ethnicities. The purpose of this study was to examine and compare the

From Leslie J. Blackhall, Gelya Frank, Sheila Murphy, and Vicki Michel, "Bioethics in a Different Tongue: The Case of Truth-Telling," *Journal of Urban Health*, vol. 78, no. 1 (March 2001), pp. 59-67, 69-71. Copyright © 2001 by The New York Academy of Medicine. Reprinted by permission of Oxford University Press.

attitudes and life experiences of people from African-American, European-American, Korean-American, and Mexican-American ethnic groups with respect to topics such as truth-telling, patient autonomy, advance care directives, and forgoing life support. This [selection] presents qualitative data from the portion of the study that dealt with the issue of truth-telling. . . .

Results

The data from this survey have been published elsewhere[1]; they are reviewed only briefly here. Almost all of the African-American and European-American subjects in our study believed that patients should be told the truth about a diagnosis of cancer (87% and 89%, respectively). Only 47% of Korean-Americans and 65% of Mexican-Americans believed in telling the truth about the diagnosis. With respect to telling the truth about a terminal prognosis, again the European-American and African-American respondents were much more likely to believe in open disclosure, with 63% of African-American and 69% of European-American subjects agreeing that a patient should be told. Only 33% of the Korean-American and 48% of the Mexican-American subjects agreed with telling a terminally ill patient about the patient's prognosis. Among the Mexican-American and Korean-American respondents, more years of education, higher income, younger age, and the ability to speak and read English predicted a positive attitude toward truth-telling.[*] Statistical analysis of the data, controlling for variables such as income, education, and access to care, revealed that ethnicity was the most important factor contributing to attitudes toward truth-telling.

Although large differences among the attitudes of our groups with respect to truth-telling are apparent from the survey data, the reasons for these differences cannot be determined from the survey responses alone. For this reason, in the ethnographic interviews, we repeated the case and asked not only whether should the patient be told, but also why. Why is it okay or not okay to tell? If it generally is not okay to tell, does that include you? Would you want to be kept in the dark? Have you ever had the experience of telling or not telling the truth to a relative or friend? The remainder of this article presents the results of our analysis of these ethnographic interviews; these results have not been published previously. The themes that emerged from the interviews are presented below; quotations from subjects are included to illustrate each point. In the sections that follow, subjects are identified by RP (research participant) number and ethnicity (EA, European-American; AA, African-American; MA, Mexican-American; KA, Korean-American).

---

[*]This was particularly important in the Mexican-American group, which was divided into two groups, one that spoke and read English and got their news from English-language media. The group generally had a higher socioeconomic status. The attitudes of those in this group on the survey tended to look more like those of the European-American group. The second group of Mexican-Americans spoke, read, and thought in Spanish; had a generally lower socioeconomic status; and had attitudes that were more negative toward truth-telling. The Korean-American group was much less diverse. In general, this group had immigrated to Los Angeles from Korea more recently, and few of them spoke English.

Themes

Patient autonomy: "Because it's me."　Among the European-American and African-American subjects, the theme that emerged most frequently was that patients in general and the subjects themselves should know the truth because, as RP 001 (EA) put it, "I'd want to know the worst because it's me; I would have to face it." For the participants holding this belief, information about their bodies is theirs to know, good or bad, simply because it is their body.

Although the knowledge of a terminal prognosis may be distressing, if you are not told, someone else is making decisions that are properly yours, and this lack of control is even more distressing than the bad news. As RP 008 (EA) said, "If there's anything wrong with me, tell me; it's my decision what to do. . . . I happen to be a person that wants to control my destiny as much as I can." Even if there is nothing that can be done to cure the disease, the knowledge itself is a form of power. To be the owner of your own body and life, you need to know about yourself. RP 259 (AA) stated this succinctly: "I want to know everything about me." It is a patient's right to know this information and the doctor's duty to tell it since "the person was intelligent enough to go to the doctor because he knew something was wrong, and he wanted to know what was wrong with him" (RP 263, AA). This complex of ideas, which is consistent with the patient autonomy model of bioethics, was mentioned by almost every African-American and European-American respondent interviewed. Many qualified their support for truth-telling with the idea that some people were not able to handle such information: "Some people, it would frighten them very much" (RP 022, EA). However, even those who worried that some were too fragile to hear the truth seemed to feel that most people could and should be told their diagnosis and prognosis, and that doctors should err on the side of truth-telling. The Korean-American and Mexican-American subjects, as we show below, were more likely to see truth-telling as cruel and potentially harmful rather than empowering, and they rarely mentioned the idea of a "right" to the truth.

You know anyway.　Related to the idea of truth as a right of the patient is the idea that patients will know, intuitively, that they are very sick or even dying, so there is no harm in telling them. RP 133 (EA) put it this way: "I think we have a sense of our bodies, and you know something's wrong, and it's better . . . to know exactly what." RP 108 (EA) said, "The person has a right to know, and I think internally a person has a feeling as to what the prognosis might be." The right to know is connected to the ability to know for these subjects. "It's my life, and I ought to know, Cause you got a feeling anyway. You know" (RP 301, AA). Ownership of your body gives you a right to truthful information; it also gives you the ability to sense this information before it is told. In comparison, some of the Korean-American and Mexican-American subjects agreed that the patient will know, but for these participants, this was a reason not to tell the patient the truth. "You don't have to tell the person about such a thing because, unless the person is a dummy, he or she will figure it out" (RP 451, KA).

Getting your things in order.   One of the most common reasons given by our European-American respondents for wanting to know the truth about a terminal prognosis was so they could get their "things" in order. This rationale was much less common in our other groups. As RP 008 (EA) put it, doctors should tell the truth because "so many people don't have wills or anything else." "We feel that you need to take care of your business . . . make provisions for those who need to have provisions made for them. To me that's simply manly" (RP 22, EA). By getting your things in order, you can ensure that your family is cared for or, at the very least, prevent them from being burdened with complex financial matters after your death:

> You settle your affairs. You've got to have a trust or a will . . . and let your wife know where everything is, and go over the things with your kids and your family so you know that by the time I'm gone this is what's here and you do this and you do that. (RP 171, EA)

A subtext here is the desire to exert control in the face of an uncontrollable process, death. In this way, one could almost link the desire to complete a will prior to death with the desire to complete a living will prior to becoming incompetent. Both are attempts to extend the reach of one's control into situations in which, by definition, one otherwise is unable to exert any control. This interpretation is supported by the fact that, when our respondents were asked about living wills or durable power of attorney for health care, they frequently discussed the concepts of living trust and durable power of attorney for financial matters. At first, it seemed that our respondents were confusing the two concepts, but when pushed by our interviewers, it became clear that these two concepts simply were linked very tightly in their minds. Both types of document usually were completed in the same place (an attorney's office), often at the same time, and were saturated with complex meanings that revolved around the themes of mortality, burdensomeness, and control.

Get it right with God.   When asked about truth-telling, some of our subjects discussed the issue as one having religious or spiritual significance. According to this idea, you should know the truth so that you can get it right with God. This theme was mentioned most frequently by our African-American respondents. If you know the truth, you have time to "get right with the good Lord . . . so when you die, your soul is saved" (RP 347, AA). "There are too many things a person has to do with his life at that point, to be in ignorance of his death . . . he has to go to his minister and . . . make whatever peace you have to make with your minister" (RP 252, AA). Even in the face of this knowledge, "When the Lord is with you, the devil can't do you no harm" (RP 289, AA).

Getting it right with God does not necessarily mean simply preparing your soul for death. If your doctor tells you that you have cancer, you have an opportunity to bring the problem to God, whose healing powers are greater than a doctor's. "I got another doctor, that's Doctor Jesus" (RP 201, AA). "[I would want him to tell me] because . . . I got another doctor I would go to that's the master of the universe, and let him tell me what to think about it"

(RP 208, AA). If you know the truth, "you can prepare for it . . . ask your God [if you can live a longer life]" (RP 280, AA). "I want to know, can he help me; if he can't, tell me. If he can't help me, I go to the next person; that's the man above" (RP 364, AA). These answers reflect the belief that doctors are fallible and frequently can not know whether a patient will live or die. Only God is capable of having that kind of knowledge. As RP 289 (AA) said, "I wouldn't care if he told me because it wouldn't make it true. . . . I believe in the Lord just because he [the doctor] said you're going to die next week, I never will believe nothing like that." "Some [doctors] they say that, and they come out of it" (RP 280, AA). Doctors have one kind of knowledge and power; God another. "The doctors say what . . . the afflictions of the righteous is, but God delivers them out of it all" (RP 201, AA).

Interestingly, this theme of needing to know the truth so that one could become closer to God either for healing or for absolution simply was not mentioned by any of the subjects in the European-American group. This was a religiously diverse group that included (in roughly equal numbers) Protestants, Catholics, and Jews. Only one of our Korean-American subjects, a deeply religious convert to Christianity, mentioned this rationale: "Yes, I would [want to know the truth]. Then, I could repent for my sins before God" (RP 409, KA). Several of the Mexican-American subjects made similar comments: "I would not want to be deceived. . . . I would put myself in God's hands; I would repent for all my sins and for the bad things I have done" (RP 607, MA).

It is cruel to tell.   In contrast to the European-American and African-American subjects, most of our Korean-American and Mexican-American subjects did not perceive the truth (especially the truth about a fatal prognosis) as empowering. Rather than envisioning the patient as an autonomous agent who needs information to make decisions and maintain control and dignity, the Mexican-American and Korean-American respondents viewed the patient as sick, weak, and in need of protection by the doctor and the family. Telling the truth in this context was seen as cruel. "Tell him [the patient] that he is getting better . . . because we should not be so cruel as to tell him, 'You are going to die, and it will be on such and such a day'" (RP 607, MA). Instead, it is kinder to "give him hope, console him . . . [so he can] always have hope that he will get better" (RP 607, MA).

> Anyway, the patient will die, so what is the use of saying you are going to die of cancer, right? The doctor should say, "You are okay; you will be fine. . . . Just take the medicine which will get you better." He shouldn't say that you have cancer so that you will die in a few months. Isn't that common sense? (RP 414, KA)

When one of our anthropologists commented to a Korean-American subject that, in America, most people were informed of their diagnosis and prognosis, the subject replied, "Yes, they are, because this allows patients to be prepared for death, but it must be very painful for those patients" (RP 447, KA). The benefit of "being prepared" here is seen as insufficient to outweigh the pain caused by knowledge of the truth. Of a son dying with liver cancer, one Korean-American respondent stated, "We just couldn't tell him because it was cruel" (RP 451, KA). She went on to illustrate this by telling how her son had guessed that he had cancer and had been very distressed:

> Holding on to me, he cried very, very sadly, saying, "Mother, I do not remember that I have done anything bad to others in my whole life. I do not know how I got stricken with this bad disease." . . . So, both he and I cried to the last drop of our tears.

This mother felt guilty that she had not been able to protect her son from the truth and did her best to make up for it: "After that, I comforted him so that he would not give up hope on himself."

Most of these subjects agreed not only that the truth should be withheld in general, but also that they would not want to know it themselves: "If they tell me . . . I have the terminal cancer, I will become more depressed because my life is coming to an end" (RP 605, MA). "I wouldn't [want to know]. . . . I would be afraid of dying" (RP 640, MA). One of our Korean-American subjects told us that, for many years, her children had hidden from her the knowledge that a surgical procedure was for cancer, and she stated, "My children did a good thing for me, not a bad thing. If I had researched what it was, then it would be bad for everyone" (RP 480, KA, after a cone biopsy).

Many of the respondents, especially the Korean-American respondents, were aware that patients often come to know the truth even if they are not told directly. As one subject put it, "The patient in critical condition could get an idea of what she or he has by the doctor's attitude. However, there is a difference in knowing about one's disease from guessing and from confirmation by others. I feel I don't want to know about my impending death . . . without hope, one cannot live. . . . So anyone who says that she or he wants to know about having a disease is out of their minds because the knowing itself is painful. If the patients have more stress, their lives are shortened" (RP 414, KA). This is discussed in more detail below; here, we just note that knowing, or rather guessing, is better than being told directly because it allows for some ambiguity and for the possibility of hope.

If you know you die faster.   The truth not only is distressing according to these respondents, but also it potentially is harmful, even fatal. "It's not good to tell people what's wrong with them because they die sooner. . . . I told the doctor not to tell him" (RP 605, MA). "If the spreading cancer didn't kill her, the fear would" (RP 640, MA). One respondent told us the story of his brother, who died of cancer in rural Mexico. The truth had been kept carefully from him until almost the end of his life, when he happened to come by a mirror and see himself. Seeing how wasted he looked, he realized his condition. After that, according to his brother, "He never recuperated. . . . That is when he gave up. I think that [noticing how grave the illness is] is very bad for a deathly ill patient. If he has something to pick him up, his life is prolonged" (RP 666, MA).

One of our Korean-American subjects brought his wife from Seoul, Korea, to Sacramento, California, for treatment without informing her of her condition: "We kept it a tight secret. . . . If she knew, she would not be able to live longer because of the fear" (RP 447, KA).

Some people can't take it.   These themes, that the truth is cruel and harmful to patients, could be found in the transcripts of European-American and African-American subjects as well. Here, it almost always took the form of a statement that the truth is harmful for *some* people: "Some people just are not able, for whatever reason, to deal with unpleasant facts" (RP 007, EA). This almost always was qualified: "But, in general, I think you've got to level with people." (This statement was made by a man who felt that he could take it, but was not sure about his wife.) In this view, some people will not be able to cope after they receive such bad news; for these few, the truth is not empowering, but disabling. "Some people fall apart over nothing. And if the doctor knows the patient at all, he should be able to determine whether this person could handle it or not" (RP 259, AA). Some even admitted that they were one of the ones who couldn't take it: "I think it depends on the person. Some people can take the news better than others. . . . I'm a worry-wart, and they tell me that; all positive things I would throw out of my mind" (RP 258, AA).

Not the truth, but hope.   Although superficially the attitudes of our Korean-American and Mexican-American subjects toward the truth seemed identical, there were differences between them. As we reviewed the data from our Mexican-American subjects, we were confused initially by what seemed to be a contradictory and ambiguous attitude toward the truth in many of the transcripts. For example, one of our Mexican-American subjects told us that, "It is my opinion that the truth must always be told [to everyone]. . . . I would want the doctor to tell me directly" (RP 658, MA). However, speaking of a cousin with cancer, she told this story:

> She suffered a lot . . . and always asked me, "Isn't it true that I have cancer?" I told her, "C'mon, what cancer? It's not cancer." . . . It would have been more suffering if she had known what she had. (RP 658, MA)

A respondent (RP 666, MA) (mentioned above), said, "I think that [noticing how grave the illness is] is very bad for a deathly ill patient," about his brother, who died after looking in a mirror. Further in that same transcript, this respondent said that, "Knowing the truth helps to make you feel better because you can look for a way to cheer up and not get to the end of the road like the doctors thought" (RP 666, MA). When asked by our anthropologist how a doctor should tell a patient the truth, he replied:

> He would tell you gently [saying], "Now, we are going to do everything in our hands so you feel better; however, we will not stop you from dying, but the 2 or 3 days you have left should be happy, and don't think about leaving because maybe it won't happen." (RP 666, MA)

That is, the doctor should tell the patient that the patient will die in 2 or 3 days, but at the same time tell the patient that maybe they aren't going to die at all.

Another subject (RP 730) answered an emphatic "Yes" to the truth-telling question and at first denied that people die faster when they are told ("Those are just rumors"), but later told us that the patient should not be told about the prognosis: "It's better not to tell them that part to encourage her so that she thinks she's going to live more than she will actually live" (RP 730, MA).

Some of these seeming contradictions simply may be an expression of the complexity of the subject. However, the perceived contradictory nature of these answers actually may be another variant of the top-down problem mentioned above. At the start of this study, the authors identified an ethical problem: truthtelling. The issue for us was whether the doctor should tell the truth. But, for these subjects, it appears that the more appropriate ethical category is "hope," and the issue is whether the doctor and family take away hope. Taking away hope is prohibited because it is cruel and because it makes the patient die faster. The truth is not the main issue; the truth can be told as long as it is told in such a way as not to remove hope. You can tell the patient that he or she is going to die as long as you tell the patient that he or she might not die. This is why telling the prognosis is so much worse than telling the diagnosis. As long as you tell the patient that the cancer can be cured, it is not so bad to tell the patient that they have cancer.

This interpretation is supported by two respondents in the Mexican-American group who actually had cancer. One of them had lung cancer. He agreed that people should be told the truth about their diagnosis, as he was. However, he admitted that he wouldn't want to know about a terminal prognosis: "No [don't tell me]. . . . It would torment me" (RP 615, MA). As far as could be determined from his description, he had only palliative (not curative) treatment (draining pleural effusions), but was convinced he was cured, or as he put it, "The tumor is dry" (RP 615, MA). . . . The patient was told the truth about his diagnosis, but given hope.

Another respondent, with head and neck cancer, had a similar story. When asked if it was appropriate to tell the truth, he stated, "Oh, yes, because then [they could] connect me to a machine instead of having surgery and giving me therapy and X-rays. . . . He [the doctor] told me that it was going to get better with the machines" (RP 754, MA). Later, when asked about being told the prognosis, he said it was okay "for the doctor to tell me, but so that I won't become discouraged, to tell me that I am [going to live longer] even though I am not." Tell me the truth about my dying, but tell it in such a way that I do not have to face it without hope that I will live. . . .

Conclusion

This study of 800 elderly subjects showed that major differences exist in the way people of different ethnicities view the issue of truth-telling. One of the core differences, around which many of the themes circled, is the question of how the truth affects the terminally ill patient. On one hand, the truth can be seen as an essential tool that allows the patient to maintain a sense of personal agency and control. Seen in this light, telling the truth, however painful, is empowering. On the other hand, the truth can be seen as traumatic and demoralizing, sapping the patient of hope and the will to live. For those who hold this view, truth-telling is an act of cruelty.

In fact, many, if not most, of our subjects held both views. They differed in the relative weight given to each view. In weighing the positive benefits of the truth versus its potential to harm, the deciding factor seems to be the way the self is understood. Are we mainly autonomous agents whose dignity and worth come from the individual choices we make with our lives, or is our most important characteristic the web of social relations in which we exist? If we hold the former view (as most of our African-American and European-American respondents did), then lack of access to the truth is almost dehumanizing since it strips us of our ability to make choices, without which we are something less than fully human. If, however, we tend to see ourselves not as individuals, but as a part of a larger social network (as was more common in the Mexican-American and Korean-American groups), then the notion of personal choice loses something of its force, and we may expect that those close to us will act on our behalf to protect and nurture us in our time of need.

The second meta-theme that emerged from these data has to do with the many meanings of telling. When we began this study, we assumed that there were two possibilities: The truth could be told to or withheld from the patient. This is how the survey instrument was designed; respondents had to answer yes or no to questions about telling the diagnosis and prognosis to a patient with terminal cancer. However, many of our subjects, particularly in the Mexican-American and Korean-American groups, had a view with more nuances of how the patient could be told, or could come to know, the truth. According to these respondents, the truth could be told vaguely, partially; could be understood without telling, by context and hints; or could be known by nunchi. These types of telling allow for ambiguity and therefore for hope. This adds another layer of complexity to the issue of truth-telling and calls into question not only whether, but also how, we should tell the truth and even what telling and the truth mean.

References

1.   Hare J, Nelson C. Will outpatients complete living wills? A comparison of two interventions. *J Gen Intern Med.* 1991;6:41–46.

2.   Sachs GA, Stocking CB, Miles SH. Empowering the older patient? A randomized controlled trial to increase discussion and use of advance directives. *J Am Geriatric Soc.* 1992;40:269–273.

3.   Caralis PV, Davis B, Wright K, Marcial E. The Influence of ethnicity and race on attitudes toward advance directives, life-prolonging treatments and euthanasia. *J Clin Ethics.* 1993;4:155–166.

4.   Teno JM, Fleishman J, Brock DW, Mor V. The use of Formal Prior Directives among patients with HIV-related diseases. *J Gen Intern Med.* 1990;5:490–494.

5. Sugarman J, Weinberger M, Samsa G. Factors associated with veterans' decisions about living wills. *Arch Intern Med.* 1992;152:343–347.

6. Murphy ST, Palmer JM, Azen S, Frank G, Michel V, Blackhall LJ. Ethnicity and advance care directives. *J Law Med Ethics.* 1996;24:108–117.

7. Blackhall LJ, Murphy S, Frank G, Michel V, Azen S. Ethnicity and attitudes toward patient autonomy. *JAMA.* 1995;274:820–825.

**Mark Kuczewski
and Patrick J. McCruden**

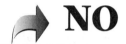 **NO**

Informed Consent: Does It Take a Village? The Problem of Culture and Truth Telling

Bioethicists have become very interested in the importance of social groups. This interest has spawned a growing literature on the role of the family[1] and the place of culture[2] in medical decisionmaking. These ethicists often argue that much of medical ethics suffers from the individualistic bias of the dominant culture and political tradition of the United States. As a result, the doctrine of informed consent has come under some scrutiny. It is believed that therein lies the source of the problem because the doctrine incorporates the assumptions of the larger society. Thus, informed consent has been reexamined, reinterpreted,[3] and even abandoned as unworkable.[4]

Our society embraces certain liberal democratic ideals such as the right of individuals to the maximum amount of freedom; that is, to do what they want, as long as they don't hurt anybody.[5] Of course, we also look for society to provide a certain equality of opportunity.[6] Otherwise one's freedom wouldn't mean much. These principles, liberty and equality, provide the foundation for the individual's pursuit of his or her particular vision of the good life. The state should remain neutral toward competing visions of the good life as long as these visions do not infringe on the rights of others. As a result, the state does not advocate a substantive morality but embraces a procedural ethic that allows each to play out his or her own life without interference from the value judgments of others.

Bioethicists have recently called our attention to the fact that this kind of ethic often works better in theory than in practice. Boundaries among individuals are sometimes not clearly demarcated. Although it is fine to speak about the rights of the individual, respecting patient autonomy usually requires a process of collaborative decisionmaking. This process involves not only the patient and physician but those who are close to the patient. Patient autonomy becomes a reality when treatment decisions are made in the way that patients typically make their other significant decisions. This often creates a legitimate role for the family in the decisionmaking schema.[7]

Similarly, some have noted that it is not only the significant interpersonal relationships that challenge medical ethics' conception of patient autonomy

From Mark Kuczewski and Patrick J. McCruden, "Informed Consent: Does It Take a Village? The Problem of Culture and Truth Telling," *Cambridge Quarterly of Healthcare Ethics,* vol. 10, no. 1 (2001), pp. 34–35, 37–41, 45–46. Copyright © 2001 by Cambridge University Press. Reprinted by permission of Cambridge University Press.

but also the patient's culture.[8] The very concept of patient autonomy is a product of our Western culture, which values individual freedom and self-determination. Insofar as these cultural assumptions are shared by the parties in the clinical encounter, medical ethics is equipped to handle the situation. However, when the patient and the patient's family are from a culture whose values are quite different, our ethic may be invalidated. If so, it is not clear how the clinician should proceed. It could follow from these premises that medical ethics is relative to culture and physician behavior would best be guided by the norms of the patient's community. In short, one could argue for a culturally relative medical ethics.[9,10]

We believe that the concerns about the individualistic nature of medical ethics are important. The rhetoric of informed consent still emphasizes self-determination despite the fact that good scholarship has expanded what bioethicists mean by that term. This scholarly trend toward a less individualistic, more process-oriented notion of informed consent and its resulting role for close others is salutary. However, it is not exactly clear what many of these critics of informed consent are seeking. Typically, compromises are called for because the "dominant Western bioethical concepts and principles are problematic" and "routine application of these concepts and principles may pose difficulties."[11] Although cautious, some argue that informed consent can be compromised. For instance, "[d]eviation from the usual formal standards of informed consent would be justified only by reference to patient-centered values."[12] And, of course, others have astutely observed that, in practice, informed consent is often compromised and truth withheld in the attempt to be culturally sensitive.[13]

Although cultural sensitivity is important, we shall argue that any suggestion that we should step outside our ethical framework entirely in favor of the ethic of the patient's culture is mistaken.[14] Such suggestions should not guide clinical behavior. We will justify this claim in two ways: (1) by reiterating the reasons our culture holds informed consent so dear and building on this foundation, and (2) by rebutting the epistemological assumptions of a culturally relative medical ethics. Furthermore, our skepticism regarding the use of culture in clinical decisionmaking might suggest that the study of culture is of no use to the clinician. We offer some preliminary speculations regarding why we believe that conclusion is overstated. . . .

The Cultural Challenge to Informed Consent

The doctrine of informed consent has certain basic features. The patient must be given information. In other words, disclosure of the diagnosis and prognosis must be made, treatment proposed, the risks and benefits of the treatment outlined, alternative options highlighted. The patient must, to some extent, grasp the information and then make a choice to accept or refuse the treatment. Certain conditions must also obtained. That is, the patient must be free from undue influence or coercion and the patient must have the cognitive and affective capacity to make the decision (i.e., the patient must be competent). Competence provides a road into the consent process for social groups.

When informed consent is a relatively straightforward onetime event, such as might occur immediately before a lifesaving emergency appendectomy, the patient may have little need of close others to provide a valid consent. However, many long-term chronic illnesses create an ongoing process of informed consent in which the patient's knowledge of treatment options and their attendant effects grows through experience. Through this experience, the patient gains insight into her illness and develops certain evaluations of the treatment options. The physician also goes through a process of refining the diagnosis and prognosis and continues to reassess her evaluations of the treatment options. The physician and patient mutually monitor each other to ascertain how their respective understandings and evaluations are proceeding.[15]

For the patient to make competent treatment choices, his or her values must be relatively stable. When consent is an event, the patient issues competent choices from existing values. But when illness demands that the patient reinterpret or develop new values to cope with the situation, close others will be needed to aid the patient in this process of reality testing and personal growth. The communitarian understanding of the interpersonal development of values through mutual self-discovery will clearly come into play. For instance, values or interpretations of values may become stable for the patient through the support of family and friends or, conversely, by standing up to the objections of these persons. Thus, the decisionmaking capacity of the patient is partially a group function. But, exactly to what degree is the person constituted by the group? Consider the following case.

Case 1

> Oscar Ramirez, a 55-year-old patient of Mexican descent, presented with a large growth in his throat. He was told that the growth was cancerous. Mr. Ramirez was also told that he would need to have the tumor removed and start an aggressive round of chemotherapy. Mr. Ramirez agreed to the proposed treatment. However, Ramirez's wife and children told the oncologist that complete truthfulness would devastate him and that it was their duty to protect him. They supported this claim by saying that their background required that "la familia" take this protective role. They added that their culture does not place the same value on the individual's control of his own life that most Americans do. Thus, when the tumor could not be completely removed, Mr. Ramirez was merely told that his recovery would be lengthy and that much treatment would be needed to keep the cancer from recurring. Because of great skill in deception and a tightly orchestrated effort to conceal the truth, Oscar Ramirez died without ever being told of his terminal illness.

Let us tease out some moral intuitions regarding this case. Case-based reasoning, also known as casuistic method, will be of help. Casuistry suggests that we should not plunge directly into a case in which our intuitions are unclear. We should look at similar cases in which the right action readily suggests itself. Then, by analogy to these paradigms, we can illuminate our path in this problematic case.

A good casuist would tell us to pursue two different paradigms; one in which it seemed correct to withhold the truth from Mr. Ramirez and one in which it was clearly wrong. We can try out a number of different scenarios in search of these paradigms, but this does not seem to be a difficult exercise. One clear paradigm case in which it would be correct to withhold the truth is one in which Mr. Ramirez would be devastated by the bad news. After hearing of the difficulties in removing the tumor, Mr. Ramirez would slip into a deep, permanent depression and lose any possible enjoyment of the remainder of his life. Similarly, we would also have a similar paradigm case in one in which Mr. Ramirez wanted the truth withheld. For a variety of reasons, he may prefer this course of action. Such reasons might include that he simply does not like negative medical news, that bad news would drain off psychological energy that could be used to fight the disease, that he wishes this situation to be managed in accord with the traditional familial roles his family outlined, and so on. But the reason seems somewhat inconsequential to the choice of the correct action. If Mr. Ramirez clearly does not want to know his diagnosis, we are obligated to withhold it. On the other hand, when we look for a paradigm of truth telling in this instance, it would usually involve a desire by Mr. Ramirez to want to know his diagnosis. Perhaps he wishes to know for any of a variety of the usual reasons, including setting his affairs in order, finishing the "unfinished business" of life, and simply managing his end-of-life decisions.

As we compare these paradigms of information withholding and truth telling, we realize that we do not consider them to be equal. We favor those paradigms that contain some direct expression of patient autonomy, either by waiver of his informed consent rights or by providing full disclosure to be more applicable. Is this merely because we are members of a liberal democratic society? Probably not. Not so long ago we thought that persons who were given bad news routinely became irreversibly depressed. Then, we became familiar with the idea that the adverse reactions patients endured were transient and that they usually reacted better in the long run if allowed to remain in control of their life and destiny. Even so, the practices of clinicians continued (and might still continue) to be less than completely truthful.[16] Nevertheless, we realize that there is no need for a paradigm to justify telling the truth. We are in need of paradigms that can justify withholding information.

It is undoubtedly true that, in the short run, Mr. Ramirez does not want bad information. But the traditional doctrine of informed consent is founded on his right to have that information, even when it's bad, and the empirical postulate that he will be better off in the long run for it. Through the normal social and psychological processes of living, Mr. Ramirez will adapt to the harsh realities and do well. In this belief, communitarian and liberal theorists agree. However, the communitarian has a deeper appreciation for the fact that such processes might be culturally relative and without a community that values taking control of one's affairs, such processes might not proceed according to the paradigm.

So the disagreement between a communitarian perspective and a liberal theorist about how to proceed in a clinical case of this type may come down to a different rebuttable presumption. The liberal rights-oriented theorist requires some direct expression of autonomy even if it be via a waiver of informed consent. A more communitarian perspective argues that this delegation of authority can also be implicit. Edmund Pellegrino writes:

> . . . among many ethnic groups in the United States . . . this delegation of authority is culturally implicit. . . . Withholding the truth from a patient demands, of course, the utmost care in responding to any occasion when the patient wishes to exert more control.[17]

If we wish to be true to the process notion of informed consent and retain its communitarian concept of the person, must this conclusion follow? If the patient is from one of the requisite cultures that do not value autonomy, should we accept the family's statement that such news would "kill him"? We think not.

Justifying the Hegemony of Informed Consent

Communitarianism and cultural sensitivity are complex phenomena. It is all too easy to fall prey to simple-minded solutions. In general, we believe that the communitarian view sketched above suffers from (1) a simple-minded epistemology and (2) a focus that excludes the culture and community of the healthcare professions. Once community membership is seen as the complex matter it is and cultural sensitivity is also extended to the culture of the clinic, we believe that it will be clear that patients must waive their right to information to justify physicians withholding it.

The epistemology of this radical communitarian position posits cultures as opaque to those outside of them. We supposedly cannot appreciate the way that a different culture sees the respective roles of the persons involved. This assumes a sharp distinction between the "inside" and "outside" of a culture. Only those on the inside can understand its working whereas those on the outside must simply accept what the insiders tell us about it. The rationality of a culture is an internal one and cannot be evaluated externally.[18] As a result, we are at the mercy of the reports Mr. Ramirez's children supply about their culture and any survey data about that culture that can confirm a dissimilarity between his culture and those of the clinicians. The opacity of the culture has been substituted for the opacity of the individual of Western liberal theory.

The main problem with this epistemology is that we have little reason to believe that cultures are, in fact, so opaque and able to enforce rigid boundaries between insiders and outsiders. Mr. Ramirez's case causes us a problem on the gut level because we have a cultural situation explained to us but are not sure how this patient relates to his own culture. Many people who seem to be clearly ensconced in a culture still pick and choose from its beliefs on many points. Mr. Ramirez does not live in one culture but in at least two. Otherwise he would not be in this particular hospital. How he relates to the beliefs of each is currently opaque. But, it need not remain so. We can simply ask him.

This would allow him to request information or to provide an explicit waiver of consent.

Second, and perhaps as important, is the fact that we have been speaking as if patients and their families come from cultures but the healthcare providers have none or one that is not authentic. This radical communitarian view caricatures them as value-free and adaptable to any culture. They normally live and die by the doctrine of informed consent because they usually encounter people from the Western liberal tradition that values freedom and individualism. Or, healthcare providers are themselves part of a culture that is value-free in valuing the autonomy of individuals. As a result, the communitarian counsels suggest that they must rein that tendency in when dealing with the contentladen value systems of other cultures. Surely, such a view is mistaken.

The clinic has its own culture and values. Typically, these are health-related values that favor treatment of illness and prolongation of life over pleasure and most other personal lifestyle choices. Clinicians, especially those engaged in clinical research or graduate medical education, also place a strong emphasis on the advancement of knowledge. Similarly, clinical practice is often thought to have an implicit ethos that varies among medical specialties or particular healthcare professions, their "standard of care." And, because healthcare professionals are highly educated and respected, they are probably likely to assume that others share these values or to overvalue the worth of their treatments. The doctrine of informed consent evolved to safeguard us from the imposition of this clinical culture on patients.

As we noted at the outset, the doctrine of informed consent requires that the physician disclose all of the pertinent facts about the diagnosis and treatment options so that the patient may decide if he or she values them to the same degree as the physician. We also saw that this required a certain process, given that it is not always obvious to the patient exactly how he or she values the proposed course of action. This process involved the relaxing of boundaries among persons as values were formed or interpreted. And, this situation can raise concerns regarding the occasional need for the healthcare provider to act as the patient's advocate in dealing with domineering family members and similar situations that may involve undue influence.[19] Clinical judgment is often strained at such moments and there are few objective signposts to guide the clinician. In these situations, some solace is found in the fact that the informed consent process is teleological in nature. That is, patient autonomy is considered the goal or outcome of the consent process. At some point, when the patient's values and preferences toward a treatment choice clearly become stable, the physician is clearly again the patient's advocate. Then, communitarian formulations recede as the patient again has an individual identity.

This teleological element is the ultimate safeguard in process models of informed consent. Concerns about the imposition of the values of family members and healthcare professionals on a vulnerable patient are assuaged by knowing that at some point, the end point, the patient will make an autonomous decision. A culturally relative medical ethics requires that we suspend this teleological element. In Mr. Ramirez's case, there was no point at which patient autonomy clearly emerged. Thus, the only safeguard against the tyranny of the culture of the clinic, a tyranny that never sought the patient's input on the level of aggressiveness of treatment, was suspended. One might attempt to argue that the clinicians and family were merely trying to respect the patient's implicit expression of autonomy, but we have absolutely no way to know whether this was more than wishful thinking. . . .

The Use of Culture in the Clinic

We are arguing for a position that recognizes the limits of healthcare professionals to step outside of their own cultural worldview and norms. We believe that it is epistemologically naïve to think otherwise as well as condescending to persons of other cultures to believe that they have no ability to engage in dialogue that stretches their limitations as well. By insisting on the doctrine of informed consent or an appropriate waiver process, we think that our healthcare system respects cultural differences rather than condescends to them. We propose that we accept these limitations and advocate the continued use of the safeguards afforded by the doctrine of informed consent and the possibilities available through explicit waivers by individuals.

If the ethics of healthcare practice are not culturally relative, then why should clinicians be concerned with culture at all? This is an interesting question. Informed consent is a conversational process and hearing what patients have to say requires some knowledge of cultures. Conversational norms are often cultural and colored by a variety of other factors such as gender. We will do well to know what norms we are likely to encounter in the clinic. But, we must never assume that a cultural generalization tells us the whole story. We should not try to get beyond our own cultural norm of informed consent that requires we ask patients what they mean.

It is also true that cultural sensitivity and understanding is worthwhile to clinicians even if it does not translate directly in behavioral change in the way things are done in the clinic. It is obvious that the encounter of other cultures increases the clinician's awareness of the culture of his or her setting. The clinician not only learns something about patients in understanding their cultures but also comes to understand himself. This reward of the practice of medicine and the healthcare specialties should not be dismissed lightly. Informed consent is, ideally, not just a process of discovery by the patient; it also holds the promise of being one of mutual self-discovery.

Notes

1.   Nelson HL, Nelson JL. *The Patient in the Family: An Ethics of Medicine and Families.* New York: Routledge, 1995.

2.   Pellegrino ED, Mazzarella P, Corsi P, eds. *Transcultural Dimensions in Medical Ethics.* Frederick, Md.: University Publishing Group, 1992.

3.   Lidz CW, Appelbaum PS, Meisel A. Two models of implementing informed consent. *Archives of Internal Medicine* 1988;148:1385–9.

4. Veatch RM. Abandoning informed consent. *Hastings Center Report* 1995;25 (2): 5–12.

5. Rawls J. *A Theory of Justice.* Cambridge, Mass.: Harvard University Press, 1971.

6. Daniels N. *Just Health Care.* New York: Cambridge University Press, 1985.

7. Kuczewski MG. Reconceiving the family: the process of consent in medical decisionmaking. *Hastings Center Report* 1996;26(2):30–7.

8. Blackhall LJ, Murphy ST, Frank G, Michel V, Azen S. Ethnicity and attitudes toward patient autonomy. *JAMA* 1995;274(10):820–5.

9. Carrese J, Rhodes L. Western bioethics on the Navajo reservation. *JAMA* 1995;274(10):826–9 at 826.

10. Pellegrino, ED. Is truth telling to the patient a cultural artifact? *JAMA* 1992; 268(13):1734–5.

11. See note 9, Carrese and Rhodes 1995:829.

12. Gostin LO. Informed consent, cultural sensitivity and respect for persons. *JAMA* 1995;274(10):844–5 at 845.

13. Freedman B. Offering truth: one ethical approach to the uninformed cancer patient. *Archives of Internal Medicine* 1993;153(5):572–6.

14. Gordon E. Decisionmaking: the notion of informed waiver. *Fordham Urban Law Journal* 1996;23(4):1321–62 at 1344.

15. See note 3, Lidz, Appelbaum, Meisel 1988: 1386.

16. Novack D, Detering B, Arnold R, Forrow L, Ladinsky M, Pezzullo J. Physicians' attitudes toward using deception to resolve difficult ethical problems. *JAMA* 1989;261(20):2980–5.

17. See note 10, Pellegrino 1992:1735.

18. This position is also known as "whole tradition communitarianism." . . .

19. See note 7, Kuczewski 1996:35.

POSTSCRIPT

Should Truth-Telling Depend on the Patient's Culture?

The classic book on truth-telling is Sissela Bok's *Lying: Moral Choice in Public and Private Life* (Pantheon Books, 1978). Written at a time when many American physicians were reluctant to tell patients the truth, she challenged that view by arguing that the harm resulting from disclosure is less than believed and is outweighed by the benefits, including the important one of giving the patient the right to choose among treatments.

Much of the literature on withholding the truth from patients concerns cancer. Mary R. Anderlik, Rebecca D. Pentz, and Kenneth R. Hess, in "Revisiting the Truth-Telling Debate: A Study of Disclosure Practices at a Major Cancer Center," *The Journal of Clinical Ethics* (Fall 2000) found that in the previous year a majority of physicians had encountered a family's request to withhold information about a prognosis or diagnosis. The majority of physicians combined a general commitment to disclosure with a willingness to be flexible in some cases, more often in prognosis than in diagnosis.

Physicians Margaret A. Drickamer and Mark S. Lachs address a different disease in their essay, "Should Patients With Alzheimer's Disease Be Told Their Diagnosis?" *The New England Journal of Medicine* (April 2, 1992). Although they favor truth-telling, they present the case for not telling, including such factors as the difficulty of conclusive diagnosis, the impaired decision-making capacity and competence of patients with Alzheimer's, and the limited therapeutic options.

An often-cited article that offers a compromise position is Benjamin Freedman's "Offering Truth: One Ethical Approach to the Uninformed Cancer Patient," *Annals of Internal Medicine* (March 8, 1993). Another article by the Blackhall team, this one with Gelya Frank as the lead author, is "Ambiguity and Hope: Disclosure Preferences of Less Acculturated Elderly Mexican Americans Concerning Terminal Cancer—A Case Story," *Cambridge Quarterly of Healthcare Ethics* (vol. 11, 2002). See also Richard Gorlin, James L. Strain, and Rosamond Rhodes, "Cultural Collisions at the Bedside: Social Expectations and Value Triage in Medical Practice," *Cambridge Quarterly of Healthcare Ethics* (no. 10, 2001). Heather J. Gert offers an alternative to complete disclosure: giving patients enough information that they will not be surprised by whatever happens—unless the physician is also surprised ("Avoiding Surprises: A Model for Informing Patients," *Hastings Center Report,* September–October 2002).

ISSUE 3

Does Direct-to-Consumer Drug Advertising Enhance Patient Choice?

YES: Alan F. Holmer, from "Direct-to-Consumer Prescription Drug Advertising Builds Bridges Between Patients and Physicians," *Journal of the American Medical Association* (January 27, 1999)

NO: Matthew F. Hollon, from "Direct-to-Consumer Marketing of Prescription Drugs," *Journal of the American Medical Association* (January 27, 1999)

ISSUE SUMMARY

YES: Alan F. Holmer, an attorney and head of the Pharmaceutical Research and Manufacturers of America, argues that advertising of medication empowers consumers by educating them about health conditions and possible treatments.

NO: Matthew F. Hollon, a physician, believes that advertising of medication is designed to increase consumer demand, rather than for educational purposes, and has little public health value.

Most uses of the term *ethical* describe a person, an action, a policy, a belief, or a theory, not a product. Yet in 1976 the Subcommittee on Health and the Environment of the U.S. House of Representatives in its "Discursive Dictionary of Health Care" defined *ethical drug* as "a *drug* which is advertised only to physicians and other *prescribing* health *professionals*. Drug manufacturers which make only or primarily such drugs are referred to as the ethical drug industry. Synonymous with *prescription drug*" (italics in original).

Less than a decade later, pharmaceutical companies began advertising directly to consumers, and now one seldom hears the term *ethical drug*. Manufacturers still advertise to physicians, and physicians must still prescribe the drugs, but consumers are now a prime marketing target, especially through television. In 1983 the Food and Drug Administration (FDA), which regulates the approval and marketing of medications, imposed a moratorium on this type of marketing but lifted it two years later. In 1997 the agency changed its guidelines to allow more flexibility in television advertising in describing medication risks. As any television viewer or magazine reader knows, the amount and intensity of drug advertising has been escalating ever since. In its November 2006 report, "Prescription Drugs: Improvements Needed in FDA's Oversight of Direct-to-Consumer Advertising," the General Accounting Office (GAO) of the U.S. House of Representatives reported that drug company spending on prescription drugs increased twice as fast from 1997 through 2005 as spending on promotion to physicians or on research and development. The FDA reviews only a small portion of the direct-to-consumer material it receives, is issuing fewer regulatory letters than it did in a 2002 GAO study, and is taking longer to issue them. The GAO concluded that the agency "cannot ensure that it is identifying or reviewing those materials that it would consider to be of the highest priority."

According to a content analysis of drug advertising in magazines from 1989 through 1998, conducted by Michael Wilkes and his colleagues at the University of California at Los Angeles, the most common medical conditions in these ads were allergies, obstetrical/gynecological, dermatological, cardiovascular, HIV/AIDS, and tobacco addiction. Women were more likely to be targeted than men.

The ads worked. The GAO report found that between 1999 and 2000 the number of prescriptions dispensed for the most heavily advertised drugs rose 25 percent but increased only 4 percent for not-so-visibly promoted drugs. Nicotine patches for tobacco addiction became an $800 million business as a result of advertising. Aggressive marketing of Claritin, produced by Schering-Plough, resulted in this drug accounting for more than half of the $1.8 billion spent in its marketing category. (In November 2002 the FDA took Claritin off the prescription drug list so that it is now available over the counter.)

A national survey conducted by *Prevention Magazine* in 1998 found that more than 53 million consumers talked to their physicians about an advertised medication, and another 49 million looked for information from another source, such as an Internet site. The GAO report estimates that about 8.5 million consumers (5 percent of the total) have both requested and received a prescription for a particular drug as a result of seeing a direct-to-consumer ad.

Although studies have found that consumers remember drug advertising, the consumers have misconceptions about a government's role in regulating this practice. Half of the respondents in a Sacramento County survey conducted by Wilkes and his UCLA colleagues believed that drug ads had to be submitted to the government for prior approval, which is not the case. Nor is it true, as 43 percent believed, that only completely safe drugs can be advertised or that drugs with serious side effects cannot be advertised, as 22 percent believed. Drug manufacturers are only required to truthfully present a fair balance of risks and effectiveness.

On balance, is direct-to-consumer advertising ethically justified or not? Does it enhance patient autonomy by giving information that in earlier decades was available only to physicians? The following selections provide two views of the debate. From an industry perspective, Alan F. Homer finds benefits to individual and public health from alerting consumers to treatable conditions. From his perspective as a physician, Matthew F. Hollon argues that drug advertising passes on costs to consumers and exposes them to risks of improper use of prescription drugs and adverse side effects.

YES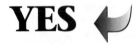

Alan F. Holmer

Direct-to-Consumer Prescription Drug Advertising Builds Bridges Between Patients and Physicians

Direct-to-consumer (DTC) advertising is an excellent way to meet the growing demand for medical information, empowering consumers by educating them about health conditions and possible treatments. By so doing, it can play an important role in improving public health.

"In health care, there is a general trend toward having consumers more responsible for their own health," according to Linda Golodner, president of the National Consumers League.[1]

The sources of user-accessible information about health care have increased exponentially just in the past few years. More than 50 consumer magazines about health care appear on the newsstands every month. Many television stations have a physician dispensing medical news. Nearly one quarter of the Internet is devoted to health care information.[2] The *Physicians' Desk Reference,* once largely confined to physicians' offices, is now available in a consumer edition at pharmacy counters.

Along with these sources, DTC advertising is a key means of informing and empowering patients. *Prevention Magazine,* in a study based on a national survey conducted during the spring of 1998 with technical assistance from the Food and Drug Administration (FDA),[3] found that:

- More than 53 million consumers talked to their physicians about a medicine they saw advertised, and an additional 49 million sought information from another source, such as the Internet.
- Thirty-eight percent of those who talked to their physicians about a medicine they saw advertised sought information about the product from at least 1 other source.
- Direct-to-consumer advertising "encouraged a projected 21.2 million consumers to talk with their doctor about a medical condition or illness they had never talked with their doctor about before seeing an advertisement."
- As many as 12.1 million consumers received a prescribed drug as a direct result of seeing a DTC advertisement.

The *Prevention Magazine* study also found that DTC advertising may improve patient compliance with drug regimens. "Many consumers who have seen advertisements for medicines they are currently taking say the advertising makes them feel better about the medicine they're taking, makes them more likely to take it and reminds them to have their prescriptions refilled," the study stated. The study concluded that DTC advertising "may play a very real role in enhancing public health."

Because DTC advertising is so new, more studies are needed to determine more definitively its cost-effectiveness and its precise impact on improving outcomes and public health. The FDA is planning a survey of consumers who have recently visited a physician to ask their views on prescription drugs they have received and their behavior regarding prescription drug advertising.

Not surprisingly, spending on DTC advertising has accelerated since the FDA changed its guidelines in August 1997 to allow manufacturers who advertise prescription medicines on television more flexibility in providing information about the risks of the drugs. IMS HEALTH, a health care information company in Plymouth Meeting, Pa, expects spending on DTC television advertising to more than double in 1998, following a large gain in 1997.

According to IMS HEALTH, spending on DTC advertising increased 46% in 1997 (to $917 million), while spending on promotion directed to physicians was about $4 billion in 1997.[4] In other words, companies spent more than 4 times as much promoting products to physicians as they spent promoting products to consumers.

Direct-to-consumer advertising that encourages millions of Americans to consult their physicians can help to improve public health because a number of leading diseases are underdiagnosed and undertreated. For example:

- An estimated 8 million undiagnosed cases of diabetes exist among adults in the United States.[5]
- Only about 10 million of the 30 million Americans with high cholesterol levels take cholesterol-lowering drugs.[6]
- Only 1 depressed person in 10 receives adequate medical treatment, and one third of people with major depression do not seek treatment.[7]
- Millions of Americans are estimated to have undiagnosed high blood pressure.[8]

For conditions such as these, which can be treated with prescription drugs, the consequences of not seeking appropriate treatment can be dire—for the individual, the family, and society. Untreated diabetes can lead to blindness or limb amputation. Unchecked high cholesterol levels can lead to heart attack or stroke, while cholesterol-lowering drugs can cut this risk by about 30%.[9] Failure to treat depression can result in suicide, and high blood pressure can lead to stroke, heart attacks, and kidney failure.

Conversely, there is a growing body of evidence that increased use of pharmaceuticals will improve public health:

- The Air Force/Texas Coronary Atherosclerosis Prevention Study concluded that use of a cholesterol-lowering drug can lower the risk of heart attacks, chest pain, and cardiac arrest by 37%, even in people with no symptoms of heart disease. The authors of the study estimate that 6 million Americans currently not recommended for this treatment could benefit.[10]

- A study by the Agency for Health Care Policy and Research found that increased use of anticoagulant drugs would prevent 40,000 strokes a year.[11]
- A study conducted at the University of Maryland Medical Center concluded that patients treated with β-blocker drugs after myocardial infarction were 40% less likely to die than those who do not receive the drug.[12] In a study from the National Cooperative Cardiovascular Project, only half the people who could be helped by a β-blocker following myocardial infarction were taking such a medicine.[13]

Direct-to-consumer advertising is a highly effective way to communicate the availability of treatments to the public. In 1992, the first DTC consumer television advertisement for a nicotine patch aired during the Super Bowl. According to the American Association of Advertising Agencies (AAAA), the public response was so great that, within weeks, demand for the patches exceeded the supply. The product had been available for months, but people who might have been interested in quitting smoking were simply not aware of it.

Advertising promoted widespread awareness overnight, prompted patient-physician conversations, and may have helped many people to stop smoking.[14] John Kamp of the AAAA stated: "Government agencies and medical professionals can use their tools until they're blue in the face and not reach the people who will be reached through television."[1] Similarly, according to data compiled by IMS HEALTH, patient visits to physicians for osteoporosis nearly doubled in the 1-year period following the debut of DTC advertisements for a new drug for the disease. In the fourth quarter of 1995, there were 409 000 visits to physicians for osteoporosis. Advertisements for the new medicine started appearing at the end of 1995. In the fourth quarter of 1996, there were 713 000 physician visits by patients seeking help for osteoporosis.[15]

An advertising campaign for a medicine for genital herpes was launched in 1997. Some 45 million people aged 12 years and older in the United States are infected with the virus that causes this disease. In a survey by the manufacturer of the medicine, 49% of the patients who had called the toll-free telephone number in the advertisement saw their physicians within 3 months after seeing the advertisement. Fifty-one percent of these patients did not receive a prescription for the medicine, indicating that the physician decided a prescription was inappropriate, even though the patient had probably asked for one (Andrew P. Witty, Glaxo Wellcome Inc, Research Triangle Park, NC, unpublished data, December 1998).

Pharmaceutical companies have both a right and a responsibility to inform people about their products under the supervision of the FDA, which regulates prescription drug advertising. Companies are committed to responsible advertising that enhances the patient-physician relationship and encourages the appropriate use of prescription drugs under a physician's supervision.

While such advertising prompts more people to seek professional help, it does not dictate the outcome of the physician visit or the kind of help patients eventually receive.

Direct-to-consumer advertising merely motivates patients to learn more about medical conditions and treatment options and to consult their physicians. Once the dialogue is started, the physician's role is preeminent. The patient has been empowered with information, not prescribing authority. In the words of Harvard Medical School Professor Jerry Avorn: "There's no detail man or pharmaceutical company or patient that puts a gun to a doctor's head to write a prescription. Ultimately, it isn't the patient's signature on the prescription—it's the doctor's."[16]

Participatory health care—consumers assuming more responsibility for their own health—is changing the nature of the patient-physician relationship. In a recent survey conducted by Yankelovich Partners, 95% of both physicians and patients described the ideal patient-physician relationship as a mutual partnership.[17] Such a partnership can lead to better health outcomes through appropriate use of safe and effective prescription medicines that save lives, cure disease, and alleviate pain and suffering.

The mortality rate for the acquired immunodeficiency syndrome (AIDS) dropped more than 3-fold from 1995 through 1997, for example, due to the increasing use of combination antiretroviral therapy.[18] Deaths due to heart disease decreased more than 30% during the 1980s, with 50% of the decline attributed to the use of new medicines.[19] Antibiotics and vaccines have virtually wiped out such diseases as diphtheria, syphilis, pertussis, measles, and polio.[20] And there are more than 1000 new medicines in development—for Alzheimer disease, cancer, heart disease, stroke, infectious diseases, AIDS, arthritis, Parkinson disease, diabetes, and many other diseases—promising even more effective treatments and better outcomes in the future.[21]

By greatly increasing the likelihood that patients will seek help for their medical problems and receive a safe and effective prescribed medicine, DTC advertising will, as the *Prevention Magazine* study stated, "play a very real role in enhancing public health."

References

1. Nordenberg T. Direct to you: TV drug ads that make sense. *FDA Consumer.* January–February 1998; 32: 7–10.

2. Kodysz M, Bower BA. Medical sites on the Internet continue to proliferate. *Mod Med.* May 1998; 66:56.

3. Prevention Magazine. *National Survey of Consumer Reactions to Direct-to-Consumer Advertising.* Emmaus, Pa: Rodale Press; 1998.

4. IMS reports pharmaceutical promotions rose 16% in 1997 [press release]. Plymouth Meeting, Pa: IMS HEALTH; March 31, 1998.

5. American Diabetes Association: Clinical Practice Recommendations 1997. *Diabetes Care.* 1997; 20(suppl 1):S1–S70.

6. Pill pushers. *Economist.* August 8, 1997;344 (8029):58–59.

7. Hirschfeld RM, Keller MB, Panico S, et al. The National Depressive and Manic-Depressive Association consensus statement on the undertreatment of depression. *JAMA.* 1997;277:333–334.

8. *National Health and Nutrition Examination Survey.* Washington, DC: National Center for Health Statistics; 1988–1994.

9. Avorn J, Monette J, Lacour A, et al. Persistence of use of lipid-lowering medications: a cross-national study. *JAMA.* 1998;279:1458–1462.

10. Downs JR, Clearfield M, Weis S, et al. Primary prevention of acute coronary events with lovastatin in men and women with average cholesterol levels: results of AFCAPS/TexCAPS. *JAMA.* 1998;279:1615–1622.

11. *Secondary and Tertiary Prevention of Stroke Patient Outcome Research Team: 9th Progress Report, March 1996.* Rockville, Md: Agency for Health Care Policy and Research; 1996.

12. Gottlieb SS, McCarter RJ, Vogel RA. Effect of beta-blockade on mortality among high-risk and low-risk patients after myocardial infarction. *N Engl J Med.* 1998;339:489–497.

13. Krumholz HM, Radford MJ, Wang Y, Chen J, Heiat A, Marciniak TA. National use and effectiveness of β-blockers for the treatment of elderly patients after acute myocardial infarction: National Cooperative Cardiovascular Project. *JAMA.* 1998;280:623–629.

14. DTC ads prompted prescriptions for 7.5 million Americans, AphA/Prevention survey concludes. *F-D-C Reports—The Pink Sheet.* October 20, 1997;59 (42):9–10.

15. National Disease and Therapeutic Index [database online]. Plymouth Meeting, Pa: IMS HEALTH; 1996.

16. Tanouye E. Drug ads spur patients to demand more prescriptions. *Wall Street Journal.* December 22, 1997;B1.

17. Executive summary. In: *A Survey of the Patient-Physician Relationship to America.* Norwalk, Conn: Yankelovich Partners Inc; April 1998:4.

18. Ventura SJ, Anderson RN, Martin JA, Smith BL. *Births and Deaths: Preliminary Data for 1997, National Vital Statistics Reports [vol 47, No. 4].* Hyattsville, Md: National Center for Health Statistics; 1998;1.

19. Hunink MGM, Goldman L, Tosteson ANA, et al. The recent decline in mortality from coronary heart disease. 1980–1990: the effect of secular trends in risk factors and treatment. *JAMA.* 1997;277:535–542.

20. Peters KD, Kochaneck KD, Murphy SL. *Deaths: Final Data for 1996: National Vital Statistics Reports [vol 47, No. 9].* Hyattsville, Md: National Center for Health Statistics, 1998:52.

21. Pharmaceutical Research and Manufacturers of America (PhRMA). New Medicines in Development Database. . . . Accessed December 1, 1998.

Matthew F. Hollon

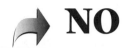 **NO**

Direct-to-Consumer Marketing of Prescription Drugs

In the early 1980s, the pharmaceutical industry began marketing prescription drugs directly to patients. The Food and Drug Administration (FDA) imposed a moratorium on this marketing strategy in 1983, then lifted it in 1985.[1] Since then, the industry has devoted increasing resources to this strategy. In a 1988 editorial on direct-to-consumer (DTC) marketing, Eric P. Cohen, MD, wrote, "Issues of regulation of advertising, cost, competition, public health, and individual well being need to be carefully examined."[2] Examination of these issues in rigorous, independent studies has not occurred. Despite the lack of studies, the FDA has relaxed regulations governing DTC marketing of prescription drugs.[3]

Proponents hypothesize that DTC marketing, by providing educational information, is valuable, notifying consumers of new therapies and motivating them to seek care. However, the pharmaceutical industry, driven in part by financial motives, is providing information of suspect quality and thus minimal benefit. Reckoning the costs, economic and otherwise, the public health value of DTC marketing is negligible. Moreover, the effects of DTC marketing are undesirable. Most important, by creating consumer demand, DTC marketing undermines the protection that is a result of requiring a physician to certify a patient's need for a prescription drug. For the benefit of patients, physicians, and the public's health, the FDA should consider stricter—not more permissive—regulations.

While providing educational information may be one of the industry's motives, the bottom-line desire for profit is undoubtedly another. In this respect, industry efforts have been successful. Advertising nicotine patches directly to consumers turned patches into "an $800 million dollar category."[4] Aggressive marketing of Claritin (Schering-Plough, Madison, NJ) captured 56% of the $1.8 billion nonsedating antihistamine market.[5] In the wake of successes, spending on DTC advertising rocketed from $13.1 million in 1989 to more than $900 million in 1997, double the $438 million spent on advertisements in medical journals.[6,7]

The pharmaceutical industry's interest in the bottom line is legitimate. The industry, which has made important medical contributions, exists because it is profitable. However, as the profit motive can affect the content of information in advertisements, the public health value of DTC marketing should be examined by comparing the benefits the public gains with the costs the public incurs.

The industry is not marketing to consumers in a health information vacuum. A vast amount of health information is accessible to and inundates the public every day.[8,9] Since "almost every drug product has some advantage for some patient," it is anecdotally true that any information the industry provides about a product has some benefit for someone.[10] However, when dumped into the ocean of available information, the sum of these anecdotes does not necessarily equal public health benefit, especially when the quality of the information provided is suspect. If studies of advertising directed at physicians offer a clue, this information, in fact, has minimal educational benefit.

In one study, Wade et al[11] asked pharmaceutical companies to supply their best evidence in support of marketing claims. Of 67 references cited, only 31 contained relevant original data and only 13 were controlled trials. These investigators concluded, "Standards of evidence used to justify advertising claims are inadequate." In a study of advertising in the leading medical journals in 18 countries, Herxheimer et al[12] reported that important warnings and precautions were missing in half of the 6700 advertisements surveyed. In yet another study, Stryer and Bero[13] concluded that advertisements contained a higher proportion of promotional material than educational material, and little of this material contained information about important therapeutic breakthroughs. In 1992, Wilkes et al[14] evaluated 109 pharmaceutical advertisements and found that 57% of these advertisements had little or no educational value.

Recently, *Consumer Reports,* evaluating the accuracy of information in prescription drug advertisements directed at patients, substantiated the conclusions drawn from studies of marketing directed at physicians.[15] Information from marketing has little educational benefit and, in general, its quality is poor. Less than half of DTC advertisements reviewed were candid about efficacy. *Consumer Reports* concluded, "the rules governing prescription drug advertising should not be loosened," and that "[advertisements] are not public service messages—they're meant to move goods."

David A. Kessler, MD, while commissioner of the FDA, wrote in response to the study by Wilkes et al, "[it] serves an important purpose. It heightens awareness of the degree to which misleading information may pervade the 'informational marketplace.'"[16] In his editorial, Kessler documented the subtle techniques used by the pharmaceutical industry to distort information including "data dredging" and making claims of "no difference" from studies with limited statistical power. Providing poor quality information in today's marketplace of health information results in little or no benefit for the public. Considering the costs, providing this information is unlikely to have public health value.

Costs can include an increase in expenditures, improper use of drugs, and harm from adverse events. Unlike many products, the use of prescription drugs can have serious consequences. The improper use of antibiotics in humans is one of the major factors accelerating antimicrobial resistance.[17,18]

Prescription drugs can and do cause harm. Consider the recent concern that the use of the combination of anorectic agents, fenfluramine and phentermine, may be associated with valvular heart disease.[19] Consider also benoxaprofen, a prescription nonsteroidal anti-inflammatory agent, launched in 1980 in the United Kingdom and subsequently the United States.[20] The product gained "a major foothold merely on the strength of a well-orchestrated marketing strategy, which included full-page advertisements in the popular press." Sixty-one drug-related deaths occurred during the 2 years in which the drug remained on the market.

Expenditures are also an important consideration. Drugs reduce expenditures by preventing complications from diseases.[21] However, this statement is not axiomatic. Expenditures may increase when marketing of prescription drugs creates need, when disease complications are rare or nonexistent, or when choices of drug therapy for a disease are available. For example, a recent survey of trends in antihypertensive drug use in the United States revealed that despite the recommendations of the Fifth Joint National Committee on the Detection, Evaluation, and Treatment of High Blood Pressure, the use of calcium antagonists and angiotensin-converting enzyme inhibitors has increased.[22] The investigators cite the effectiveness of pharmaceutical promotion practices as one of the possible reasons for this. They note, "the cost implications of these practice patterns are enormous."

If DTC marketing affects physicians' prescribing practices, then DTC marketing has no public health value because the public ostensibly incurs costs that exceed the minimal benefits. Some argue that physicians serve as the system's safety net, preventing the inappropriate use of prescription drugs. This argument, however, rests on a number of questionable assumptions. It assumes that physicians are always rational in prescribing. It assumes that such things as patients' demands do not influence physicians' prescribing practices. It assumes that, at a population level, physicians are nearly infallible. Available evidence casts doubt on these assumptions.

Variability not explained solely by the pharmacological needs of patients exists in physicians' prescribing practices.[23,24] Examining this variability, Schwartz et al[25] identified physicians who prescribed 3 drugs "at a rate far greater than that warranted by scientific evidence of their effectiveness." In this study, patient demand was the most commonly cited motivation for prescribing the target drugs. In a study of antibiotic use for upper respiratory tract infections, Hamm et al[26] documented that the patient's expectation for an antibiotic is an important factor in the decision to prescribe the drug. Moreover, 2 recent studies concur with previous findings that patients who expect a prescription are "many times more likely to receive one."[27] At the population level, Willcox et al[28] found that 23.5% of Americans aged 65 years or older living in the community receive at least 1 of 20 inappropriate drugs. These authors call for broader educational and regulatory initiatives. Finally, preliminary evidence from a study by Hueston et al[29] suggests managed care organizations have not reduced inappropriate prescribing.

The act of issuing a prescription is the culmination of a complex set of decisions; certainly, physicians' decisions can improve. What effect does DTC marketing have on these decisions? Consumer advocates of DTC marketing argue that this strategy, highlighting the evolving relationship between physicians and patients, shifts control over prescription decisions from physicians to patients, giving patients greater command over their health care.[30] In reality, the principal effect of DTC marketing is to create consumer demand, changing the physician-patient relationship to a physician-consumer relationship. The consequences of this change are open for debate, but the impact is noticeable.

In 1992, physicians reported that 88% of patients asked for a drug by brand name, up from 45% in 1989.[6] At the same time, a survey revealed that 63% of consumers do not believe they can tell if they are being misled by advertisements for prescription drugs.[31] An advertising industry executive concludes, "Creating consumer demand [among patients] for prescription pharmaceuticals is now an attainable marketing objective."[32] Physicians' prescribing decisions can improve, but creating consumer demand does not help. Rather, by influencing these decisions, consumer demand undermines the protection that is a result of requiring a physician to consider seriously a patient's need for a drug, then certify that need.

Neither physicians nor patients are immune to the effects of marketing. However, while physicians are not immune, their education and knowledge presumably make them more competent than consumers in interpreting promotional material for prescription drugs. Additionally, unlike consumers who hear of just 1 drug, physicians are capable of offering sound advice to patients about a range of therapeutic options. If the value of DTC marketing is negligible and the primary effect of this strategy is to create consumer demand, then, unlike the truly valuable contributions of the pharmaceutical industry, DTC marketing is not good for patients, physicians, or the public's health.

An industry consultant predicts, "The winners in the prescription drug category are not going to be the ones with the best patents or products, but those that are the best marketers."[5] Currently the industry is pursuing the next steps in DTC marketing, including using broadcast media and the Internet. The industry is moving beyond mass media vehicles to more focused efforts such as direct marketing through databases to targeted consumers.[32] Until well-designed, independent studies based on available observational data prove the information from DTC marketing has public health value and desirable effects, the FDA should consider stricter—not more permissive—regulations.

References

1. Food and Drug Administration. Direct-to-consumer advertising of prescription drugs: withdrawal of moratorium. *Federal Register.* September 9, 1985; 50:36677–36678.

2. Cohen EP. Direct-to-the-public advertisement of prescription drugs. *N Engl J Med.* 1988;318:373–376.

3. US Department of Health and Human Services, Public Health Service, Food and Drug Administration. FDA to review standards for all direct-to-consumer Rx drug promotion. . . . Accessed August 25, 1997.

4. Weber J, Carey J. Drug ads: a prescription for controversy. *Business Week.* January 18, 1993:58-59.

5. Freeman L. Aggressive strategy helps propel Claritin to top slot. *Advertising Age.* March 16, 1998;69(11):S6-S7.

6. Liebman H. Consumer, heal thyself: ads for prescription drugs are popping up more frequently in consumer media. *Mediaweek.* July 5, 1993;3(27):12.

7. Wilke M. Prescription for profit. *Advertising Age.* March 16, 1998;69(11):S1, S26.

8. Why do Americans resist a healthy lifestyle? *USA Today Magazine.* October 1994;123(2593):1-2.

9. Harper J. Information overload may be making some Americans sick. *Insight on the News.* September 15, 1997;13(34):40-41.

10. Peck CC, Rheinstein PH. FDA regulation of prescription drug advertising. *JAMA.* 1990;264:2424-2425.

11. Wade VA, Mansfield PR, McDonald PJ. Drug companies' evidence to justify advertising. *Lancet.* 1989;2:1261-1264.

12. Herxheimer A, Lundborg CS, Westerholm B. Advertisements for medicines in leading medical journals in 18 countries: a 12-month survey of information content and standards. *Int J Health Serv.* 1993;23:161-172.

13. Stryer D, Bero LA. Characteristics of materials distributed by drug companies. *J Gen Intern Med.* 1996;11:575-583.

14. Wilkes MS, Doblin BH, Shapiro MF. Pharmaceutical advertisements in leading medical journals: experts' assessments. *Ann Intern Med.* 1992;116: 912-919.

15. Drug advertising: is this good medicine? *Consumer Reports.* June 1996;61(6): 62-63.

16. Kessler DA. Addressing the problem of misleading advertising. *Ann Intern Med.* 1992;116:950-951.

17. Williams RJ, Heymann DL. Containment of antibiotic resistance. *Science.* 1998; 279:1153-1154.

18. Low DE, Scheld WM. Strategies for stemming the tide of antimicrobial resistance. *JAMA.* 1998;279:394-395.

19. Connolly HM, Crary JL, McGoon MD, et al. Valvular heart disease associated with fenfluramine-phentermine. *N Engl J Med.* 1997;337:581-588.

20. Gerber P. Mass product-liability litigation. *Med J Aust.* 1988;148:485-488.

21. US Department of Health and Human Services, Public Health Service, Food and Drug Administration. FDA public hearing: direct-to-consumer promotion. . . . Accessed June 21, 1997.

22. Siegel D, Lopez J. Trends in antihypertensive drug use in the United States: do the JNC V recommendations affect prescribing? *JAMA.* 1997;278:1745-1748.

23. Hemminki E. Review of literature on the factors affecting drug prescribing. *Soc Sci Med.* 1975;9:111-115.

24. Weiss MC, Fitzpatrick R, Scott DK, Goldacre MJ. Pressures on the general practitioner and decisions to prescribe. *Fam Pract.* 1996;13:432-438.

25. Schwartz RK, Soumerai SB, Avorn J. Physician motivations for nonscientific drug prescribing. *Soc Sci Med.* 1989;28:577-582.

26. Hamm RM, Hicks RJ, Bemben DA. Antibiotics and respiratory infections: are patients more satisfied when expectations are met? *J Fam Pract.* 1996;43: 56-62.

27. Greenhalgh T, Gill P. Pressure to prescribe. *BMJ.* 1997;315:1482-1483.

28.   Willcox SM, Himmelstein DU, Woolhandler S. Inappropriate drug prescribing for the community-dwelling elderly. *JAMA.* 1994;272: 292–296.

29.   Hueston WJ, Mainous AG III, Brauer N, Mercuri J. Evaluation and treatment of respiratory infections: does managed care make a difference? *J Fam Pract.* 1997;44:572–577.

30.   National Consumers League, Golodner LF. Consumer group responds to FDA's draft guidance on direct-to-consumer advertising on television. . . . Accessed August 26, 1997.

31.   Whyte J. Direct consumer advertising of prescription drugs. *JAMA.* 1993; 269:146, 150.

32.   Wilke M, Teinowitz I, Kelly KJ. Ad fever sweeps healthcare industry. *Advertising Age.* January 13, 1997;68(2):1, 18–19.

POSTSCRIPT

Does Direct-to-Consumer Drug Advertising Enhance Patient Choice?

In June 2005, the American Medical Association (AMA) asked the Food and Drug Administration (FDA) to place stricter controls on prescription drug advertising. Under the AMA proposal, a newly approved drug could not be advertised to consumers for a period of six to 12 months. This moratorium would give physicians a chance to learn about the drug, its appropriate use, and its side effects before patients started demanding it. Some drug companies already wait this length of time voluntarily. The AMA also suggested guidelines for using actors to portray physicians in TV ads.

Researchers from Harvard University/Massachusetts General Hospital and Harris Interactive conducted a national telephone survey of consumers in 2002 asking about their experience with direct-to-consumer drug advertising. About 35 percent reported that an ad prompted them to have a discussion with a physician about the drug or the condition. A quarter of these patients received a new diagnosis, and nearly three-quarters were given a prescription, with about 43 percent getting a prescription for the advertised drug. About four out of five consumers who got a drug and took it as prescribed reported feeling much or somewhat better (Joel S. Weissman, et. al., "Consumers' Reports on the Health Effects of Direct-to-Consumer Drug Advertising," *Health Affairs,* February 2003). The same team also surveyed physicians on this issue. They pointed to improved communication and education as a benefit of direct-to-consumer advertising but also felt it led patients to seek unnecessary treatments. When the advertised drug was prescribed, 46 percent of physicians said it was the most effective treatment, and 48 percent said that other drugs were equally effective. Among the most common new diagnoses were impotence (15.5 percent), anxiety (9 percent), and arthritis (6.8 percent) (Joel Weissman, et al., "Physicians Report on Patient Encounters Involving Direct-to-Consumer Advertising," *Health Affairs,* April 28, 2004).

For more information on direct-to-consumer advertising, see Michael W. Wilkes, Robert A. Bell, and Richard L. Kravitz, "Direct-to-Consumer Prescription Drug Advertising: Trends, Impact, and Implications," *Health Affairs* (March–April 2000). A point-counterpoint exchange in the *Western Journal of Medicine* (December 2001) addresses the question, Have drug companies hyped social anxiety disorder to increase sales? David Healy says marketing hinders discovery of long-term solutions, while David V. Sheehan argues that efforts to relieve human suffering deserve rewards.

At present only the United States and New Zealand allow direct-to-consumer advertising. Barbara Mintzes supports the view that European consumers should have access to direct-to-consumer advertising while Silvia N. Bonaccorso and Jeffrey L. Sturchio offer the opposing view in "Direct-to-Consumer Advertising Is Medicalising Normal Human Experience," *British Medical Journal* (April 13, 2002). Writing from a European perspective, Andreas Hasman and Søren Holm believe that an outright ban on direct-to-consumer advertising inhibits the free market in healthcare information but support a regulated market to protect patients who are particularly vulnerable ("Direct-to-Consumer Advertising: Should There Be a Free Market in Healthcare Information?" *Cambridge Quarterly of Healthcare Ethics,* vol. 15, 2006). In his essay "To Inform or Persuade? Direct-to-Consumer Advertising of Prescription Drugs," Ernst R. Berndt points to the considerable public health potential of this practice, but asserts that "industry needs to respond to consumers and physicians, who seek more balanced communication of risks and benefits" (*New England Journal of Medicine,* January 27, 2005).

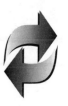

Internet References . . .

Euthanasia and Physician-Assisted Suicide:
All Sides of the Issues

This site offers a general overview of the controversy concerning physician-assisted suicide as well as statisics and a list of Web sites that represent both sides of the debate.

http://www.religioustolerance.org/
euthanas.htm

National Hospice and Palliative Care Organization

This organization's Web site has information about each state's advance directive rules as well as aspects of care of dying people.

http://www.nhpco.org

Death and Dying

*W*hat are the ethical responsibilities associated with death? Doctors are sworn "to do no harm," but this proscription is open to many different interpretations. Death is a natural event that can, in some instances, be hastened to put an end to suffering. Is it ethically necessary to prolong life at all times under all circumstances? Medical personnel as well as families often face these agonizing questions. They are made more agonizing in disaster conditions, when ordinary resources are not available. The right of an individual to decide his or her own fate may conflict with society's interest in maintaining the value of human life or in not wasting valuable resources that could be used to save other lives. This conflict is apparent in the matter of physician-assisted suicide and, in a different way, in the question of "futile" treatment. This section examines some of these anguishing questions.

- Do Some Advance Directives Limit Patients' Rights?

- Do Standard Medical Ethics Apply in Disaster Conditions?

- Should Physicians Be Allowed to Assist in Patient Suicide?

- Should Doctors Be Able to Refuse Demands for "Futile" Treatment?

ISSUE 4

Do Some Advance Directives Limit Patients' Rights?

YES: Christopher James Ryan, from "Betting Your Life: An Argument Against Certain Advance Directives," *Journal of Medical Ethics* (vol. 22, 1996)

NO: Steven Luttrell and Ann Sommerville, from "Limiting Risks by Curtailing Rights: A Response to Dr. Ryan," *Journal of Medical Ethics* (vol. 22, 1996)

ISSUE SUMMARY

YES: Psychiatrist Christopher James Ryan argues that advance directives that refuse active treatment in situations when a patient's incompetence is potentially reversible should be abolished because healthy people are likely to underestimate their desire for treatment should they become ill.

NO: Geriatricians Steven Luttrell and Ann Sommerville assert that respect for the principle of autonomy requires that individuals be permitted to make risky choices about their own lives and that ignoring autonomous choices made by competent adults reinstates the outmoded notion of medical paternalism.

Since ancient times people have drawn up wills to determine what should be done with their property, or who should take custody of their children, after they die. In 1969 Luis Kutner, a law professor, proposed a "living will," a document that would determine the course of medical treatment should the signer become unable to express his or her wishes. A typical living will stated, "If I am permanently unconscious or there is no reasonable expectation for my recovery from a serious incapacitating or lethal illness or condition, I do not wish to be kept alive by artificial means." The proposal came at a time when the public was just beginning to be aware of the use of machines to keep people breathing and their hearts beating even though there was no possibility of regaining consciousness. In 1975 the Karen Ann Quinlan case, involving a young, permanently unconsciousness woman on a ventilator, focused ethical and legal attention on the unwanted use of medical technology.

In 1976, following the Quinlan case, California enacted the nation's first law approving the use of living wills. Nearly every state in the United States followed suit. Sometimes called "natural death acts," these laws and the wills they approved were so vaguely worded and so difficult to interpret that they were hardly ever effective in achieving their goals. It was difficult, for example, to determine what was meant by "reasonable expectation," "artificial means," or even "lethal illness."

In 1983 the President's Commission for the Study of Ethical Problems in Medicine and Biomedical and Behavioral Research recommended an alternative approach. Rather than signing a document that specified certain treatments that should be forgone, patients were encouraged to name a person who would make health care decisions in their place.

There are several types of advance directives. They can be formally written and legally authorized, or they can be informal communications with family members or health care providers. Much of the legal wrangling about withdrawal of life supports has turned on whether or not the patient expressed such desires while competent. The case of Nancy Cruzan, which eventually went to the U.S. Supreme Court, is one example. The parents of this young Missouri woman, who was permanently unconscious after an automobile accident, sued the state to have her life supports removed, claiming that this is what Nancy herself would have wanted. The state argued that there was no clear and convincing evidence that Nancy would have made the same decision. In 1990 the U.S. Supreme Court ruled that states had an interest in preserving life and could require a high standard of evidence of the patient's expressed preference for withdrawing treatment. The case then went back to the Missouri courts, which this time found the evidence convincing and agreed to allow withdrawal of life support.

To add to the weight of the Supreme Court's decision, in 1991 Congress passed the Patient Self-Determination Act (PSDA), which requires all health care providers reimbursed by Medicare to inform patients about their right to sign advance directives. By this measure Congress intended to promote the use of advance directives in hospitals and nursing homes where elderly patients are often treated.

Despite legislative and judicial approval of advance directives and widespread public opinion supporting them, such documents are still rarely signed by competent patients, and even when signed they are still rarely consulted or implemented. Studies have documented barriers such as lack of appropriate communication and physicians' disregard of the wishes expressed in the directives.

The following selections address a more basic issue: the ethical acceptability of a particular kind of advance directive. Christopher James Ryan favors the abolition of advance directives in which a healthy patient chooses withdrawal of active treatment in a future situation in which he or she is incompetent but where the incompetence is potentially reversible. Steven Luttrell and Ann Sommerville assert that advance directives are mostly made by ill patients, who do have a good idea of what they want, and that their autonomous decisions, even when risky, should be respected.

YES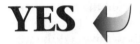

Christopher James Ryan

Betting Your Life: An Argument Against Certain Advance Directives

Along time ago, in a country far far away, there lived a very wise old king. The king was a very ethical man and his subjects were very happy. Everyone lived together in perfect harmony and times were generally regarded as good.

One day the king introduced a new law. The law allowed his subjects to enter into a mysterious wager. Those who won the wager would receive a rich reward, but those who lost would be put to death. Entry into the wager was entirely voluntary and despite the dire consequences of losing many took up the challenge. To win, a contestant had only correctly to answer an apparently straightforward question. The question was known to all participants before they entered and all who took up the challenge were sure that they knew the answer and could not lose. Strangely, even the king's ethicists had no objection to the introduction of the law and in fact praised the king for his wisdom and progressiveness. The ethicists also believed that the answer to the question was obvious and focused only on the rich reward.

Unfortunately, however, many contestants got the answer wrong. They lost the wager and were put to an early and needless death. The question, that caused so much difficulty, was this: "Even though you are now well and healthy, imagine yourself in a situation where you have a terminal illness and are temporarily confused or unconscious. Imagine that whilst you are in this state your doctors give you a choice; either they will treat you to the best of their ability and you may recover some of your health for some undefined period, or they will treat you conservatively and, though they will ensure that you are in no pain, they will not attempt to save your life. If you were in this situation what would you want the doctors to do?"

Advance directives or living wills frequently require their users to undertake the kind of task set out above; that is, to imagine themselves in a situation where they are required to make a decision about whether or not they should receive active treatment but are incompetent to do so. These have become increasingly popular over the last decade. Legislation giving statutory status to these directives has been enacted in many parts of the Western world and planned in many others. In places where no such legislation exists living wills are thought to have increasing weight in common law.[1-3]

From Christopher James Ryan, "Betting Your Life: An Argument Against Certain Advance Directives," *Journal of Medical Ethics*, vol. 22 (1996), pp. 95–99. Copyright © 1996 by The British Medical Association. Reprinted by permission.

In this paper I oppose a common form of advance directive on ethical grounds. The basis of my argument is my contention that, like the citizens of the country above, many people who take out advance directives do so under the belief that they know the answer to the question above, when in fact they do not. In order [to] support my position I will first provide evidence which supports this contention and then demonstrate the ethical difficulties this creates for advocates of living wills.

I do not intend to provide opposition to all forms of advance directive, but will restrict my discussion to a fairly narrow but not uncommon set of criteria. I will examine only cases where an advance directive demands that the user receive only conservative or palliative care in a situation where he or she is incompetent to consent to such treatment but where that incompetence is potentially reversible.

Getting the Answer Wrong

My argument hinges on the notion that people are likely grossly to under-estimate their desire to have medical intervention should they become ill; I will therefore explain why this is likely to be so on theoretical grounds and then provide some empirical evidence that suggests that this actually occurs.

Denial is a strong and largely successful mechanism for dealing with the stressors of everyday life. For the healthy person considering a terminal illness it involves the subconscious decision to reject the possibility that one will suffer in the way one might be expected to if one were to succumb to such an illness. There are two standard ways of going about this. The first is simply to tell yourself that terminal illnesses are things that happen to other people and that they will not happen to you. This method works reasonably well whilst one is still young and all, or most, of the people that get such illnesses are not like you at all. It starts to lose its power, however, as you grow older and terminal illnesses begin to befall your peers. Now the other people begin to look a lot like you and the only-happens-to-others strategy looks increasingly anaemic.

The second option is to use denial in a slightly more complicated manner and when confronted by the suffering of another in the midst of a terminal illness to say that this would not happen to you because, if you were in that situation, you would kill yourself before the suffering became too great. Here you have traded the real and very distressing possibility that you may develop, and suffer at the hands of, a terminal illness for the hypothetical notion of a future early death. As a hypothetical abstract your early death is unpleasant but much more bearable than the realisation that you could become so ill.

Of course once you have developed a terminal illness, this coping strat-egy will no longer be successful. Now the possibility of your death is no longer hypothetical and you are faced with balancing real dying with the pos-sibility of real suffering. While there is no doubt that some individuals now decide that they would still be better off dead, I believe that the vast majority of people now decide to battle it out. Most people with terminal illnesses do not want to die and are prepared to put up with a certain amount of suffering in order to live a little longer. Now that death is no longer a hypothetical it holds little appeal and frequently denial is used again, this time to maintain hope that a cure will be found.[4]

Human beings are, I suggest, very poor at determining their attitudes to treatment for some hypothetical future terminal illness and very frequently grossly under-estimate their future desire to go on living.

Though based on psychological theorising, there is some evidence to support this contention. The first piece of evidence is admittedly anecdotal but none the less quite powerful. Healthy people frequently believe that if they were suffering a terminal illness and required various forms of medical intervention they would rather be allowed to slip away. This view is so common among healthy people that it can be regarded as perfectly normal. Among terminally ill people, however, the sustained expression of a preference not to receive treatment is very rare. Most palliative care specialists will readily recall one or two patients who persistently requested that they be allowed to die. Some will recall several. However, palliative care physicians do not report that this sustained desire is very common and certainly do not report that it is the norm. This strongly suggests that many people who, when healthy, predict they would refuse treatment in the future, will change their mind when they develop a terminal illness.

This anecdotal evidence is supported by a number of studies in the psychiatric literature. One such study by Owen *et al* found that among patients with cancer the strongest interest in euthanasia was among those patients being offered potentially curative treatment. Patients with poorer prognoses, who were only being offered palliative care, tended to reject the idea of euthanasia as a future option (p < 0.05).[5] Similarly, a 1994 study by Danis *et al*, which examined the stability of future treatment preferences, found that while preferences for most remained stable over the study's two-year duration, people that had been hospitalised, had an accident or had become immobile were likely to change their health care preferences to opt for more intervention.[6] Both studies suggest that having had an episode of serious illness or a deterioration of an existing illness may make people more likely to want more intervention.

Seale and Addington-Hall asked relatives and friends of people who had died whether the dead person would have benefited from an earlier death. They found that respondents, who were not spouses, were frequently willing to say that an earlier death would have been better for the person even though the person who had died had not expressed a desire to die sooner. That is, the healthy relatives and friends were keener on euthanasia than the terminally ill patient had been. This again suggests that healthy people may view euthanasia differently from terminally ill people or at least that it is hard to empathise with the position of the terminally ill.[7]

Though it is not possible directly to equate suicide with a desire for euthanasia, one might expect that if terminally ill people increasingly wanted to die as they became sicker and sicker then suicide among patients with terminal illness would peak towards the end of their illnesses. This would be the time when pain and suffering was at its worst and when there was little to look forward to. In fact, however, completed suicide is most common in the first year after diagnosis in the terminally ill.[8] It may be that in this situation suicide more often represents an irrational reaction to the crisis of diagnosis than a reasoned decision that life has become intolerable.

Further evidence that a desire for euthanasia is uncommon in the terminally ill comes from a study by Brown and co-workers who found that among forty-four terminally ill patients, the only patients who had experienced a desire for an early death were those who were suffering from a clinical depressive illness.[9]

Arguments in Support of Advance Directives

Advocates of this form of advance directive argue for the documents along two lines. Firstly, they take a deontological position that the directives maximise the affected person's autonomy by allowing her some control over her medical management. They argue that since maximisation of autonomy is a legitimate aim and since living wills seem to facilitate the maximisation of autonomy, then living wills are not only ethically justified but beneficial.[10-12] Second, advocates may take a utilitarian line and argue that the directives help to facilitate the death of people who believe they would be better off dead than alive. By facilitating these deaths the directives not only end people's suffering, but spare them an undignified death. In addition the directive may ease the burden on medical staff and family of the ill individual who may find making these decisions painful. Through all these means, they argue, the directive increases the net utility of the community.[10]

Opponents of this form of advance directive usually base their opposition upon an opposition to euthanasia.[13] However, since most living will legislation throughout the world facilitates only passive euthanasia and since passive euthanasia is rarely objected to, there has been little solid opposition to this form of advance directive legislation.

My objections to these advance directives do not rely on an objection to either active or passive euthanasia. Rather my objections are based on the proposition that these living wills do not necessarily increase the user's autonomy nor society's net utility in the unproblematic way they are imagined to do, because people are much more likely to refuse treatment when faced with a future hypothetical scenario than when faced with a real here and now choice. If this contention is accepted it has a number of consequences for arguments used in support of living wills.

Consequences for the Argument from Autonomy

The principle of a right to autonomy holds that adult human beings have the right to make decisions about their lives and so direct the course of their own fate. The right to autonomy is a powerful maxim. It is the right to autonomy that underlies the notions of consent, the right to freedom and democracy itself. By grounding their support for directives in this principle proponents of living wills set up a strong case.

It is an accepted part of the principle, however, that one cannot properly exercise one's autonomy if one is not in possession of all available information that might influence one's decisions. A patient's consent to a procedure, for example, is only valid if she has been informed of all the risks and consequences. If the psychological reasoning and empirical evidence above is accepted, then a person currently using a living will does not have access to a vital piece of information that may radically alter her decision. Specifically, she does not know that it is highly likely that her decision, made now, that she would rather die if faced with a hypothetical future scenario is not what her decision would have been if she were actually faced with that scenario.

Almost everyone assumes that he knows his own mind and that he would know the choices he would make in the event of a crisis. While there is little doubt that the individual alone is in the best position to know how he would act and it is also true that some people must correctly guess how they would act, nevertheless evidence strongly suggests that many people simply get it wrong. They believe they would not opt for treatment in a hypothetical future circumstance but were they actually to face the circumstance they would opt for treatment. Most people have no experience of their reactions to a life-threatening illness, they can only guess at their reaction and they frequently guess wrong. More importantly for my argument, people do not believe in, or even know of the possibility of, an inaccurate guess. If users of advance directives do not know of the distinct possibility that their choices may be inaccurate, they lack a vital piece of information and that lack prohibits a fully informed and autonomous choice.

Consequences for the Utilitarian Argument

The possibility that a large number of people are dying when they would not have wanted to because of the introduction of advance directives, directly threatens the utilitarian argument offered in support of these directives.

The utilitarian argument draws its strength from the hope that the existence of advance directives will end the suffering of people with terminal illnesses who have decided that they would be better off dead. It is assumed that they have come to this opinion by weighing up the benefits of their continued existence with the pain and suffering of their terminal illness. There is an additional hidden assumption that the affected individuals can accurately estimate this balance from the safety of health and happiness prior to their illness. If this additional assumption is unjustified then the utilitarian argument is undermined.

Conclusions Regarding Living Wills

With the argument from autonomy and the utilitarian argument both undermined, ethical support for living wills of this sort is seriously diminished. The effect this diminution will have upon one's attitudes to living wills will depend on both the seriousness with which one takes the evidence for the inaccuracy of people's choices and one's beliefs about how well this inaccuracy can be addressed through changes to legislation and education.

At a minimum one should require significant changes in legislation to address users' ignorance of their likelihood of wrong decisions. The principle of autonomy demands that the individual making the choice be given all available relevant information, therefore those making living wills must be informed of the apparent likelihood that their decision to refuse treatment now may not accurately reflect the decision they would make in the future, were they competent at the time. To my knowledge, no piece of living will legislation currently refers to this likelihood. Though there are numerous published advance directive forms and more publications to assist in filling them in, none of them inform the potential user of the likely inaccuracy of their current decision. [10, 11, 14, 15]

While such a change may satisfy strong advocates of advance directives that autonomy is now again maximised, I would remain dubious that this were the case. The logistics of giving such warnings to all people filling in living wills will necessarily mean that the warnings will be scant and superficial. The belief that one knows one's own mind now and in the future is understandably held with some vehemence by most of the community. The psychological needs met by the belief that one would rather be dead in a future tragic situation are strong and deeply ingrained. An insignificant warning is unlikely to have any impact upon this belief and many people will continue falsely to believe they definitely know what they would want in the hypothetical scenario.

This kind of reasoning leads me to believe that it will be practically impossible to allow people to make an autonomous choice about this kind of advance directive and therefore on the grounds that such directives will neither increase autonomy nor increase the community's level of utility I believe that this type of living will should be abolished.

It is important to note that this line of argument will not demand the abandonment of all varieties of advance directive. It will not, for example, apply to advance directives where the ability to consent to treatment is irreversibly lost. In this situation there will be no possibility of the person recovering to give carers a more accurate report of her current desire for treatment. Carers would then be justified in taking their best guess as to the affected individual's preferences, no matter how inaccurate it is likely to be. Moreover, this best guess will be substantially improved if the person has taken out a living will. Neither will it affect advance directives made by people who are already critically ill and who are, for example, giving instruction that they should not be resuscitated in the event of cardiac arrest. These people are already critically ill and therefore are able to correctly determine their preferences for what is essentially their current situation.

The argument applies only to advance directives made by essentially healthy individuals who opt for withdrawal of active care in a situation where their inability to consent is potentially reversible. In these situations, patients should be resuscitated and their opinions regarding future treatment sought again now that they are in the scenario that they had previously only imagined. For some no doubt this will lead to considerable hardship, as they must again state their preference that they would rather be allowed to die, but for others, perhaps the majority, it will provide a safety net and a chance to reconsider their decision with all available information.

Those who would have wished to see the King's wager abolished because of the needless deaths it seemed to cause must be similarly troubled by this form of living will.

References

1.   Mendelson D. The Medical Treatment (Enduring Power of Attorney) Act and assisted suicide: the legal position in Victoria. *Bioethics News* 1993; **12**: 34–42.

2.   Stern K. Living wills in English law. *Palliative Medicine* 1993; **7**: 283–8.

3.   Greco PJ, Schulman KA, Lavizzo-Mourey R, Hansen-Flaschen J. The Patient Self-Determination Act and the future of advance directives. *Annals of Internal Medicine* 1991; **115**: 639–43.

4.   Kübler-Ross E. *On death and dying.* New York: Macmillan, 1969.

5.   Owen C, Tennant C, Levis J, Jones M. Suicide and euthanasia: patient attitudes in the context of cancer. *Psycho-Oncology* 1992; **1**: 79–88.

6.   Danis M, Garrett J, Harris R, Patrick DL. Stability of choices about life-sustaining treatments. *Annals of Internal Medicine* 1994; **120**: 567–73.

7.   Dillner L. Relatives keener on euthanasia than patients. *British Medical Journal* 1994; *309:* 1107.

8.   Allebeck P, Bolund C, Ringback G. Increased suicide rate in cancer patients. *Journal of Clinical Epidemiology* 1989; **42**: 611–6.

9.   Brown JH, Henteleff P, Barakat S, Rowe CJ. Is it normal for terminally ill patients to desire death? *American Journal of Psychiatry* 1986; **143**: 208–11.

10.   Molloy W, Mepham V, Clarnette R. *Let me decide.* Melbourne: Penguin, 1993.

11.   Quill TE. *Death and dignity. Making choices and taking charge.* New York: WW Norton, 1993.

12.   Charlesworth M. A good death. In: Kuhse H, ed. *Willing to listen—waiting to die.* Melbourne: Penguin, 1994: 203–16.

13.   Marker R. *Deadly compassion. The death of Ann Humphry and the case against euthanasia.* London: Harper Collins, 1994.

14.   Humphry D. *Dying with dignity: understanding euthanasia.* New York: Birch Lane Press, 1992.

15.   Kennedy L. *Euthanasia.* London: Chatto & Windus, 1990.

Steven Luttrell and
Ann Sommerville

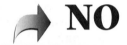 **NO**

Limiting Risks by Curtailing Rights: A Response to Dr. Ryan

Decisions about life-sustaining medical treatment should really be left to doctors. That is the core message of "betting your life" by Dr C J Ryan.[1] Although he focuses on only one type of decision—when the patient's mental incompetence is potentially reversible—the implication is that healthy people cannot validly appreciate the dimensions of the risk involved when they seek to limit in advance the scope of their own medical treatment. The danger of such miscalculation is said to be so profound that their right to take the risk must be curtailed for their own good. The general argument is not new. As the House of Lords Select Committee on Medical Ethics noted: "Disabled individuals are commonly more satisfied with their life than able-bodied people expect to be with the disability. The healthy do not choose in the same way as the sick."[2] But does this mean healthy people are to be deprived of the opportunity to make the attempt?

Some of the existing criticism of advance decision-making has been preoccupied with personal identity and the continuity of mind and mental state as the important criteria. According to such arguments, the rupture caused by loss of competence is so great that it makes nonsense of the concept of personal continuity. A competent individual is not making advance decisions for herself but for the future relict of who she once was. Dr Ryan's argument is a variation on this theme and seeks to prove that in advance of disability, people are in such a totally different mind-set that they are "likely to grossly under-estimate their desire for medical intervention should they become ill."[1]

We do not agree with Dr Ryan's view that advance directives dealing with situations where the deterioration in mental capacity is potentially reversible should be abolished and take issue with him on the following points:

(i) His argument hinges on the notion that people are likely to under-estimate substantially their desire to have medical intervention should they become ill. The evidence for this is not convincing. Emanuel *et al* following a prospective study of 495 HIV-positive or oncology out-patients and 102 members of the public concluded that most people made moderately stable treatment choices and that recent hospitalisation did not decrease that stability.[3]

From Steven Luttrell and Ann Sommerville, "Limiting Risks by Curtailing Rights: A Response to Dr. Ryan," *Journal of Medical Ethics*, vol. 22 (1996), pp. 100–104. Copyright © 1996 by The British Medical Association. Reprinted by permission.

Even if it is the case that in general the sick do not make the same choices as the healthy, there is evidence that this does not apply to people who have completed an advance directive. Although Danis *et al* found that patients who were hospitalised one or more times between baseline and follow-up interviews were more likely to change their choices and desire more treatment, patients who had a living will were more likely to maintain stable preferences. Indeed, patients who had living wills and chose the least amount of care at their initial interview had extremely stable preferences (96 percent unchanged).[4]

There appears to be little evidence that healthy people consider making treatment decisions in advance. Even in the United States, where living wills have been in existence much longer than in Britain, there is a wide disparity between the large percentage of people who indicate a desire to die without heroic measures and the small percentage who have made advance directives.[5] The scant UK evidence[6] supports American findings that interest in living wills is primarily shown by people who are educated, articulate and already have a diagnosis. (In the USA, the obligation for hospitals to raise the subject of advance decision-making arose only with patients who were checking in for treatment and therefore, by definition, were not a healthy population.) Part of the increased interest in this mechanism in the UK has been as a result of a small but well-informed population of HIV-positive patients witnessing the terminal treatment of friends and partners. Indeed, one of the limitations of advance statements is their lack of ready accessibility to people with differing levels of education, experience and literacy.

(ii) Dr Ryan states that it is an accepted principle that one cannot properly exercise one's autonomy if one is not in possession of all available information that might influence one's decisions and that a patient's consent to a procedure is only valid if she has been informed of all the risks and consequences. We take issue with this view. It implicitly denies the option of consciously deciding from a knowingly incomplete knowledge base and the option to decide validly to allow another person to decide on one's behalf. It is not necessarily obligatory for an individual to know each and every one of the risks implicit in a course of action. Indeed, if this were the case, no person could ever make a valid decision. As human beings, our motivation is often intuitive or emotional as well as cognitive and we sometimes exercise autonomy by choosing not to know or at least not to recognise the full import of our actions. It is arguably not necessary to examine all the implications in order for a person to be clear that she does not want to go on living indefinitely with a restricted range of competency or mobility, even if some small improvement is possible. If applied to other spheres of medicine, Dr Ryan's principle would mean that people cannot make valid decisions about childbearing without taking account of potentially available genetic information or pre-natal testing.

Arguably, therefore, it cannot be assumed that in real life, people who make advance refusals want to know everything or, if having chosen not to be fully informed of every detail, are incapable of understanding the implications of their decision. Nevertheless, the *Code of Practice on Advance Statements,* published by the British Medical Association, sees health professionals as obliged to make all appropriate efforts to raise patients' awareness at the drafting stage about the risks and disadvantages, as well as the benefits, of advance statements.[7] As a matter of law in the UK, a patient's consent to a procedure is valid if he understands in general terms the nature of the intervention. There is no legal obligation to explain *all* the risks and benefits.[8]

(iii) Even if people do make unwise choices, we believe that this should not be used as a reason to curtail their autonomy. Society generally recognises that individuals sometimes make bad or risky choices in the way they shape their lives. In our society, the libertarian legacy of Mill, however, assumes that individual choices should be permitted, unless they impinge on the rights of others. Mill's famous dictum was that "the sole end for which mankind are warranted, individually or collectively, in interfering with the liberty of action of any of their number is self-protection" and that an individual "cannot rightfully be compelled to do or forbear because it will be better for him to do so, because it will make him happier, because in the opinions of others to do so would be wise or even right."[9] So, does it damage the fabric of society or the rights of other people to allow Jehovah's Witnesses, for example, the right to refuse in advance the administration of blood products in all circumstances, even when their condition is curable? Or should they, as Dr Ryan suggests, be forcibly treated and only then "their opinions regarding future treatment be sought again now that they are in the scenario that they had previously only imagined"?[1]

Common Sense

It is trite to observe that people's views change with their circumstances. The philosopher, Parfit, for example, discussing different stages of individual development, talks about "my most recent self," "one of my earlier selves" and "one of my distant selves"; each of these showing a different degree of psychological connectedness with the present self.[10] From a practical perspective, would this mean that greater weight must automatically be attached to an advance directive made comparatively recently by an individual who is still more or less the same self? Common sense would seem to support such a view even if the individual was completely healthy when making the directive and now is in an altered psychological state. Simply acknowledging varying degrees of psychological continuity or disparity with regard to former and future selves does not answer the question of whether it is morally correct for subsequent selves to be treated in contravention of an advance directive reflecting their former interests.

(iv) We believe that a retreat to medical paternalism is not a practical option in societies increasingly aware of patient charters and consumer rights. Many forms of advance directives offer the drafter a choice of specifying personal instructions and/or nominating a proxy to decide. American surveys show that the option most commonly chosen is for people to select decision-making by a family member or other proxy despite the evidence of a variable correlation between the judgments of nominated proxy decision-makers and the patients' own prior wishes.[11] One study indicated that of 104 patients with life-threatening illness who were offered advance directives, 69 took up the offer and most asked for non-aggressive treatment if "the burdens of treatment outweigh the expected benefits." None, however, gave any other personal instructions,[12] although evidence suggests that proxies are more likely than patients themselves to opt for life-prolonging treatment, ie, to support more conservative choices than the individual would have made if competent and in that situation.[13]

Dr Ryan contests one specific type of advance directive on grounds of utility and autonomy. He argues that it is contrary to utility to permit people to die when their lives could be prolonged and their condition improved. This might be true if utility were a matter of simply prolonging life rather than also a question of maximising happiness and choice and reducing misery, including the misery of families who may see their relative being resuscitated contrary to an informed and competent advance refusal.

Two Autonomies

Nor is autonomy a simple matter. When an individual is conscious but mentally incapacitated, in Dworkin's view, "two autonomies are in play: the autonomy of the demented patient and the autonomy of the person who became demented. These two autonomies can conflict, and the resulting problems are complex and difficult."[14] Of course, some philosophers solve this by attributing no autonomy to the demented person and recognising the "residual interests" of the previously competent individual as paramount. A range of psychological and philosophical questions arise here about our ability to decide now life and death matters for the people we will be in the future when some part of what makes us the individuals we are—our awareness of ourselves, our past and continuity—has been lost. Dworkin seems to support Dr Ryan's approach in seeing the competent person who makes the anticipatory decision as fundamentally different from and other to the incapacitated individual who lives out (or not) the consequences of the decision. It is widely accepted that individuals can only make advance directives for "themselves." A person who becomes severely mentally disordered, however, is in some sense no longer "herself." Nevertheless, despite the lack of continuity, the former, competent "self" should arguably still retain moral rights about how the later, incompetent self is treated.[15] Even if acknowledged as being not quite the same person, the claim of the competent to decide on behalf of the later incompetent self still appears stronger than the claims of other players, especially bearing in mind the above-mentioned tendency for proxy decision-makers to choose options inconsistent with the individual's own values.

There is a danger that health professionals and nominated proxies will not take full account of the complex mixture of reasoning which leads some people to choose to forego treatment even in situations where medicine can offer them an extension of life. Although doctors' decisions about lifesaving treatment correlate with their own estimate of subsequent quality of life, they significantly underestimate their elderly patients' quality of life compared with the views of the patients themselves.[16] For some people, medical views of quality of life or possibility of improvement may not be a central issue. Just as Dr Ryan points out that it is difficult for healthy people convincingly to imagine themselves with disability, so it is often hard for the young or middle-aged to envisage that there may be a stage when we have simply lived long enough and the burdens of further treatment no longer outweigh the benefits. We may then wish to opt out even at the risk of potentially missing out on a slightly prolonged lifespan.

(v) We do not agree that advance directives for conditions of temporary mental incapacity should be less valid than advance directives for conditions of permanent mental incapacity. We question the logic of such a distinction. Dr Ryan concedes that his argument does not apply where loss of mental capacity is permanent. He distinguishes this situation as there "will be no possibility of the person recovering to give carers a more accurate report of her current desire for treatment"[1] and therefore they should be guided by an existing living will. He recognises that an accurate report of individual wishes is of value and therefore should be respected. If, however, a Jehovah's Witness, for example, repeatedly states that under no circumstances does he want a transfusion with blood products, Dr Ryan would urge us to ignore this directive if mental incapacity is temporarily impaired. There is no logical reason why the situation where mental incapacity is temporary should be treated in a different way from the situation where the incapacity is permanent. We feel that in both cases an appropriately worded advance directive should be equally applicable.

Information-Sharing

(vi) Even if Dr Ryan's arguments are accepted, we do not agree that "there is the possibility of large numbers of people dying when they would not have wanted to" although it may be that some will die when doctors would prefer to keep them alive. Doctors hostile to the concept of advance decision-making can limit or otherwise influence patients' choices. The acceptance or refusal of treatment is highly dependent on the amount and manner of information-sharing about the treatment options.[17] Discussion with elderly out-patients about limiting treatment rarely occurs[18] and in Emanuel's survey of patient and public opinion, the lack of physician initiative was the most frequently mentioned perceived barrier to the making of advance directives. In this survey of 405 out-patients and 102 members of the public, 93 per cent of the former and 89 per cent of the latter claimed to desire advance directives but considered their doctors to be reluctant.[19] Yet it is to be strongly advised that advance directives are only made in conjunction with advice and information from health professionals.[20]

Dr Ryan's arguments only apply to advance directives which withhold consent to treatment where there has been a temporary loss of mental capacity. We agree that the greatest value of advance directives is their use in situations where the loss of mental capacity is not reversible, such as in cases of dementia, chronic stroke or chronic brain injury due to trauma.

Nevertheless, we refute his thesis that large numbers of people will die unnecessarily since we believe it unlikely that many people will draft advance directives specifically indicating that they would not want treatment if they were to suffer temporary mental incapacity. Examples of common clinical situations where a reduction in mental capacity is potentially reversible include the acute confusional state in an older person, the early phase of recovery from an acute stroke, and the early stage of recovery from head trauma and psychiatric illness. We agree that the advance directive is of more limited application in these situations as it may be very difficult to envisage what degree of recovery will occur. Certainly, with respect to mental illness, if a patient is detained under a section of the Mental Health Act 1983, treatment under the Act will override any refusal of treatment of mental disorder set out in an advance directive.

If one examines the standard forms for advance directives in the UK, many emphasise that for the decision to be implementable the deterioration in mental capacity must be considered permanent or where life is nearing its end due to a terminal physical illness. People may draft their decisions in any form but many use standard documents which direct attention to irreversible conditions. One of the most common living wills, the Terrence Higgins Trust model, is not unique in allowing drafters the option of choosing to have all available treatment as well as refusing interventions in three situations:

- When there is a life-threatening illness *from which there is no likelihood of recovery* and it is so serious that life is nearing its end;
- When *mental functions become permanently impaired with no likelihood of improvement* and the impairment is so severe that the drafter does not understand what is happening and medical treatment is needed to keep him alive;
- When the drafter is *permanently unconscious* with no likelihood of regaining consciousness.[21]

Dr Ryan's argument is based on the fact that the sick do not make the same choices as the healthy. He does not point out, however, that in many instances advance directives are made by people who are already sick. Indeed, the mechanism is probably most useful for those people who have already been diagnosed as having a chronic illness for which there is no adequate curative treatment and where there is likely to be a predictable pattern of deterioration, for example, patients with AIDS or dementia. Moreover, even if an advance directive is made while the drafter is healthy, he or she will often have the opportunity of revoking or changing it when illness occurs as long as mental capacity is retained.

Conclusion

For the reasons outlined in this paper, we maintain that advance directives refusing treatment during periods of temporary incapacity should be respected. We acknowledge, however, that there are difficulties for healthy people trying to make decisions for future events. It is important that patients are made aware of these difficulties and not discouraged by medical reluctance to discuss the matter so that they draft directives in isolation. Emanuel found that those patients who had discussions with their physicians made the most stable decisions.[3] We would therefore urge any person making an advance directive about medical therapy to discuss the directive with a medical practitioner.

References

1. Ryan J. Betting your life: an argument against certain advance directives. *Journal of Medical Ethics* 1996; **22**: 95-9.

2. House of Lords Select Committee on Medical Ethics. *Report from the Select Committee on Medical Ethics.* London: HMSO, 1994: **1**: 41.

3. Emanuel L, Emanuel E, Stoeckle, *et al.* Advance directives, stability of patient's treatment choices. *Archives of Internal Medicine* 1994; **154**: 209-17.

4. Danis M, Garret J, Harris R, *et al.* Stability of choices about life sustaining treatments. *Annals of Internal Medicine* 1994; **120**: 567-73.

5. Menikoff JA, Sachs GA, Seigler M. Beyond advance directives: health care surrogate laws. *New England Journal of Medicine* 1992; **327**: 1165-9.

6. Meadows P. Use of living wills in HIV infection and AIDS. *Lancet* 1994; **334**: 1509. Calvert GM. The completion of living wills: an examination of the demographics, completion and issues raised by the living will. London: Terrence Higgins Trust, 1994. Schlyter C. *Advance directives and AIDS: an empirical study of the interest in living wills and proxy decision making in the context of HIV/AIDs care.* London: Centre of Medical Law and Ethics, Kings College, 1992.

7. Sommerville A. *Advance statements about medical treatment.* London: BMJ Publishing Group, 1995: 23.

8. Sidaway v Board of Governors of the Bethlem Royal Hospital and the Maudsley Hospital [1985] AC 871.

9. Mill JS. *On liberty.* London: Parker and Son, 1859: 68.

10. Parfit D. Personal identity. In: Honderich T, Burnyeat M, eds. *Philosophy as it is.* Harmondsworth: Pelican, 1979: 186-211.

11. For example see Seckler AB, Meier DE, Mulvihill M, Cammer Paris BE: Substituted judgement: how accurate are proxy predictions? *Annals of Internal Medicine* 1991; **115**: 92-8. Ouslander JG, Tymchuk AJ, Rhabar B. Health care decisions among elderly long care residents and their potential proxies. *Archives of Internal Medicine* 1989; **149**: 1367-72. Emanuel BJ, Emanuel LL. Proxy decision making for incompetent patients: an ethical and empirical analysis. *Journal of the American Medical Association* 1992; **267**: 2067-71.

12. Schneiderman L, *et al.* Effects of offering advance directives on medical treatments and costs. *Annals of Internal Medicine* 1992; **117**: 599-606.

13. See reference 11: Seckler AB, *et al.*

14. Dworkin R. *Life's dominion.* London: Harper Collins, 1993.

15. Sommerville A. Are advance directives the answer? In: Maclean S, ed. *Death, dying and the law.* Aldershot: Dartmouth Press, 1996.

16. Uhlmann RF, Pearlman RA. Perceived quality of life and preferences for life sustaining treatment in older adults. *Archives of Internal Medicine* 1991; **151**: 495-7.

17.   Ainslie A, Beisecker A. Changes in treatment decisions by elderly persons based on treatment descriptions. *Archives of Internal Medicine* 1994; **154**: 2225–33. Malloy TR, Wigton RS, Meeske J, Tape TG. The influence of treatment descriptions on advance directive decisions. *Journal of the American Geriatric Society* 1992; **40**: 1255–60.

18.   Goold SD, Arnold RM, Siminoff LA. Discussion about limiting treatment in a geriatric clinic. *Journal of the American Geriatric Society* 1993; **41**: 277–81.

19.   Emanuel LL, Barry MJ, Stoeckle JD, *et al.* Advance directives for medical care—a case for greater use. *New England Journal of Medicine* 1991; **324**: 889–95.

20.   Mower WR, Baraff LJ. Advance directives, effect of type of directive on physicians' therapeutic decisions. *Archives of Internal Medicine* 1993; **153**: 375–81.

21.   Living will drawn up by Terrence Higgins Trust and King's College Centre for Medical Ethics and Law.

POSTSCRIPT

Do Some Advance Directives Limit Patients' Rights?

The case of Terri Schiavo, a Florida woman who was in a persistent vegetative state from 1990 until her death in March 2005, garnered more media attention and political involvement than did the similar case of Nancy Cruzan, 30 years earlier. Cruzan's family was united in their effort to remove her feeding tube. In contrast, Schiavo's husband Michael began efforts to remove her feeding tube in 1998, declaring that this was his wife's wish should she be in a permanent nonresponsive condition, but her parents, Robert and Mary Schindler, vehemently opposed this action. The case was tried in the legal system and in the court of public opinion through extensive media coverage and political actions. In the end Michael Schiavo prevailed and the feeding tube was removed, but Terri Schiavo's death did not end the controversy. In March 2006, three books were published presenting different sides of the controversy: Michael Schiavo and Michael Hirsh published *Terri: The Truth* (Dutton); "Terri's Family" (her parents, brother, and sister) published *A Life That Matters: The Legacy of Terri Schiavo—A Lesson for Us All* (Warner Books); and Arthur L. Caplan, James J. McCartney, and Dominic A. Sisti published *The Case of Terri Schiavo: Ethics at the End of Life* (Prometheus).

All 50 states and the District of Columbia have laws on advance directives; however, they differ in the limits they place on the substitute decision maker's power to refuse life-sustaining treatment, specifically artificial nutrition and hydration. See Muriel T. Gillick, "Advance Care Planning," *New England Journal of Medicine* (February 11, 2005) for a review.

Angela Fagerlin and Carl E. Schneider argue that the living will (but not durable powers of attorney) should be abandoned because it has not produced results ("Enough: The Failure of the Living Will," *Hastings Center Report,* March–April 2004).

The President's Council on Bioethics' 2006 report *Taking Care: Ethical Caregiving in an Aging Society* argues that advance directives do not account for the possibility that a person might change his or her mind, and that surrogate decision makers should not be bound by patients' prior declarations. The report is available at: http://bioethics.gov/reports/taking_care/index.html.

Nancy M. P. King argues in favor of advance directives in *Making Sense of Advance Directives,* rev. ed. (Georgetown University Press, 1996). Among her major points are that advance directives are only one procedural mechanism for implementing an individual's constitutional right to make decisions concerning his or her own body. See also Robert S. Olick, *Taking*

Advance Directives Seriously: Prospective Autonomy and Decisions Near the End of Life (Georgetown University Press, 2001) and Lawrence P. Ulrich and Mark J. Hanson, eds., *The Patient Self-Determination Act: Meeting the Challenge in Patient Care* (Georgetown University Press, 2001).

ISSUE 5

Do Standard Medical Ethics Apply in Disaster Conditions?

YES: **Robert W. Donnell,** from "A Bright Line," *Medscape* (October 3, 2006)

NO: **Mary Faith Marshall,** from "Oh, the Water . . . It Stoned Me to My Soul," *University of Minnesota Bioethics Examiner* (Summer 2006)

ISSUE SUMMARY

YES: Physician Robert W. Donnell believes that the medical profession must apply moral absolutes in matters of life and death, no matter what the conditions, and one of those absolutes is never to administer fatal doses of medication.

NO: Philosopher Mary Faith Marshall argues for compassion, not absolutism, when tragic choices have to be made.

August is hurricane season in the southern and eastern regions of the United States. By any measure, 2005 was a particularly deadly year. Hurricane Katrina, the costliest hurricane ever to hit the Gulf Coast states of Louisiana and Mississippi and the costliest natural disaster in U.S. history, was the third Category 5 storm (the next to highest designation) in that season. As the nation watched, unforgettable images unfold on television, Katrina took over 1,800 lives and caused an estimated $81.2 billion in property damages. Efforts to rebuild are still underway and will take years to complete. The losses and disruptions to individuals and families are incalculable as more than a million people were evacuated to other states, many still unable to return.

Many individuals performed heroically in their attempts to save lives and bring needed supplies to the dispossessed and suffering. Nevertheless, it was clear at the time and has become even more compelling in hindsight that there were inadequate emergency rescue and evacuation preparations for a storm of such huge dimensions. Local, state, and federal agencies were not equipped to handle the population's desperate needs. This was as true of medical facilities as it was of other critical support systems. In New Orleans, hospital capacity was reduced by 80 percent and safety-net clinics by 75 percent.

Dr. Tyler J. Curiel, chief of hematology and medical oncology at the Tulane University Hospital and Clinic in New Orleans, wrote that in the previous year his hospital had announced a "code gray," a process by which staff would be assigned specific duties when a hurricane struck. "As it turned out," he wrote, "there was no real system for code-gray assignments. . . . [H]ospitals generally enlisted whichever doctors happened to be on duty during a potential hurricane strike."

Katrina's floodwaters, he says, "crippled emergency power generators, transforming hospitals into dark, fetid, dangerous shells. . . . We were under tremendous strain: in addition to the dire medical circumstances of many of our patients, we confronted uncertainty about our own evacuation, exacerbated by the tensions of threatened violence and frazzled soldiers and guards."

Against this background the events in Memorial Medical Center in New Orleans during that period have come to symbolize the conflict between standard medical ethics, which prohibits administering fatal doses of medications, and disaster conditions. Thirty-four patients at Memorial died in the days following the hurricane. In July 2006, a physician and two nurses were arrested and accused of second-degree murder in four of these cases. Dr. Anna Pou, a cancer specialist, and nurses Cheri A. Landry and Lori L. Budo are accused of administering lethal doses of morphine and midazolam, known as Versed, to these patients.

Charles Foti, Jr., Louisiana's attorney general, called the deaths "plain and simple homicide," he said, by "people that pretended that maybe they were God." Outraged by the arrests, physicians and others declared that the drugs were probably administered to reduce pain and anxiety in seriously ill patients in at atmosphere of incredible crisis when government failed to fulfill its most basic responsibilities.

In the following selections, the two positions are starkly opposed. Dr. Robert W. Donnell believes that the medical profession must adhere to moral absolutes in cases of life and death, regardless of the situation. Philosopher Mary Faith Marshall, on the other hand, advises compassion and respect for ambiguity. Using a title taken from a Van Morrison song, she cites historical analogies of tragic choices between painless and brutal deaths.

YES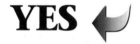

Robert W. Donnell

A Bright Line

Soon after Hurricane Katrina hit in 2005, news media reported instances of "mercy killing" of stranded victims, severely ill, or injured beyond hope of recovery.[1] Many observers, doubting the veracity of the reports, dismissed the story as urban legend. But months later, Louisiana authorities leveled second-degree murder accusations against a doctor and 2 nurses for allegedly euthanizing patients confined to a New Orleans hospital in the wake of the disaster.[2] Few details are available, and it would be premature to render judgment on these allegations. The episode does, however, raise a broader question: Can euthanasia be justified in extreme conditions such as disaster or combat?

Although relatively little seems to have been written about this particular aspect of euthanasia, we have much to guide us about general issues involved in physician-assisted death. Increasing acceptance of euthanasia and assisted suicide is relatively recent in the history of medical ethics, representing a significant departure from historic traditions that hold life as a non-negotiable value.

The Hippocratic Oath states, "I will not give a lethal drug to anyone if I am asked, nor will I advise such a plan . . ." The Christian Medical and Dental Associations (CMDA) proscribe physician-assisted death with this statement: "We oppose active intervention with the intent to produce death for the relief of suffering, economic considerations or convenience of patient, family or society." CMDA recognizes the responsibility of physicians to relieve suffering, but not at any cost.[3]

Dr. Mark Siegler, Director of the MacLean Bioethics Center at the University of Chicago, summed it up best when interviewed by *The New York Times:* "We begin with the general rule that doctors don't kill patients." He went on to say that even in extreme conditions, doctors have a responsibility to relieve pain and suffering, "but not to the point of putting patients to death."[4]

Two examples from the combat setting are worth considering, one from ancient history and one from recent headlines. In the Old Testament, II Samuel 1, we read that a soldier, hoping to win favor with David, claimed the mercy killing of King Saul. According to the soldier's account, the mortally wounded King Saul said, "Come, stand over me and kill me; for convulsions have seized me, and yet my life still lingers." The soldier continued: "So I stood over him, and killed him, for I knew that he could not live after he had

From Medscape.com, vol. 8, no. 2, Summer 2006. Copyright © 2006 by Medscape, LLC.

fallen." David, however, considered the act to be murder and ordered the soldier punished.

On May 21, 2005, an Iraqi insurgent severely wounded in a clash with the First Armored Division tank company was shot by Capt. Rogelio Maynulet, to "put him out of his misery."[5] Reports indicate that the Iraqi was wounded so severely that doctors viewing footage of the event disagreed on whether the victim was still alive at the time of the mercy killing. Maynulet was convicted of assault with intent to commit voluntary manslaughter. What is unusual is that this episode was caught on tape. We can only speculate how many mercy killings on the battle field go undocumented. Nevertheless, the US military justice system condemns euthanasia, even in such extreme circumstances.

The story of Captain Maynulet affords a vivid example with which to test our question, "Can euthanasia ever be justified in unusual situations?" What could have been more extreme? A portion of the victim's skull was blown away, and the medic advised Captain Maynulet that nothing could be done. If a case for euthanasia ever existed, can we imagine a more compelling one? Yet, over time, doubts began to surface. The medic gave conflicting testimony and later expressed second thoughts. A seemingly open-and-shut case began to crumble as conflicting testimony unfolded.[5]

If we allow exceptions to the prohibition of euthanasia, how should the exceptions be defined and applied? Endless questions would naturally arise, setting the stage for unintended consequences and a dangerous slippery slope. R. Alta Charo, professor of law and bioethics at the University of Wisconsin, speaking of the alleged New Orleans mercy killings, told *The New York Times*: "But if the killing was intentional, even if it was meant to be merciful, it is something that society draws a 'bright line' against for fear that it will get out of hand."[4]

I make no claim to the high ground in this debate. But I believe that our profession must apply moral absolutes in matters of life and death. Absolutes are needed to guide future actions, not to point fingers or to condemn individuals. None of us can be certain of how we would act in extreme conditions. We are morally frail creatures. Good intentions do not always lead to correct actions. That's why we need a bright line.

References

1. Graham C, Knowsley J. We had to kill our patients. *The Daily Mail*. September 11, 2005. . . .

2. Nossiter A, Dewan S. Patient deaths in New Orleans bring arrests. *The New York Times*. July 19, 2006. . . .

3. Euthanasia ethics statement. Christian Medical & Dental Associations. . . .

4. Grady D. Medical and ethical questions raised on deaths of critically ill patients. *The New York Times*. July 20, 2006. . . .

5. U.S. Army court-martials captain for mercy killing. . . . March 30, 2005. . . .

Mary Faith Marshall 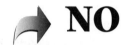 **NO**

Oh, the Water . . .
It Stoned Me to My Soul

Years ago, when I was writing a chapter on micro and macro allocation for the first edition of *Introduction to Clinical Ethics*, I thought long and hard about tragic choices. I wanted to open the chapter with a paradigm case; with a seemingly impossible dilemma. A case that even Solomonic wisdom couldn't resolve, because the options seemed morally bankrupt, or worse. I wanted to assert, from the get-go and in a graphic way, the nature of moral dilemmas, the fact that they don't involve, as Joseph Fletcher put it, "Sunday school ethics." To put forth Hegel's notion that tragedy is not the simplistic collision of good and evil, but involves the "headachy" business of choosing between competing goods, or competing evils. To apprise students of John Fletcher's cautionary aphorism that clinical ethics "isn't the happiness business." I wanted to ensure that those who might "do" clinical ethics in an applied way understood the emotional and personal liabilities for all concerned in ethics case consultation—to veer prospective consultants away from the pitfalls of hubris, complacency, and self-satisfaction.

I settled on William Styron's *Sophie's Choice*—primarily because it is difficult to imagine anything more painful or impossible than deciding which of one's children to send to the gas chamber. What earthly criteria could obtain? How could one possibly bear the psychic burden of such a choice for a moment, much less for a lifetime? Styron depicted this horrific scenario (a real one during the Holocaust, even though Sophie herself is fictional) with stark and mind-numbing pathos. His artistic mastery surfaces in the slight tenderness that tempers the scene, rendering it all the more morally obscene: "Mama!" she heard Eva's thin but soaring cry at the instant that she thrust the child away from her and rose from the concrete with a clumsy stumbling motion. 'Take the baby!' she called out. 'Take my little girl!'

At this point the aide—with a careful gentleness that Sophie would try without success to forget—tugged at Eva's hand and led her away into the waiting legion of the damned. She would forever retain a dim impression that the child had continued to look back, beseeching. But because she was now almost completely blinded by salty, thick, copious tears, she was spared whatever expression Eva wore, and she was always grateful for that. For in the bleak honesty of her heart she knew that she would never have been able to tolerate

From *University of Minnesota Bioethics Examiner*, vol. 9, issue 4, Summer 2006, pp. 1–3. Copyright © 2006 by Center for Bioethics, University of Minnesota. Reprinted by permission.

it, driven nearly mad as she was by her last glimpse of that vanishing small form."[2]

Sophie comes to mind when I happen across situations where life has gotten suddenly and twistedly sideways on the unexpectant. When, for example, I read of the Sri Lankan tsunami; of a mother's tale of immersion in the deluge, clinging to her husband and child; and of losing the strength to hold fast to both of them, of having to let one go. Sophie emerged, too, when I read of children taken hostage at their school in Beslan, Russia, and of parents with multiple captive children being allowed to remove only one. How do you decide which hand to release, which name to give?

Or when, as a doctor or a nurse at Memorial Medical Center in Katrina-ravaged New Orleans, you are faced with a different sort of dilemma: how to deliver care to critically ill and dying patients when your hospital is surrounded by floodwater, has no electricity, water or sanitation, and the indoor temperature exceeds one hundred degrees. When the floodwaters have shorted out the generators that power the mechanical ventilators, the dialysis machines and other life sustaining equipment. When you fear for your patients' safety and for your own in a context of seeming social anarchy—of looting and worse. When it is now four days since the hurricane, and only an infrequent boat or helicopter happens along to evacuate patients. When the sickest patients have do-not-resuscitate orders and are *in extremis*, suffering, frightened, dying.

Do you palliate their physical and psychic pain as best you can with comfort and morphine? Do you step further down the path and decide what kind of death these patients will, and will not, have? Do you euthanize them with morphine, engage in mercy killing?

You do. Such, at least has been alleged in the popular press. An allegation that has prompted an investigation by the Louisiana Attorney General's office, with findings due imminently.

As many as 140 patients in hospitals and nursing homes in the New Orleans area died during or shortly after the storm. The Orleans Parish Coroner listed "Katrina-related" causes of death for over 40 patients at Memorial Medical Center, and for 34 residents at St. Rita's Nursing Home. As many as six hospitals and thirteen nursing homes in Louisiana, including Memorial and St. Rita's, may be under investigation by the Attorney General.

The allegations themselves, and the subsequent investigation have occasioned widespread moral outrage; both among those who believe that physicians should never kill, and those who believe that mercy killing under such brutal circumstances is an act of courage and compassion and should not be punished.

Most of us in the worlds of bioethics and philosophy are wary of moral absolutes. We might maintain that there are few, if any, of them. There is no public or professional consensus in the United States on proscriptions against physician assisted dying, or euthanasia.

One paradigm that might enlighten our consideration of the Memorial Medical Center allegations is the traditional "lifeboat ethics" case. In such cases, a choice in one individual's favor or interest is inherently not in the interest of, and imposes a detriment on another person. *United States v. Holmes* is the American classic in this family of cases. Considering it may prove illustrative not because of the nature of the case itself, but because of the social and moral ambivalence reflected in its final outcome.

In 1841, the American ship, the William Brown, foundered off the coast of Newfoundland after striking an iceberg. All of the crew, and thirty-four of sixty-five passengers escaped in the ship's two lifeboats. Twenty-four hours later, when one of the boats appeared to be sinking in the frigid waters, the crew threw fourteen men overboard, all of whom perished. The survivors in the boat were rescued some hours later. Holmes, the sole crewman who did not disappear after the crew landed in Philadelphia, was charged with manslaughter. He was subsequently convicted, the court finding that his duty as a seaman was to "protect, not sacrifice" those entrusted to his care. In sympathy with Holmes, and the desperate circumstances under which he had acted, the judge sentenced him to a term of only six months, and fined him twenty dollars.

When I hear the absolutistic statement, "doctors should never kill," or "euthanasia is always wrong," I am reminded of Adina Blady Szwajger's story. She is a pediatrician, who, during the Holocaust, worked as a twenty-two year old nurse (she had by then completed two years of medical school) at the Warsaw Childrens' Hospital in the Warsaw ghetto. Most of the children in the hospital were dying of some combination of starvation, typhus, or tuberculosis. In her bleak, heartbreaking reminiscence, *I Remember Nothing More*, Szwajger tells of naked and starving children crying and begging to be admitted to the hospital and shows photographs of children wrapped in newspaper and lying in the gutter, dead from starvation or infectious disease. And she tells of euthanizing an entire children's ward with morphine so that dying children could not be loaded onto trucks to be taken and killed elsewhere, or murdered in their beds by Ukrainian guards:

"I took the morphine upstairs. Dr. Margolis was there and I told her what I wanted to do. So we took a spoon and went to the infants' room. And just as, during those two years of real work in the hospital, I had bent down over the little beds, so now I poured this last medicine into those tiny mouths. Only Dr. Margolis was with me. And downstairs, there was screaming because the Szaulis and the Germans were already there, taking the sick from the wards to the cattle trucks."[3]

Adina Blady Szwajger and Dr. Margolis made a fundamental decision about what kind of death their young patients were due. Some critics would (and have in the New Orleans Memorial Medical Center case), argue the absolute stance—that extreme circumstances never occasion or justify mercy killing by physicians. It is an understandable position to take. A more cogent outlook, I believe, would allow for exceptions, for contingencies. I would rather that my child die the gentle death administered by Szwajger at Warsaw Children's Hospital, than die a violent death at the hands of soldiers. What I would have wanted for a loved one at Memorial Medical Center I cannot say, not having been there, and not knowing the facts being unearthed in the investigation. But I am sympathetic to those who face impossible choices. What can you do but your best?

This isn't the happiness business. Let us hope that when the Louisiana Attorney General makes his findings, and as the case plays out, that compassion, not absolutism, is the order of the day.

Notes

1. Morrison V. It Stoned Me.
2. Styron W. *Sophie's Choice* (New York, NY: Random House, 1979):483.
3. Szwajger A. *I Remember Nothing More* (New York, NY: Pantheon Books, 1988):56–57.

POSTSCRIPT

Do Standard Medical Ethics Apply in Disaster Conditions?

$\mathbf{A}$t the end of 2006, no formal charges had been filed against Dr. Pou and nurses Landry and Budo. No grand jury had been convened to hear the case. During a hearing on whether documents in the case should be made public, Orleans Parish District Judge Calvin Johnson said, "This case needs to either go forward or end" (Associated Press, November 20, 2006). In another case, Salvadore and Mabel Mangano, co-owners of St. Rita's Nursing Home in St. Bernard's Parish, were accused of negligent homicide after 34 residents drowned. This case has also failed to go forward.

For the full text of Dr. Curiel's essay, see "Murder or Mercy? Hurricane Katrina and the Need for Disaster Training," *New England Journal of Medicine*, November 16, 2006. In "Federal Health Policy Response to Hurricane Katrina: What It Was and What It Could Have Been," Jeanne M. Lambrew and Donna E. Shalala , both former federal officials, cite three major faults: the assistance provided by Congress and the White House was inadequate to meet immediate and subsequent needs; the long period of uncertainty before funding was agreed upon reduced the states' willingness to help evacuees; and the disaster highlighted flaws in the decision-making process. These authors call for system-wide reform so that in future disasters the response can be appropriate to the need.

The November 2006 issue of the *American Journal of the Medical Sciences* contains "Hurricane Katrina Symposium," a collection of 12 articles by physicians who experienced the disaster.

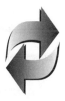

ISSUE 6

Should Physicians Be Allowed to Assist in Patient Suicide?

YES: **Marcia Angell**, from "The Supreme Court and Physician-Assisted Suicide—The Ultimate Right," *The New England Journal of Medicine* (January 2, 1997)

NO: **Kathleen M. Foley**, from "Competent Care for the Dying Instead of Physician-Assisted Suicide," *The New England Journal of Medicine* (January 2, 1997)

ISSUE SUMMARY

YES: Physician Marcia Angell asserts that a physician's main duties are to respect patient autonomy and to relieve suffering, even if that sometimes means assisting in a patient's death.

NO: Physician Kathleen M. Foley counters that if physician-assisted suicide becomes legal, it will begin to substitute for interventions that otherwise might enhance the quality of life for dying patients.

Since the early 1980s physicians, lawyers, philosophers, and judges have examined questions about withholding life-sustaining treatment. Their deliberations have resulted in a broad consensus that competent adults have the right to make decisions about their medical care, even if those decisions seem unjustifiable to others and even if they result in death. Furthermore, the right of individuals to name others to carry out their prior wishes or to make decisions if they should become incompetent is now well established. Thirty-eight states now have legislation allowing advance directives (commonly known as "living wills").

The debate in specific cases continues (see, for example, the issue on withholding food and nutrition), but on the whole, patients' rights to self-determination have been bolstered by 80 or more legal cases, dozens of reports, and statements made by medical societies and other organizations.

As often occurs in bioethical debate, the resolution of one issue only highlights the lack of resolution about another. There is clearly no consensus about either euthanasia or physician-assisted suicide.

Like truth telling, euthanasia is an old problem given new dimensions by the ability of modern medical technology to prolong life. The word itself is Greek (literally, *happy death*) and the Greeks wrestled with the question of whether, in some cases, people would be better off dead. But the Hippocratic Oath in this instance was clear: "I will neither give a deadly drug to anybody if asked for it, nor will I make a suggestion to that effect." On the other hand, if the goal of medicine is not simply to prolong life but to reduce suffering, at some point the question of what measures should be taken or withdrawn will inevitably arise. The problem is: When death is inevitable, how far should one go in hastening it?

The majority of cases in which euthanasia is raised as a possibility are among the most difficult ethical issues to resolve, for they involve the conflict between a physician's duty to preserve life and the burden on the patient and the family that is created by fulfilling that duty. One common distinction is between *active* euthanasia (that is, some positive act such as administering a lethal injection) and *passive* euthanasia (that is, an inaction such as deciding not to administer antibiotics when the patient has a severe infection). Another common distinction is between *voluntary* euthanasia (that is, the patient wishes to die and consents to the action that will make it happen) and *involuntary*—or better, *nonvoluntary*—euthanasia (that is, the patient is unable to consent, perhaps because he or she is in a coma).

The two selections that follow address a particularly controversial aspect of this issue. Is it ethical for a physician to assist in a hopelessly ill patient's suicide? Marcia Angell argues that sometimes hastening death should be an option for physicians although "reluctantly as a last resort." Angell states that a physician must consider patient autonomy and suffering when deciding upon care. Kathleen M. Foley contends that the medical profession should take the lead in developing guidelines for the end of life. This means that one must not confuse compassion for a patient's suffering with competence in care.

YES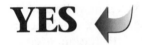

Marcia Angell

The Supreme Court and Physician-Assisted Suicide—The Ultimate Right

The importance and contentious issue of physician-assisted suicide, now being argued before the U.S. Supreme Court, is the subject of the following two editorials. Writing in favor of permitting assisted suicide under certain circumstances is the Journal's executive editor, Dr. Marcia Angell. Arguing against it is Dr. Kathleen Foley, co-chief of the Pain and Palliative Care Service of Memorial Sloan-Kettering Cancer Center in New York. We hope these two editorials, which have in common the authors' view that care of the dying is too often inadequate, will help our readers in making their own judgments.

—Jerome P. Kassirer, M.D.

The U.S. Supreme Court will decide later this year whether to let stand decisions by two appeals courts permitting doctors to help terminally ill patients commit suicide.[1] The Ninth and Second Circuit Courts of Appeals last spring held that state laws in Washington and New York that ban assistance in suicide were unconstitutional as applied to doctors and their dying patients.[2,3] If the Supreme Court lets the decisions stand, physicians in 12 states, which include about half the population of the United States, would be allowed to provide the means for terminally ill patients to take their own lives, and the remaining states would rapidly follow suit. Not since *Roe* v. *Wade* has a Supreme Court decision been so fateful.

The decision will culminate several years of intense national debate, fueled by a number of highly publicized events. Perhaps most important among them is Dr. Jack Kevorkian's defiant assistance in some 44 suicides since 1990, to the dismay of many in the medical and legal establishments, but with substantial public support, as evidenced by the fact that three juries refused to convict him even in the face of a Michigan statute enacted for that purpose. Also since 1990, voters in three states have considered ballot initiatives that would legalize some form of physician-assisted dying, and in 1994 Oregon became the first state to approve such a measure.[4] (The Oregon law was stayed pending a court challenge.) Several surveys indicate that roughly two thirds of the American public now support physician-assisted suicide,[5,6] as do more than half the doctors in the United States,[6,7] despite the fact that influential physicians' organizations are opposed. It seems clear that many

Americans are now so concerned about the possibility of a lingering, high-technology death that they are receptive to the idea of doctors' being allowed to help them die.

In this editorial I will explain why I believe the appeals courts were right and why I hope the Supreme Court will uphold their decisions. I am aware that this is a highly contentious issue, with good people and strong arguments on both sides. The American Medical Association (AMA) filed an amicus brief opposing the legalization of physician-assisted suicide,[8] and the Massachusetts Medical Society, which owns the *Journal,* was a signatory to it. But here I speak for myself, not the *Journal* or the Massachusetts Medical Society. The legal aspects of the case have been well discussed elsewhere, to me most compellingly in Ronald Dworkin's essay in the *New York Review of Books.*[9] I will focus primarily on the medical and ethical aspects.

I begin with the generally accepted premise that one of the most important ethical principles in medicine is respect for each patient's autonomy, and that when this principle conflicts with others, it should almost always take precedence. This premise is incorporated into our laws governing medical practice and research, including the requirement of informed consent to any treatment. In medicine, patients exercise their self-determination most dramatically when they ask that life-sustaining treatment be withdrawn. Although others may sometimes consider the request ill-founded, we are bound to honor it if the patient is mentally competent—that is, if the patient can understand the nature of the decision and its consequences.

A second starting point is the recognition that death is not fair and is often cruel. Some people die quickly, and others die slowly but peacefully. Some find personal or religious meaning in the process, as well as an opportunity for a final reconciliation with loved ones. But others, especially those with cancer, AIDS, or progressive neurologic disorders, may die by inches and in great anguish, despite every effort of their doctors and nurses. Although nearly all pain can be relieved, some cannot, and other symptoms, such as dyspnea, nausea, and weakness, are even more difficult to control. In addition, dying sometimes holds great indignities and existential suffering. Patients who happen to require some treatment to sustain their lives, such as assisted ventilation or dialysis, can hasten death by having the life-sustaining treatment withdrawn, but those who are not receiving life-sustaining treatment may desperately need help they cannot now get.

If the decisions of the appeals courts are upheld, states will not be able to prohibit doctors from helping such patients to die by prescribing a lethal dose of a drug and advising them on its use for suicide. State laws barring euthanasia (the administration of a lethal drug by a doctor) and assisted suicide for patients who are not terminally ill would not be affected. Furthermore, doctors would not be *required* to assist in suicide; they would simply have that option. Both appeals courts based their decisions on constitutional questions. This is important, because it shifted the focus of the debate from what the majority would approve through the political process, as exemplified by the Oregon initiative, to a matter of fundamental rights, which are largely immune from the political process. Indeed, the Ninth Circuit Court drew an explicit analogy between suicide and abortion, saying that both were personal choices protected by the Constitution and that forbidding doctors to assist would in effect nullify these rights. Although states could regulate assisted suicide, as they do abortion, they would not be permitted to regulate it out of existence.

It is hard to quarrel with the desire of a greatly suffering, dying patient for a quicker, more humane death or to disagree that it may be merciful to help bring that about. In those circumstances, loved ones are often relieved when death finally comes, as are the attending doctors and nurses. As the Second Circuit Court said (in the case of *Quill v. Vacco*), the state has no interest in prolonging such a life. Why, then, do so many people oppose legalizing physician-assisted suicide in these cases? There are a number of arguments against it, some stronger than others, but I believe none of them can offset the overriding duties of doctors to relieve suffering and to respect their patients' autonomy. Below I list several of the more important arguments against physician-assisted suicide and discuss why I believe they are in the last analysis unpersuasive.

Assisted suicide is a form of killing, which is always wrong. In contrast, withdrawing life-sustaining treatment simply allows the disease to take its course. There are three methods of hastening the death of a dying patient: withdrawing life-sustaining treatment, assisting suicide, and euthanasia. The right to stop treatment has been recognized repeatedly since the 1976 case of Karen Ann Quinlan[10] and was affirmed by the U.S. Supreme Court in the 1990 Cruzan decision[11] and the U.S. Congress in its 1990 Patient Self-Determination Act.[12] Although the legal underpinning is the right to be free of unwanted bodily invasion, the purpose of hastening death was explicitly acknowledged. In contrast, assisted suicide and euthanasia have not been accepted; euthanasia is illegal in all states, and assisted suicide is illegal in most of them.

Why the distinctions? Most would say they turn on the doctor's role: whether it is passive or active. When life-sustaining treatment is withdrawn, the doctor's role is considered passive and the cause of death is the underlying disease, despite the fact that switching off the ventilator of a patient dependent on it looks anything but passive and would be considered homicide if done without the consent of the patient or a proxy. In contrast, euthanasia by the injection of a lethal drug is active and directly causes the patient's death. Assisting suicide by supplying the necessary drugs is considered somewhere in between, more active than switching off a ventilator but less active than injecting drugs, hence morally and legally more ambiguous.

I believe, however, that these distinctions are too doctor-centered and not sufficiently patient-centered. We should ask ourselves not so much whether the doctor's role is passive or active but whether the *patient's* role is passive or active. From that perspective, the three methods of hastening death line up quite differently. When life-sustaining treatment is withdrawn from an incompetent patient at the request of a proxy or when euthanasia is performed, the patient may be utterly passive. Indeed, either act can be performed even if the patient is unaware of the decision. In sharp contrast, assisted suicide, by definition, cannot occur without the patient's knowledge and participation. Therefore, it must be active—that is to say, voluntary. That is a crucial distinction, because it provides an inherent safeguard against abuse that is not present with the other two methods of hastening death. If the loaded term "kill" is to be used, it is not the doctor who kills, but the patient. Primarily because euthanasia can be performed without the patient's participation, I oppose its legalization in this country.

Assisted suicide is not necessary. All suffering can be relieved if care givers are sufficiently skillful and compassionate, as illustrated by the hospice movement. I have no doubt that if expert palliative care were available to everyone who needed it, there would be few requests for assisted suicide. Even under the best of circumstances, however, there will always be a few patients whose suffering simply cannot be adequately alleviated. And there will be some who would prefer suicide to any other measures available, including the withdrawal of life-sustaining treatment or the use of heavy sedation. Surely, every effort should be made to improve palliative care, as I argued 15 years ago,[13] but when those efforts are unavailing and suffering patients desperately long to end their lives, physician-assisted suicide should be allowed. The argument that permitting it would divert us from redoubling our commitment to comfort care asks these patients to pay the penalty for our failings. It is also illogical. Good comfort care and the availability of physician-assisted suicide are no more mutually exclusive than good cardiologic care and the availability of heart transplantation.

Permitting assisted suicide would put us on a moral "slippery slope." Although in itself assisted suicide might be acceptable, it would lead inexorably to involuntary euthanasia. It is impossible to avoid slippery slopes in medicine (or in any aspect of life). The issue is how and where to find a purchase. For example, we accept the right of proxies to terminate life-sustaining treatment, despite the obvious potential for abuse, because the reasons for doing so outweigh the risks. We hope our procedures will safeguard patients. In the case of assisted suicide, its voluntary nature is the best protection against sliding down a slippery slope, but we also need to ensure that the request is thoughtful and freely made. Although it is possible that we may someday decide to legalize voluntary euthanasia under certain circumstances or assisted suicide for patients who are not terminally ill, legalizing assisted suicide for the dying does not in itself make these other decisions inevitable. Interestingly, recent reports from the Netherlands, where both euthanasia and physician-assisted suicide are permitted, indicate that fears about a slippery slope there have not been borne out.[14,15,16]

Assisted suicide would be a threat to the economically and socially vulnerable. The poor, disabled, and elderly might be coerced to request it. Admittedly, overburdened families or cost-conscious doctors might pressure vulnerable patients to request suicide, but similar wrongdoing is at least as likely in the case of withdrawing life-sustaining treatment, since that decision can be made by proxy. Yet, there is no evidence of widespread abuse. The Ninth Circuit Court recalled that it was feared *Roe* v. *Wade* would lead to coercion of poor and uneducated women to request abortions, but that did not happen. The concern that coercion is more likely in this era of managed care, although understandable, would hold suffering patients hostage to the deficiencies of our health care system. Unfortunately, no human endeavor is immune to abuses. The question is not whether a perfect system can be devised, but whether abuses are likely to be sufficiently rare to be offset by the benefits to patients who otherwise would be condemned to face the end of their lives in protracted agony.

Depressed patients would seek physician-assisted suicide rather than help for their depression. Even in the terminally ill, a request for assisted suicide might signify treatable depression, not irreversible suffering. Patients suffering greatly at the end of life may also be depressed, but the depression does not necessarily explain their decision to commit suicide or make it irrational. Nor is it simple to diagnose depression in terminally ill patients. Sadness is to be expected, and some of the vegetative symptoms of depression are similar to the symptoms of terminal illness. The success of antidepressant treatment in these circumstances is also not ensured. Although there are anecdotes about patients who changed their minds about suicide after treatment,[17] we do not have good studies of how often that happens or the relation to antidepressant treatment. Dying patients who request assisted suicide and seem depressed should certainly be strongly encouraged to accept psychiatric treatment, but I do not believe that competent patients should be *required* to accept it as a condition of receiving assistance with suicide. On the other hand, doctors would not be required to comply with all requests; they would be expected to use their judgment, just as they do in so many other types of life-and-death decisions in medical practice.

Doctors should never participate in taking life. If there is to be assisted suicide, doctors must not be involved. Although most doctors favor permitting assisted suicide under certain circumstances, many who favor it believe that doctors should not provide the assistance.[6,7] To them, doctors should be unambiguously committed to life (although most doctors who hold this view would readily honor a patient's decision to have life-sustaining treatment withdrawn). The AMA, too, seems to object to physician-assisted suicide primarily because it violates the profession's mission. Like others, I find that position too abstract.[18] The highest ethical imperative of doctors should be to provide care in whatever way best serves patients' interests, in accord with each patient's wishes, not with a theoretical commitment to preserve life no matter what the cost in suffering.[19] If a patient requests help with suicide and the doctor believes the request is appropriate, requiring someone else to provide the assistance would be a form of abandonment. Doctors who are opposed in principle need not assist, but they should make their patients aware of their position early in the relationship so that a patient who chooses to select another doctor can do so. The greatest harm we can do is to consign a desperate patient to unbearable suffering—or force the patient to seek out a stranger like Dr. Kevorkian. Contrary to the frequent assertion that permitting physician-assisted suicide would lead patients to distrust their doctors, I believe distrust is more likely to arise from uncertainty about whether a doctor will honor a patient's wishes.

Physician-assisted suicide may occasionally be warranted, but it should remain illegal. If doctors risk prosecution, they will think twice before assisting with suicide. This argument wrongly shifts the focus from the patient to the doctor. Instead of reflecting the condition and wishes of patients, assisted suicide would reflect the courage and compassion of their doctors. Thus, patients with doctors like Timothy Quill, who described in a 1991 *Journal* article how he helped a patient take her life,[20] would get the help they need and want, but similar patients with less steadfast doctors would not. That makes no sense.

People do not need assistance to commit suicide. With enough determination, they can do it themselves. This is perhaps the cruelest of the arguments against physician-assisted suicide. Many patients at the end of life are, in fact, physically unable to commit suicide on their own. Others lack the resources to do so. It has sometimes been suggested that they can simply stop eating and drinking and kill themselves that way. Although this method has been described as peaceful under certain conditions,[21] no one should count on that. The fact is that this argument leaves most patients to their suffering. Some, usually men, manage to commit suicide using violent methods. Percy Bridgman, a Nobel laureate in physics who in 1961 shot himself rather than die of metastatic cancer, said in his suicide note, "It is not decent for Society to make a man do this to himself."[22]

My father, who knew nothing of Percy Bridgman, committed suicide under similar circumstances. He was 81 and had metastatic prostate cancer. The night before he was scheduled to be admitted to the hospital, he shot himself. Like Bridgman, he thought it might be his last chance. At the time, he was not in extreme pain, nor was he close to death (his life expectancy was probably longer than six months). But he was suffering nonetheless—from nausea and the side effects of antiemetic agents, weakness, incontinence, and hopelessness. Was he depressed? He would probably have freely admitted that he was, but he would have thought it beside the point. In any case, he was an intensely private man who would have refused psychiatric care. Was he overly concerned with maintaining control of the circumstances of his life and death? Many people would say so, but that was the way he was. It is the job of medicine to deal with patients as they are, not as we would like them to be.

I tell my father's story here because it makes an abstract issue very concrete. If physician-assisted suicide had been available, I have no doubt my father would have chosen it. He was protective of his family, and if he had felt he had the choice, he would have spared my mother the shock of finding his body. He did not tell her what he planned to do, because he knew she would stop him. I also believe my father would have waited if physician-assisted suicide had been available. If patients have access to drugs they can take when they choose, they will not feel they must commit suicide early, while they are still able to do it on their own. They would probably live longer and certainly more peacefully, and they might not even use the drugs.

Long before my father's death, I believed that physician-assisted suicide ought to be permissible under some circumstances, but his death strengthened my conviction that it is simply a part of good medical care—something to be done reluctantly and sadly, as a last resort, but done nonetheless. There should be safeguards to ensure that the decision is well considered and consistent, but they should not be so daunting or violative of privacy that they become obstacles instead of protections. In particular, they should be directed not toward reviewing the reasons for an autonomous decision, but only toward ensuring that the decision is indeed autonomous. If the Supreme Court upholds the decisions of the appeals courts, assisted suicide will not be forced on either patients or doctors, but it will be a choice for those patients who need it and those doctors willing to help. If, on the other hand, the Supreme Court overturns the lower courts' decisions, the issue will continue to be grappled with state by state, through the political process. But sooner or later, given the need and the widespread public support, physician-assisted suicide will be demanded of a compassionate profession.

References

1. Greenhouse L. High court to say if the dying have a right to suicide help. New York Times. October 2, 1996:A1.

2. Compassion in Dying v. Washington, 79 F.3d 790 (9th Cir. 1996).

3. Quill v. Vacco, 80 F.3d 716 (2d Cir. 1996).

4. Annas GJ. Death by prescription—the Oregon initiative. N Engl J Med 1994;331:1240-3.

5. Blendon RJ, Szalay US, Knox RA. Should physicians aid their patients in dying? The public perspective. JAMA 1992;267:2658-62.

6. Bachman JG, Alcser KH, Doukas DJ, Lichtenstein RL, Corning AD, Brody H. Attitudes of Michigan physicians and the public toward legalizing physician-assisted suicide and voluntary euthanasia. N Engl J Med 1996;334:303-9.

7. Lee MA, Nelson HD, Tilden VP, Ganzini L, Schmidt TA, Tolle SW. Legalizing assisted suicide—views of physicians in Oregon. N Engl J Med 1996;334: 310-5.

8. Gianelli DM. AMA to court: no suicide aid. American Medical News. November 25, 1996:1, 27, 28.

9. Dworkin R. Sex, death, and the courts. New York Review of Books. August 8, 1996.

10. In re: Quinlan, 70 N.J. 10, 355 A.2d 647 (1976).

11. Cruzan v. Director, Missouri Department of Health, 497 U.S. 261, 110 S.Ct. 2841 (1990).

12. Omnibus Budget Reconciliation Act of 1990, P.L. 101–508, sec. 4206 and 4751, 104 Stat. 1388, 1388-115, and 1388-204 (classified respectively at 42 U.S.C. 1395cc(f) (Medicare) and 1396a(w) (Medicaid) (1994)).

13. Angell M. The quality of mercy. N Engl J Med 1982;306:98-9.

14. van der Maas PJ, van der Wal G, Haverkate I, et al. Euthanasia, physician-assisted suicide, and other medical practices involving the end of life in the Netherlands, 1990–1995. N Engl J Med 1996;335:1699–705.

15. van der Wal G, van der Maas PJ, Bosma JM, et al. Evaluation of the notification procedure for physician-assisted death in the Netherlands. N Engl J Med 1996;335:1706–11.

16. Angell M. Euthanasia in the Netherlands—good news or bad? N Engl J Med 1996;335:1676–8.

17. Chochinov HM, Wilson KG, Enns M, et al. Desire for death in the terminally ill. Am J Psychiatry 1995;152:1185–91.

18. Cassel CK, Meier DE. Morals and moralism in the debate over euthanasia and assisted suicide. N Engl J Med 1990;323:750–2.

19. Angell M. Doctors and assisted suicide. Ann R Coll Physicians Surg Can 1991;24:493–4.

20. Quill TE. Death and dignity—a case of individualized decision making. N Engl J Med 1991;324:691–4.

21. Lynn J, Childress JF. Must patients always be given food and water? Hastings Cent Rep 1983;13(5):17–21.

22. Nuland SB. How we die. New York: Alfred A. Knopf, 1994:152.

Kathleen M. Foley

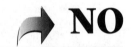 **NO**

Competent Care for the Dying Instead of Physician-Assisted Suicide

While the Supreme Court is reviewing the decisions by the Second and Ninth Circuit Courts of Appeals to reverse state bans on assisted suicide, there is a unique opportunity to engage the public, health care professionals, and the government in a national discussion of how American medicine and society should address the needs of dying patients and their families. Such a discussion is critical if we are to understand the process of dying from the point of view of patients and their families and to identify existing barriers to appropriate, humane, compassionate care at the end of life. Rational discourse must replace the polarized debate over physician-assisted suicide and euthanasia. Facts, not anecdotes, are necessary to establish a common ground and frame a system of health care for the terminally ill that provides the best possible quality of living while dying.

The biased language of the appeals courts evinces little respect for the vulnerability and dependency of the dying. Judge Stephen Reinhardt, writing for the Ninth Circuit Court, applied the liberty-interest clause of the Fourteenth Amendment, advocating a constitutional right to assisted suicide. He stated, "The competent terminally ill adult, having lived nearly the full measure of his life, has a strong interest in choosing a dignified and humane death, rather than being reduced to a state of helplessness, diapered, sedated, incompetent."[1] Judge Roger J. Miner, writing for the Second Circuit Court of Appeals, applied the equal-rights clause of the Fourteenth Amendment and went on to emphasize that the state "has no interest in prolonging a life that is ending."[2] This statement is more than legal jargon. It serves as a chilling reminder of the low priority given to the dying when it comes to state resources and protection.

The appeals courts' assertion of a constitutional right to assisted suicide is narrowly restricted to the terminally ill. The courts have decided that it is the patient's condition that justifies killing and that the terminally ill are special—so special that they deserve assistance in dying. This group alone can receive such assistance. The courts' response to the New York and Washington cases they reviewed is the dangerous form of affirmative action in the name of compassion. It runs the risk of further devaluing the lives of terminally ill patients and may provide the excuse for society to abrogate its responsibility for their care.

From *New England Journal of Medicine,* January 2, 1997, pp. 54–58. Copyright © 1997 by Massachusetts Medical Society. Reprinted by permission.

Both circuit courts went even further in asserting that physicians are already assisting in patients' deaths when they withdraw life-sustaining treatments such as respirators or administer high doses of pain medication that hasten death. The appeals courts argued that providing a lethal prescription to allow a terminally ill patient to commit suicide is essentially the same as withdrawing life-sustaining treatment or aggressively treating pain. Judicial reasoning that eliminates the distinction between letting a person die and killing runs counter to physicians' standards of palliative care.[3] The courts' purported goal in blurring these distinctions was to bring society's legal rules more closely in line with the moral value it places on the relief of suffering.[4]

In the real world in which physicians care for dying patients, withdrawing treatment and aggressively treating pain are acts that respect patients' autonomous decisions not to be battered by medical technology and to be relieved of their suffering. The physician's intent is to provide care, not death. Physicians do struggle with doubts about their own intentions.[5] The courts' arguments fuel their ambivalence about withdrawing life-sustaining treatments or using opioid or sedative infusions to treat intractable symptoms in dying patients. Physicians are trained and socialized to preserve life. Yet saying that physicians struggle with doubts about their intentions in performing these acts is not the same as saying that their intention is to kill. In palliative care, the goal is to relieve suffering, and the quality of life, not the quantity, is of utmost importance.

Whatever the courts say, specialists in palliative care do not think that they practice physician-assisted suicide or euthanasia.[6] Palliative medicine has developed guidelines for aggressive pharmacologic management of intractable symptoms in dying patients, including sedation for those near death.[3,7,8] The World Health Organization has endorsed palliative care as an integral component of a national health care policy and has strongly recommended to its member countries that they not consider legalizing physician-assisted suicide and euthanasia until they have addressed the needs of their citizens for pain relief and palliative care.[9] The courts have disregarded this formidable recommendation and, in fact, are indirectly suggesting that the World Health Organization supports assisted suicide.

Yet the courts' support of assisted suicide reflects the requests of the physicians who initiated the suits and parallels the numerous surveys demonstrating that a large proportion of physicians support the legalization of physician-assisted suicide.[10,11,12,13,14,15] A smaller proportion of physicians are willing to provide such assistance, and an even smaller proportion are willing to inject a lethal dose of medication with the intent of killing a patient (active voluntary euthanasia). These survey data reveal a gap between the attitudes and behavior of physicians; 20 to 70 percent of physicians favor the legalization of physician-assisted suicide, but only 2 to 4 percent favor active voluntary euthanasia, and only approximately 2 to 13 percent have actually aided patients in dying, by either providing a prescription or administering a lethal injection. The limitations of these surveys, which are legion, include inconsistent definitions of physician-assisted suicide and euthanasia, lack of information about non-respondents, and provisions for maintaining confidentiality that have led to inaccurate reporting.[13,16] Since physicians' attitudes toward alternatives to assisted suicide have not been studied, there is a void in our knowledge about the priority that physicians place on physician-assisted suicide.

The willingness of physicians to assist patients in dying appears to be determined by numerous complex factors, including religious beliefs, personal values, medical specialty, age, practice setting, and perspective on the use of financial resources.[13,16,17,18,19] Studies of patients' preferences for care at the end of life demonstrate that physicians' preferences strongly influence those of their patients.[13] Making physician-assisted suicide a medical treatment when it is so strongly dependent on these physician-related variables would result in a regulatory impossibility.[19] Physicians would have to disclose their values and attitudes to patients to avoid potential conflict.[13] A survey by Ganzini et al. demonstrated that psychiatrists' responses to requests to evaluate patients were highly determined by their attitudes.[13] In a study by Emanuel et al., depressed patients with cancer said they would view positively those physicians who acknowledged their willingness to assist in suicide. In contrast, patients with cancer who were suffering from pain would be suspicious of such physicians.[11]

In this controversy, physicians fall into one of three groups. Those who support physician-assisted suicide see it as a compassionate response to a medical need, a symbol of nonabandonment, and a means to reestablish patients' trust in doctors who have used technology excessively.[20] They argue that regulation of physician-assisted suicide is possible and, in fact, necessary to control the actions of physicians who are currently providing assistance surreptitiously.[21] The two remaining groups of physicians oppose legalization.[19,22,23,24] One group is morally opposed to physician-assisted suicide and emphasizes the need to preserve the professionalism of medicine and the commitment to "do no harm." These physicians view aiding a patient in dying as a form of abandonment, because a physician needs to walk the last mile with the patient, as a witness, not as an executioner. Legalization would endorse justified killing, according to these physicians, and guidelines would not be followed, even if they could be developed. Furthermore, these physicians are concerned that the conflation of assisted suicide with the withdrawal of life support or adequate treatment of pain would make it even harder for dying patients, because there would be a backlash against existing policies. The other group is not ethically opposed to physician-assisted suicide and, in fact, sees it as acceptable in exceptional cases, but these physicians believe that one cannot regulate the unregulatable.[19] On this basis, the New York State Task Force on Life and the Law, a 24-member committee with broad public and professional representation, voted unanimously against the legalization of physician-assisted suicide.[24] All three groups of physicians agree that a national effort is needed to improve the care of the dying. Yet it does seem that those in favor of legalizing physician-assisted suicide are disingenuous in their use of this issue as a wedge. If this form of assistance with dying is legalized, the courts will be forced to broaden the assistance to include active voluntary euthanasia and, eventually, assistance in response to requests from proxies.

One cannot easily categorize the patients who request physician-assisted suicide or euthanasia. Some surveys of physicians have attempted to determine retrospectively the prevalence and nature of these requests.[10] Pain, AIDS, and neurodegenerative disorders are the most common conditions in patients requesting assistance in dying. There is a wide range in the age of such patients, but many are younger persons with AIDS.[10] From the limited data available, the factors most commonly involved in requests for assistance are concern about future loss of control, being or becoming a burden to others, or being unable to care for oneself and fear of severe pain.[10] A small number of recent studies have directly asked terminally ill patients with cancer or AIDS about their desire for death.[25,26,27] All these studies show that the desire for death is closely associated with depression and that pain and lack of social support are contributing factors.

Do we know enough, on the basis of several legal cases, to develop a public policy that will profoundly change medicine's role in society?[1,2] Approximately 2.4 million Americans die each year. We have almost no information on how they die and only general information on where they die. Sixty-one percent die in hospitals, 17 percent in nursing homes, and the remainder at home, with approximately 10 to 14 percent of those at home receiving hospice care.

The available data suggest that physicians are inadequately trained to assess and manage the multifactorial symptoms commonly associated with patients' requests for physician-assisted suicide. According to the American Medical Association's report on medical education, only 5 of 126 medical schools in the United States require a separate course in the care of the dying.[28] Of 7048 residency programs, only 26 percent offer a course on the medical and legal aspects of care at the end of life as a regular part of the curriculum. According to a survey of 1068 accredited residency programs in family medicine, internal medicine, and pediatrics and fellowship programs in geriatrics, each resident or fellow coordinates the care of 10 or fewer dying patients annually.[28] Almost 15 percent of the programs offer no formal training in terminal care. Despite the availability of hospice programs, only 17 percent of the training programs offer a hospice rotation, and the rotation is required in only half of those programs; 9 percent of the programs have residents or fellows serving as members of hospice teams. In a recent survey of 55 residency programs and over 1400 residents, conducted by the American Board of Internal Medicine, the residents were asked to rate their perception of adequate training in care at the end of life. Seventy-two percent reported that they had received adequate training in managing pain and other symptoms; 62 percent, that they had received adequate training in telling patients that they are dying; 38 percent, in describing what the process will be like; and 32 percent, in talking to patients who request assistance in dying or a hastened death (Blank L: personal communication).

The lack of training in the care of the dying is evident in practice. Several studies have concluded that poor communication between physicians and patients, physicians' lack of knowledge about national guidelines for such care, and their lack of knowledge about the control of symptoms are barriers to the provision of good care at the end of life.[23,29,30]

Yet there is now a large body of data on the components of suffering in patients with advanced terminal disease, and these data provide the basis for treatment algorithms.[3] There are three major factors in suffering: pain and other physical symptoms, psychological distress, and existential distress (described as the experience of life without meaning). It is not only the patients who suffer but also their families and the health care professionals attending them. These experiences of suffering are often closely and inextricably related. Perceived distress in any one of the three groups amplifies distress in the others.[31,32]

Pain is the most common symptom in dying patients, and according to recent data from U.S. studies, 56 percent of outpatients with cancer, 82 percent of outpatients with AIDS, 50 percent of hospitalized patients with various diagnoses, and 36 percent of nursing home residents have inadequate management of pain during the course of their terminal illness.[33,34,35,36] Members of minority groups and women, both those with cancer and those with AIDS, as well as the elderly, receive less pain treatment than other groups of patients. In a survey of 1177 physicians who had treated a total of more than 70,000 patients with cancer in the previous six months, 76 percent of the respondents cited lack of knowledge as a barrier to their ability to control pain.[37] Severe pain that is not adequately controlled interferes with the quality of life, including the activities of daily living, sleep, and social interactions.[33,38]

Other physical symptoms are also prevalent among the dying. Studies of patients with advanced cancer and of the elderly in the year before death show that they have numerous symptoms that worsen the quality of life, such as fatigue, dyspnea, delirium, nausea, and vomiting.[36,38]

Along with these physical symptoms, dying patients have a variety of well-described psychological symptoms, with a high prevalence of anxiety and depression in patients with cancer or AIDS and the elderly.[27,39] For example, more than 60 percent of patients with advanced cancer have psychiatric problems, with adjustment disorders, depression, anxiety, and delirium reported most frequently. Various factors that contribute to the prevalence and severity of psychological distress in the terminally ill have been identified.[39] The diagnosis of depression is difficult to make in medically ill patients[3,26,40]; 94 percent of the Oregon psychiatrists surveyed by Ganzini et al. were not confident that they could determine, in a single evaluation, whether a psychiatric disorder was impairing the judgment of a patient who requested assistance with suicide.[13]

Attention has recently been focused on the interaction between uncontrolled symptoms and vulnerability to suicide in patients with cancer or AIDS.[41] Data from studies of both groups of patients suggest that uncontrolled pain contributes to depression and that persistent pain interferes with patients' ability to receive support from their families and others. Patients with AIDS have a high risk of suicide that is independent of physical symptoms. Among New York City residents with AIDS, the relative risk of suicide in men between the ages of 20 and 59 years was 36 times higher than the risk among men without AIDS in the same age group and 66 times higher than the risk in the general population.[41] Patients with AIDS who committed suicide generally did so within nine months after receiving the diagnosis; 25 percent had made a previous suicide attempt, 50 percent had reported severe depression, and 40 percent had seen a psychiatrist within four days before committing suicide. As previously noted, the desire to die is most closely associated with the diagnosis of depression.[26,27] Suicide is the eighth leading cause of death in the United States, and the incidence of suicide is higher in patients with cancer or AIDS and in elderly men than in the general population. Conwell and Caine reported that depression was underdiagnosed by primary care physicians in a cohort of elderly patients who subsequently committed suicide; 75 percent of the patients had seen a primary care physician during the last month of life but had not received a diagnosis of depression.[22]

The relation between depression and the desire to hasten death may vary among subgroups of dying patients. We have no data, except for studies of a small number of patients with cancer or AIDS. The effect of treatment for depression on the desire to hasten death and on requests for assistance in doing so has not been examined in the medically ill population, except for a small study in which four of six patients who initially wished to hasten death changed their minds within two weeks.[26]

There is also the concern that certain patients, particularly members of minority groups that are estranged from the health care system, may be reluctant to receive treatment for their physical or psychological symptoms because of the fear that their physicians will, in fact, hasten death. There is now some evidence that the legalization of assisted suicide in the Northern Territory of Australia has undermined the Aborigines' trust in the medical care system[42]; this experience may serve as an example for the United States, with its multicultural population.

The multiple physical and psychological symptoms in the terminally ill and elderly are compounded by a substantial degree of existential distress. Reporting on their interviews with Washington State physicians whose patients had requested assistance in dying, Back et al. noted the physicians' lack of sophistication in assessing such nonphysical suffering.[10]

In summary, there are fundamental physician-related barriers to appropriate, humane, and compassionate care for the dying. These range from attitudinal and behavioral barriers to educational and economic barriers. Physicians do not know enough about their patients, themselves, or suffering to provide assistance with dying as a medical treatment for the relief of suffering. Physicians need to explore their own perspectives on the meaning of suffering in order to develop their own approaches to the care of the dying. They need insight into how the nature of the doctor-patient relationship influences their own decision making. If legalized, physician-assisted suicide will be a substitute for rational therapeutic, psychological, and social interventions that might otherwise enhance the quality of life for patients who are dying. The medical profession needs to take the lead in developing guidelines for good care of dying patients. Identifying the factors related to physicians, patients, and the health care system that pose barriers to appropriate care at the end of life should be the first step in a national dialogue to educate health care professionals and the public on the topic of death and dying. Death is an issue that society as a whole faces, and it requires a compassionate response. But we should not confuse compassion with competence in the care of terminally ill patients.

References

1. Reinhardt, Compassion in Dying v. State of Washington, 79 F. 3d 790 9th Cir. 1996.

2. Miner, Quill v. Vacco 80 F. 3d 716 2nd Cir. 1996.

3. Doyle D, Hanks GWC, MacDonald N. The Oxford textbook of palliative medicine. New York: Oxford University Press, 1993.

4. Orentlicher D. The legalization of physician-assisted suicide. N Engl J Med 1996;335:663–7.

5. Wilson WC, Smedira NG, Fink C, McDowell JA, Luce JM. Ordering and administration of sedatives and analgesics during the withholding and withdrawal of life support from critically ill patients. JAMA 1992;267:949–53.

6. Foley KM. The relationship of pain and symptom management to patient requests for physician-assisted suicide. J Pain Symptom Manage 1991;6:289–97.

7. Cherny NI, Coyle N, Foley KM. Guidelines in the care of the dying patient. Hematol Oncol Clin North Am 1996;10:261–86.

8. Cherny NI, Portenoy RK. Sedation in the management of refractory symptoms: guidelines for evaluation and treatment. J Palliat Care 1994;10(2): 31–8.

9. Cancer pain relief and palliative care. Geneva: World Health Organization, 1989.

10. Back AL, Wallace JI, Starks HE, Pearlman RA. Physician-assisted suicide and euthanasia in Washington State: patient requests and physician responses. JAMA 1996;275:919–25.

11. Emanuel EJ, Fairclough DL, Daniels ER, Clarridge BR. Euthanasia and physician-assisted suicide: attitudes and experiences of oncology patients, oncologists, and the public. Lancet 1996;347:1805–10.

12. Lee MA, Nelson HD, Tilden VP, Ganzini L, Schmidt TA, Tolle SW. Legalizing assisted suicide—views of physicians in Oregon. N Engl J Med 1996;334: 310–5.

13. Ganzini L, Fenn DS, Lee MA, Heintz RT, Bloom JD. Attitudes of Oregon psychiatrists toward physician-assisted suicide. Am J Psychiatry 1996; 153:1469–75.

14. Cohen JS, Fihn SD, Boyko EJ, Jonsen AR, Wood RW. Attitudes toward assisted suicide and euthanasia among physicians in Washington State. N Engl J Med 1994;331:89–94.

15. Doukas DJ, Waterhouse D, Gorenflo DW, Seid J. Attitudes and behaviors on physician-assisted death: a study of Michigan oncologists. J Clin Oncol 1995;13:1055–61.

16. Morrison S, Meier D. Physician-assisted dying: fashioning public policy with an absence of data. Generations. Winter 1994:48–53.

17. Portenoy RK, Coyle N, Kash K, et al. Determinants of the willingness to endorse assisted suicide: a survey of physicians, nurses, and social workers. Psychosomatics (in press).

18. Fins J. Physician-assisted suicide and the right to care. Cancer Control 1996; 3:272–8.

19. Callahan D, White M. The legalization of physician-assisted suicide: creating a regulatory Potemkin Village. U Richmond Law Rev 1996;30:1–83.

20. Quill TE. Death and dignity—a case of individualized decision making. N Engl J Med 1991;324:691–4.

21. Quill TE, Cassel CK, Meier DE. Care of the hopelessly ill—proposed clinical criteria for physician-assisted suicide. N Engl J Med 1992;327:1380–4.

22. Conwell Y, Caine ED. Rational suicide and the right to die—reality and myth. N Engl J Med 1991;325:1100–3.

23. Foley KM. Pain, physician assisted suicide and euthanasia. Pain Forum 1995;4:163–78.

24. When death is sought: assisted suicide and euthanasia in the medical context. New York: New York State Task Force on Life and the Law, May 1994.

25. Brown JH, Henteleff P, Barakat S, Rowe CJ. Is it normal for terminally ill patients to desire death? Am J Psychiatry 1986;143:208–11.

26. Chochinov HM, Wilson KG, Enns M, et al. Desire for death in the terminally ill. Am J Psychiatry 1995;152:1185–91.

27. Breitbart W, Rosenfeld BD, Passik SD. Interest in physician-assisted suicide among ambulatory HIV-infected patients. Am J Psychiatry 1996;153:238–42.

28. Hill TP. Treating the dying patient: the challenge for medical education. Arch Intern Med 1995;155:1265–9.

29. Callahan D. Once again reality: now where do we go? Hastings Cent Rep 1995;25(6):Suppl:S33–S36.

30. Solomon MZ, O'Donnell L, Jennings B, et al. Decisions near the end of life: professional views on life-sustaining treatments. Am J Public Health 1993;83:14–23.

31. Cherny NI, Coyle N, Foley KM. Suffering in the advanced cancer patient: definition and taxonomy. J Palliat Care 1994;10(2):57–70.

32. Cassel EJ. The nature of suffering and the goals of medicine. N Engl J Med 1982;306:639–45.

33. Cleeland CS, Gonin R, Hatfield AK, et al. Pain and its treatment in outpatients with metastatic cancer. N Engl J Med 1994;330:592–6.

34. Breitbart W, Rosenfeld BD, Passik SD, McDonald MV, Thaler H, Portenoy RK. The undertreatment of pain in ambulatory AIDS patients. Pain 1996; 65:243–9.

35. The SUPPORT Principal Investigators. A controlled trial to improve care for seriously ill hospitalized patients. JAMA 1995;274:1591–8.

36. Seale C, Cartwright A. The year before death. Hants, England: Avebury, 1994.

37. Von Roenn JH, Cleeland CS, Gonin R, Hatfield AK, Pandya KJ. Physician attitudes and practice in cancer pain management: a survey from the Eastern Cooperative Oncology Group. Ann Intern Med 1993;119:121–6.

38. Portenoy RK. Pain and quality of life: clinical issues and implications for research. Oncology 1990;4:172–8.

39. Breitbart W. Suicide risk and pain in cancer and AIDS patients. In: Chapman CR, Foley KM, eds. Current and emerging issues in cancer pain. New York: Raven Press, 1993.

40. Chochinov H, Wilson KG, Enns M, Lander S. Prevalence of depression in the terminally ill: effects of diagnostic criteria and symptom threshold judgments. Am J Psychiatry 1994;151:537–40.

41. Passik S, McDonald M, Rosenfeld B, Breitbart W. End of life issues in patients with AIDS: clinical and research considerations. J Pharm Care Pain Symptom Control 1995;3:91–111.

42. NT "success" in easing rural fear of euthanasia. The Age. August 31, 1996:A7.

POSTSCRIPT

Should Physicians Be Allowed to Assist in Patient Suicide?

In 1997 Oregon became the only state to implement a law legalizing physician-assisted suicide. The Death with Dignity Act was originally passed in 1994, but its implementation was delayed until 1997, when it was upheld by a large majority of voters. Under this law, a person who is mentally competent and suffering from a terminal illness (likely to die within 6 months) may receive lethal drugs from a physician. The person has to consult two doctors and wait 15 days before obtaining the drugs.

In 2001 Attorney General John Ashcroft issued a U.S. Justice Department rule that declared that, under the federal Controlled Substance Act (CSA), dispensing or prescribing controlled substances is not a legitimate medical practice and is illegal. This rule was intended to make the Oregon law unworkable. A challenge to the rule went to the U.S. Supreme Court. In the case of *Gonzalez v. Oregon,* the Court ruled in February 2006 that the CSA does not allow the attorney general to override state law in prescribing controlled drugs. The Court said, "The structure of the CSA, then, conveys unwillingness to cede medical judgments to an Executive official who lacks medical expertise." In "Physician-Assisted Suicide: A Legitimate Medical Practice?" law professor Lawrence O. Gostin analyzes the Court's ruling and its implications (*Journal of the American Medical Association,* April 26, 2006).

Very few patients in Oregon actually use the option of requesting physician-assisted suicide. The number has remained relatively stable since 2002. In 2005, for example, 38 Oregon residents died after taking medications prescribed under the Death with Dignity Act, including six who had received medications in 2004. In 2005, 39 physicians wrote a total of 64 prescriptions for lethal doses of medications. In that year there were an estimated 12 deaths under the Death with Dignity Act for every 10,000 deaths from other causes. Those most likely to request drugs were divorced, never married, more highly educated, and had amyotrophic lateral sclerosis (Lou Gehrig's disease), HIV/AIDS, or cancer. Physicians reported that patient requests stemmed from concerns related to loss of autonomy, decreasing ability to participate in enjoyable activities, and loss of dignity, not to mention unbearable pain. The full report from the Oregon Department of Human Services is available at http://oregon.gov/DHS/ph/pas/docs/year8.pdf.

Researchers led by Susan Tolle in Oregon found that, regardless of legalization, many more people consider physician-assisted suicide than follow through with it. The complexity of the process to obtain a lethal drug—a safeguard against misuse—also may be a barrier to those who do not fulfill their intentions (Susan W. Tolle, et. al., "Characteristics and Proportion of Dying

Oregonians Who Personally Consider Physician-Assisted Suicide," *Journal of Clinical Ethics*, Summer 2004).

In the Netherlands, euthanasia—defined as "the intentional termination of the life of a patient at his or her request by a physician"—was legalized in 2002. The practice had occurred before then without repercussions for the physician. About 9,700 requests are made each year. Those who oppose the practice claim that not all requests are voluntary.

Physician-Assisted Dying: The Case for Palliative Care and Patient Choice, edited by Timothy E. Quill and Margaret P. Battin, is a collection of articles that present the case for the legalization of physician-assisted dying (Johns Hopkins University Press, 2004). Opposing the practice are the authors in *The Case Against Assisted Suicide,* edited by Kathleen E. Foley and Herbert Hendin (Johns Hopkins University Press, 2002). See also Arthur L. Caplan, Lois Snyder, and Kathy Feber-Langendoen, "The Role of Guidelines in the Practice of Physician-Assisted Suicide," *Annals of Internal Medicine* (March 21, 2000). The entire issue is devoted to this subject.

ISSUE 7

Should Doctors Be Able to Refuse Demands for "Futile" Treatment?

YES: Steven H. Miles, from "Informed Demand for 'Non-Beneficial' Medical Treatment," *The New England Journal of Medicine* (August 15, 1991)

NO: Felicia Ackerman, from "The Significance of a Wish," *Hastings Center Report* (July–August 1991)

ISSUE SUMMARY

YES: Physician Steven H. Miles maintains that physicians' duty to follow patients' wishes ends when the requests are inconsistent with what medical care can reasonably be expected to achieve, when they violate community standards of care, and when they consume an unfair share of collective resources.

NO: Philosopher Felicia Ackerman contends that it is ethically inappropriate for physicians to decide what kind of life is worth prolonging and that decisions involving personal values should be made by the patient or family.

In the typical controversy involving life-prolonging treatment, it is the patient or patient's family who wants to stop treatment and the doctor or hospital administrator who wants to continue it. That line of cases began, most prominently, with *In re Quinlan* (1976) and was decided again in *Cruzan v. Director of Missouri Department of Health* (1990). Another scenario, however, is emerging. What happens when the patient or family demands that treatment be continued past the point that doctors or hospital administrators feel it is warranted? Families may hope for a miracle and want "everything possible" done to preserve life. In the case of "Baby L," described by John Paris, Robert K. Crone, and Frank Reardon in *The New England Journal of Medicine* (April 5, 1990), pediatricians refused a mother's request to start ventilator treatment for a severely compromised, blind, deaf, and neurologically impaired child who had spent all 28 months of her life in intensive care.

In other cases, patients or families may act out of religious convictions that life is a God-given gift that must be preserved at all costs. In her book

Ethics on Call (Crown Publishers, 1992), Nancy Dubler describes the case of "Joseph," a devoutly religious man who interpreted Jewish law to mean that life can be taken only by God, and that he must take whatever measures are available to sustain his life, no matter what suffering was entailed. There may even be cases in which a criminal prosecution may hinge on whether a patient dies or not, or there may be financial motivations to preserving life.

These cases stretch the limits of patient autonomy and come to a full stop when they reach the boundaries of professional responsibility. Just as patients are moral agents, so too are physicians. Their professional ethic begins with the Hippocratic injunction "First, do no harm." Beyond avoiding harm, they are guided by the obligation to do good—to provide benefit to patients within the limits of their expertise. Since ancient times physicians have felt it is their prerogative to determine whether or not treatment is justified. The writings of Hippocrates and Plato warn physicians to acknowledge when their art is doomed to fail.

In modern times the Vatican's 1980 *Declaration on Euthanasia* places a strong emphasis on physician judgment, pointing out that "[doctors] may . . . judge that the investment in instruments and personnel is disproportionate to the results foreseen; they may also judge that the techniques applied impose on the patient strain or suffering out of proportion with the benefits." The U.S. President's Commission for the Study of Bioethical Problems in Medicine concluded in 1983 that "health care professionals or institutions may decline to provide a particular option because that choice may violate their conscience or professional judgement, though, in doing so they may not abandon a patient." Even more recently (December 1990), the Society of Critical Care Medicine declared that "treatments that offer no benefit and serve to prolong the dying process should not be employed."

As frequently happens in bioethics, one case—not necessarily the first to arise—serves to focus the arguments. In the area of demands for "nonbeneficial" treatment, that case involved the treatment of Helga Wanglie, an elderly Minnesota woman who suffered a series of medical problems, culminating in a year and a half spent unconscious on a respirator in a persistent vegetative state. Her physicians asked her husband to consent to withdrawing treatment; his refusal set off a chain of events described in the following selections.

Steven H. Miles, a gerontologist and ethics consultant to Mrs. Wanglie's physicians, argues that Mrs. Wanglie was "overmastered" by her disease and that continued intensive care was inappropriate and inconsistent with reasonable medical expectations of benefit. Felicia Ackerman maintains that decisions about what lives are worth living properly fall to those who share the values of the patient—in this case, the family.

YES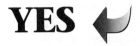

Steven H. Miles

Informed Demand for "Non-Beneficial" Medical Treatment

An 85-year-old woman was taken from a nursing home to Hennepin County Medical Center on January 1, 1990, for emergency treatment of dyspnea [shortness of breath] from chronic bronchiectasis [widening of the air passages]. The patient, Mrs. Helga Wanglie, required emergency intubation [insertion of a tube] and was placed on a respirator. She occasionally acknowledged discomfort and recognized her family but could not communicate clearly. In May, after attempts to wean her from the respirator failed, she was discharged to a chronic care hospital. One week later, her heart stopped during a weaning attempt; she was resuscitated and taken to another hospital for intensive care. She remained unconscious, and a physician suggested that it would be appropriate to consider withdrawing life support. In response, the family transferred her back to the medical center on May 31. Two weeks later, physicians concluded that she was in a persistent vegetative state. . . . She was maintained on a respirator, with repeated courses of antibiotics, frequent airway suctioning, tube feedings, an air flotation bed, and biochemical monitoring.

In June and July of 1990, physicians suggested that life-sustaining treatment be withdrawn since it was not benefiting the patient. Her husband, daughter, and son insisted on continued treatment. They stated their view that physicians should not play God, that the patient would not be better off dead, that removing life support showed moral decay in our civilization, and that a miracle could occur. Her husband told a physician that his wife had never stated her preferences concerning life-sustaining treatment. He believed that the cardiac arrest would not have occurred if she had not been transferred from Hennepin County Medical Center in May. The family reluctantly accepted a do-not-resuscitate order based on the improbability of Mrs. Wanglie's surviving a cardiac arrest. In June, an ethics committee consultant recommended continued counseling for the family. The family declined counseling, including the counsel of their own pastor, and in late July asked that the respirator not be discussed again. In August, nurses expressed their consensus that continued life support did not seem appropriate, and I, as the newly appointed ethics consultant, counseled them.

In October 1990, a new attending physician consulted with specialists and confirmed the permanence of the patient's cerebral and pulmonary

From *New England Journal of Medicine*, August 15, 1991, pp. 512–515. Copyright © 1991 by Massachusetts Medical Society. Reprinted by permission.

conditions. He concluded that she was at the end of her life and that the respirator was "non-beneficial," in that it could not heal her lungs, palliate her suffering, or enable this unconscious and permanently respirator-dependent woman to experience the benefit of the life afforded by respirator support. Because the respirator could prolong life, it was not characterized as "futile."[1] In November, the physician, with my concurrence, told the family that he was not willing to continue to prescribe the respirator. The husband, an attorney, rejected proposals to transfer the patient to another facility or to seek a court order mandating this unusual treatment. The hospital told the family that it would ask a court to decide whether members of its staff were obliged to continue treatment. A second conference two weeks later, after the family had hired an attorney, confirmed these positions, and the husband asserted that the patient had consistently said she wanted respirator support for such a condition.

In December, the medical director and hospital administrator asked the Hennepin County Board of Commissioners (the medical center's board of directors) to allow the hospital to go to court to resolve the dispute. In January, the county board gave permission by a 4-to-3 vote. Neither the hospital nor the county had a financial interest in terminating treatment. Medicare largely financed the $200,000 for the first hospitalization at Hennepin County; a private insurer would pay the $500,000 bill for the second. From February through May of 1991, the family and its attorney unsuccessfully searched for another health care facility that would admit Mrs. Wanglie. Facilities with empty beds cited her poor potential for rehabilitation.

The hospital chose a two-step legal procedure, first asking for the appointment of an independent conservator to decide whether the respirator was beneficial to the patient and second, if the conservator found it not, for a second hearing on whether it was obliged to provide the respirator. The husband crossfiled, requesting to be appointed conservator. After a hearing in late May, the trial court on July 1, 1991, appointed the husband, as best able to represent the patient's interests. It noted that no request to stop treatment had been made and declined to speculate on the legality of such an order.[2] The hospital said that it would continue to provide the respirator in the light of continuing uncertainty about its legal obligation to provide it. . . .

Discussion

This sad story illustrates the problem of what to do when a family demands medical treatment that the attending physician concludes cannot benefit the patient. Only 600 elderly people are treated with respirators for more than six months in the United States each year.[3] Presumably, most of these people are actually or potentially conscious. It is common practice to discontinue the use of a respirator before death when it can no longer benefit a patient.[4,5]

We do not know Mrs. Wanglie's treatment preferences. A large majority of elderly people prefer not to receive prolonged respirator support for irreversible unconsciousness.[6] Studies show that an older person's designated family proxy overestimates that person's preference for life-sustaining treatment in a hypothetical coma.[7-9] The implications of this research for clinical decision making have not been cogently analyzed.

A patient's request for a treatment does not necessarily oblige a provider or the health care system. Patients may not demand that physicians injure them (for example, by mutilation), or provide plausible but inappropriate therapies (for example, amphetamines for weight reduction), or therapies that have no value (such as laetrile for cancer). Physicians are not obliged to violate their personal moral views on medical care so long as patients' rights are served. Minnesota's Living Will law says that physicians are "legally bound to act consistently within my wishes within limits of reasonable medical practice" in acting on requests and refusals of treatment.[10] Minnesota's Bill of Patients' Rights says that patients "have the right to appropriate medical . . . care based on individual needs . . . [which is] limited where the service is not reimbursable."[11] Mrs. Wanglie also had aortic insufficiency. Had this condition worsened, a surgeon's refusal to perform a life-prolonging valve replacement as medically inappropriate would hardly occasion public controversy. As the Minneapolis *Star Tribune* said in an editorial on the eve of the trial,

> The hospital's plea is born of realism, not hubris. . . . It advances the claim that physicians should not be slaves to technology—any more than patients should be its prisoners. They should be free to deliver, and act on, an honest and time-honored message: "Sorry, there's nothing more we can do."[12]

Disputes between physicians and patients about treatment plans are often handled by transferring patients to the care of other providers. In this case, every provider contacted by the hospital or the family refused to treat this patient with a respirator. These refusals occurred before and after this case became a matter of public controversy and despite the availability of third-party reimbursement. We believe they represent a medical consensus that respirator support is inappropriate in such a case.

The handling of this case is compatible with current practices regarding informed consent, respect for patients' autonomy, and the right to health care. Doctors should inform patients of all medically reasonable treatments, even those available from other providers. Patients can refuse any prescribed treatment or choose among any medical alternatives that physicians are willing to prescribe. Respect for autonomy does not empower patients to oblige physicians to prescribe treatments in ways that are fruitless or inappropriate. Previous "right to die" cases address the different situations of a patient's right to choose to be free of a prescribed therapy. This case is more about the nature of the patient's choice in using that entitlement.

The proposal that this family's preference for this unusual and costly treatment, which is commonly regarded as inappropriate, establishes a right to such treatment is ironic, given that preference does not create a right to other needed, efficacious, and widely desired treatments in the United States. We could not afford a universal health care system based on patients' demands. Such a system would irrationally allocate health care to socially powerful people with strong preferences for immediate treatment to the disadvantage of those with less power or less immediate needs.

After the conclusion was reached that the respirator was not benefiting the patient, the decision to seek a review of the duty to provide it was based on an ethic of "stewardship." Even though the insurer played no part in this case, physicians' discretion to prescribe requires responsible handling of requests for inappropriate treatment. Physicians exercise this stewardship by counseling against or denying such treatment or by submitting such requests to external review. This stewardship is not aimed at protecting the assets of insurance companies but rests on fairness to people who have pooled their resources to insure their collective access to appropriate health care. Several citizens complained to Hennepin County Medical Center that Mrs. Wanglie was receiving expensive treatment paid for by people who had not consented to underwrite a level of medical care whose appropriateness was defined by family demands.

Procedures for addressing this kind of dispute are at an early stage of development. Though the American Medical Association[13] and the Society of Critical Care Medicine[14] also support some decisions to withhold requested treatment, the medical center's reasoning most closely follows the guidelines of the American Thoracic Society.[15] The statements of these professional organizations do not clarify when or how a physician may legally withdraw or withhold demanded life-sustaining treatments. The request for a conservator to review the medical conclusion before considering the medical obligation was often misconstrued as implying that the husband was incompetent or ill motivated. The medical center intended to emphasize the desirability of an independent review of its medical conclusion before its obligation to provide the respirator was reviewed by the court. I believe that the grieving husband was simply mistaken about whether the respirator was benefiting his wife. A direct request to remove the respirator seems to center procedural oversight on the soundness of the medical decision making rather than on the nature of the patient's need. Clearly, the gravity of these decisions merits openness, due process, and meticulous accountability. The relative merits of various procedures need further study.

Ultimately, procedures for addressing requests for futile, marginally effective, or inappropriate therapies require a statutory framework, case law, professional standards, a social consensus, and the exercise of professional responsibility. Appropriate ends for medicine are defined by public and professional consensus. Laws can, and do, say that patients may choose only among medically appropriate options, but legislatures are ill suited to define medical appropriateness. Similarly, health-facility policies on this issue will be difficult to design and will focus on due process rather than on specific clinical situations. Public or private payers will ration according to cost and overall efficacy, a rationing that will become more onerous as therapies are misapplied in individual cases. I believe there is a social consensus that intensive care for a person as "overmastered" by disease as this woman was is inappropriate.

Each case must be evaluated individually. In this case, the husband's request seemed entirely inconsistent with what medical care could do for his wife, the standards of the community, and his fair share of resources that many people pooled for their collective medical care. This case is about limits to what can be achieved at the end of life.

References

1. Tomlinson T, Brody H. Futility and the ethics of resuscitation. JAMA 1990; 264:1276–80.

2. In re Helga Wanglie, Fourth Judicial District (Dist. Ct., Probate Ct. Div.) PX-91-283. Minnesota, Hennepin County.

3. Office of Technology Assessment Task Force. Life-sustaining technologies and the elderly. Washington, D.C.: Government Printing Office, 1987.

4. Smedira NG, Evans BH, Grais LS, et al. Withholding and withdrawal of life support from the critically ill. N Engl J Med 1990; 322:309–15.

5. Lantos JD, Singer PA, Walker RM, et al. The illusion of futility in clinical practice. Am J Med 1989; 87:81–4.

6. Emanuel LL, Barry MJ, Stoeckle JD, Ettelson LM, Emanuel EJ. Advance directives for medical care—a case for greater use. N Engl J Med 1991; 324:889–95.

7. Zweibel NR, Cassel CK. Treatment choices at the end of life: a comparison of decisions by older patients and their physician-selected proxies. Gerontologist 1989; 29:615–21.

8. Tomlinson T, Howe K, Notman M, Rossmiller D. An empirical study of proxy consent for elderly persons. Gerontologist 1990; 30:54–64.

9. Danis M, Southerland LI, Garrett JM, et al. A prospective study of advance directives for life-sustaining care. N Engl J Med 1991; 324:882–8.

10. Minnesota Statutes. Adult Health Care Decisions Act. 145b.04.

11. Minnesota Statutes. Patients and residents of health care facilities: Bill of rights. 144.651:Subd.6.

12. Helga Wanglie's life. Minneapolis Star Tribune. May 26, 1991:18A.

13. Council on Ethical and Judicial Affairs. American Medical Association. Guidelines for the appropriate use of do-not-resuscitate orders. JAMA 1991; 265: 1868–71.

14. Task Force on Ethics of the Society of Critical Care Medicine. Consensus report on the ethics of foregoing life-sustaining treatments in the critically ill. Crit Care Med 1990; 18:1435–9.

15. American Thoracic Society. Withholding and withdrawing life-sustaining therapy. Am Rev Respir Dis (in press).

Felicia Ackerman

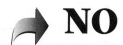

NO

The Significance of a Wish

The case of Helga Wanglie should be seen in the general context of conflicts that can arise over whether a patient should be maintained on life-support systems. Well-publicized conflicts of this sort usually involve an institution seeking to prolong the life of a patient diagnosed as terminally ill and/or permanently comatose, versus a family that claims, with varying degrees of substantiation, that the patient would not have wanted to be kept alive under these circumstances. But other sorts of conflicts about prolonging life also occur. Patients who have indicated a desire to stay alive may face opposition from family or medical staff who think these patients' lives are not worth prolonging. Such cases can go badly for patients, who may have difficulty getting their preferences even believed, let alone respected.[1]

Helga Wanglie's case is not as clear cut. But in view of the fact that keeping her on a respirator will prolong her life, that there is more reason to believe she would have wanted this than to believe she would not have wanted it, that medical diagnoses of irreversible unconsciousness are not infallible, and that her private health insurance plan has not objected to paying for her respirator support and in fact has publicly taken the position that cost should not be a factor in treatment decisions, I believe HCMC [Hennepin County Medical Center] should continue to maintain Mrs. Wanglie on a respirator. This respirator support is medically and economically feasible, and it serves a recognized medical goal—that of prolonging life and allowing a chance at a possible, albeit highly unlikely, return to consciousness.

The Significance of Medical Expertise

Dr. Steven Miles, ethics consultant at HCMC, has argued that continued respirator support is "medically inappropriate" for Mrs. Wanglie. The argument is based on a criterion of medical appropriateness that allows doctors to prescribe respirators for any of three purposes: to allow healing, to alleviate suffering, and to enable otherwise disabled persons to continue to enjoy life. Since keeping Mrs. Wanglie on a respirator serves none of these ends, it is argued, such treatment is medically inappropriate.

But just what does "medically inappropriate" mean here? A clear case of medical inappropriateness would be an attempt to cure cancer with laetrile, since medicine has presumably shown that laetrile cannot cure cancer.

From *Hastings Center Report,* vol. 21, no. 4, July August 1991. Copyright © 1991 by Hastings Center Report. Reprinted by permission.

Moreover, since laetrile's clinical ineffectiveness is a technical medical fact about which doctors are supposed to have professional expertise, it is professionally appropriate for doctors to refuse to grant a patient's request to have laetrile prescribed for cancer. But HCMC's disagreement with Mrs. Wanglie's family is not a technical dispute about a matter where doctors can be presumed to have greater expertise than laymen. The parties to the dispute do not disagree about whether maintaining Mrs. Wanglie on a respirator is likely to prolong her life; they disagree about whether her life is worth prolonging. This is not a medical question, but a question of values. Hence the term "medically inappropriate," with its implication of the relevance of technical medical expertise, is itself inappropriate in this context. It is as presumptuous and *ethically* inappropriate for doctors to suppose that their professional expertise qualifies them to know what kind of life is worth prolonging as it would be for meteorologists to suppose their professional expertise qualifies them to know what kind of destination is worth a long drive in the rain.

It has also been argued that continued respirator support does not serve Mrs. Wanglie's interests since a permanently unconscious person cannot "enjoy any realization of the quality of life."[2] Yet were this approach to be applied consistently, it would undermine the idea frequently advanced in other life-support cases that it is in the interests of the irreversibly comatose to be "allowed" to die "with dignity." Such people are not suffering or even conscious, so how can death benefit them or serve their interests? The obvious reply in both cases is that there is a sense in which it is in a permanently comatose person's interests to have his or her previous wishes and values respected. And there is some evidence that Mrs. Wanglie would want to be kept alive.

But why suppose doctors are any more obliged to serve this want than they would be to help gratify some nonmedical desire such as a desire to be remembered in a certain way? An obvious answer is that prolonging life is a medical function, as is allowing a possible return to consciousness. Medical diagnoses of irreversible coma are not infallible, as the recent case of Carrie Coons clearly demonstrates. The court order to remove her feeding tube, requested by her family, was rescinded after Mrs. Coons regained consciousness following five and a half months in what was diagnosed as an irreversible vegetative state.[3] Such cases cast additional light on the claim that respirator support is medically inappropriate and not in Mrs. Wanglie's interests. When the alternative is death, the question of whether going for a long-shot chance of recovering consciousness is worth it is quite obviously a question of values, rather than a technical medical question doctors are especially professionally qualified to decide.

The Significance of Quality of Life

Medical ethicists who take into account the possibility that seemingly irreversibly comatose patients might regain consciousness have offered further general arguments against maintaining such patients on life-support systems. One such argument relies on the fact that "the few patients who have recovered consciousness after a prolonged period of unconsciousness were severely disabled,"[4] with disabilities including blindness, inability to speak, permanent distortion of limbs, and paralysis. Since many blind, mute, and/or paralyzed people seem to find their lives well worth living, however, the assumption that disability is a fate worse than death seems highly questionable. Moreover, when the patient's views on the matter are unknown, maintaining him on a respirator to give him a chance to regain consciousness and then decide whether to continue his disabled existence seems preferable to denying him even the possibility of a choice by deciding in advance that he would be better off dead. Keeping alive someone who would want to die and "allowing" to die someone who would want a chance of regained consciousness are not parallel wrongs. While both obviously go against the patient's values, only the latter has the additional flaw of doing this in a way that could actually affect his conscious experience.

The other argument asserts that since long-term treatment imposes emotional and often financial burdens on the comatose patient's family and most patients, before losing consciousness, place a high value on their families' welfare, presumably these patients would rather die than be a burden to their loved ones.[5] Though very popular nowadays, this latter sort of argument is cruel because it attributes extreme self-abnegation to those unable to speak for themselves. It is also biased because it assumes great sacrificial love on the part of the patient, but not the family. Why not argue instead that a loving family will not want to deny a beloved member a last chance at regained consciousness and hence that it is *not* in the interest of the patient's loved ones to withdraw life supports? Mrs. Wanglie's family clearly wants her kept alive.[6]

The Significance of a Gesture

Mrs. Wanglie's family claims that she would want to be kept alive. Yet Dr. Cranford suggests that her family at first denied having previously discussed the matter with her, and that it was only after the HCMC committed itself to going to court that the family claimed Mrs. Wanglie had said she would want to be kept alive. Dr. Miles mentions that during the months when she was on a respirator before becoming unconscious, Mrs. Wanglie at times pulled at her respirator tubing.

I agree that Mrs. Wanglie's views are less than certain. Yet for reasons given above and also because death is irrevocable, there should be a presumption in favor of life when a patient's views are unclear or unknown. Pulling at a respirator tube is obviously insufficient evidence of even a fleeting desire to die; it may simply be a semi-automatic attempt to relieve discomfort, like pulling away in a dentist's chair even when one has an overriding desire that the dental work be performed. Basically, although the circumstances of the family's claim about Mrs. Wanglie's statement of her views make the claim questionable, it is their word against nobody's. No one claims that she ever said she would prefer *not* to be kept alive, despite her months of conscious existence on a respirator.

It has also been argued that we should not allow patients to demand medically inappropriate care when the costs of that care are borne by others who have not consented to do so. I have already discussed the question of medical appropriateness. And a private health plan is paying for Mrs. Wanglie's care, a plan whose officials have publicly stated that cost should not be a factor in treatment decisions. The pool of subscribers to the plan, whose premiums are what indirectly subsidize Mrs. Wanglie's care, have, by being members of this plan, committed themselves to a practice of medicine that does not take cost into account. It would be unfair to make cost a factor in Mrs. Wanglie's treatment decision now. Public statements by health insurance plan officials are expected to be taken into account by consumers selecting health insurance and must not be reneged upon. Mrs. Wanglie's insurer is not seeking to renege. Instead, it is her *doctors* who have decided that her life is not worth prolonging.

Moreover, to say it would be the underlying disease rather than the act of removing the respirator that would cause Helga Wanglie's death is not helpful. If Mrs. Wanglie is, as the HCMC staff claims, irreversibly respirator-dependent, then saying that removing the respirator would cause her death is just as logical as saying that withdrawing a rope from a drowning man would cause his death, even if his death is to be "attributed" to his drowning. If the person in either case has an interest in living, one violates his interest by withdrawing the necessary means. This is what HCMC is seeking court permission to do to Mrs. Wanglie.

References

1. For example, consider the case of seventy-eight-year-old Earl Spring, whose mental deterioration did not prevent him from saying that he did not want to die. The statement of this preference was not considered conclusive reason to keep him on dialysis over his family's objections. Similarly, the *New York Times Magazine* recently described the situation of a severely disabled, elderly woman whose explicit advance directive that she wanted everything possible done to keep her alive was apparently ignored by both her husband and the hospital's ethics committee (K. Bouton, "Painful Decisions: The Role of the Medical Ethicist," 5 August 1990).

2. This argument comes from an unpublished letter from Dr. Steven Miles, made available to me by the *Hastings Center Report* at his request.

3. The Coons case was widely reported in newspapers. For example, see C. DeMare, "'Hopeless' Hospital Patient, 86, Comes Out of Coma," *Albany Times Union*, 12 April 1989. Additional cases of this sort are cited in President's Commission for the Study of Ethical Problems in Medicine and Biomedical and Behavioral Research, *Deciding to Forego Life-Sustaining Treatment* (Washington, D.C.: U.S. Government Printing Office, 1983).

4. President's Commission, *Deciding to Forego Life-Sustaining Treatment*, p. 182.

5. President's Commission, *Deciding to Forego Life-Sustaining Treatment*, p. 183.

6. I have given this sort of argument in a letter to the *New York Times*, 4 November 1987, as well as in a short story about terminal illness, "The Forecasting Game," in *Prize Stories 1990: The O. Henry Awards*, ed. W. Abrahams (New York: Doubleday, 1990), pp. 315–35, and in an op-ed "No Thanks, I Don't Want to Die with Dignity," *Providence Journal-Bulletin*, 19 April 1990 (reprinted in other newspapers under various different titles).

POSTSCRIPT

Should Doctors Be Able to Refuse Demands for "Futile" Treatment?

T hree days after the Minnesota court named Oliver Wanglie as his wife's legal conservator, thus preserving his right to make decisions about her treatment, Helga Wanglie died of multisystem organ failure. Her aggressive treatment had been continued throughout.

A series of cases involving infants has extended the debate on medical futility. The most publicized case is that of "Baby K," who was born in 1992 with most of her brain missing. In most cases of this condition (anencephaly), babies die within a few days. Baby K's mother, however, insisted that Fairfax Hospital in Falls Church, Virginia, provide ventilator support to help the baby breathe, which kept her alive in a nursing home. In February 1994 the hospital's request to stop this treatment was denied by a federal appeals court. Despite continued treatment, Baby K died in April 1995 at the age of three.

Lawrence J. Schneiderman and Alexander Morgan Capron ask "How Can Hospital Futility Practices Contribute to Establishing Standards of Practice?" *Cambridge Quarterly of Healthcare Ethics* (vol. 9, 2000) and conclude that hospitals are likely to find courts willing to defer to well-defined and procedurally scrupulous processes for internal resolutions of futility disputes. In 1999, Texas became the first state to adopt a law providing a process for resolving medical futility disputes without court involvement. The law was updated in 2003. In "Resolution of Futility by Due Process: Early Experience with the Texas Advance Directives Act," Robert L. Fine and Thomas Wm. Mayo conclude that the law is a first step toward practical resolution of this controversial area (*Annals of Internal Medicine*, May 6, 2003).

In describing their hospital's medical futility policy, Robert D. Truog and Christine Mitchell, from Boston Children's Hospital, express concern that the Texas law takes power away from patients and families and endorses unilateral decision making by medical professionals ("Futility: From Hospital Policies to State Laws," *American Journal of Bioethics,* September–October, 2006). In 2006 two of the few challenges to the Texas law so far received wide publicity. Andrea Clark, a 54-year-old woman with congenital heart disease, suffered serious complications after surgery at St. Luke's Episcopal Hospital in Houston. She and her family wanted treatment continued even though doctors and the hospital's ethics committee determined that it would be futile under the law. The hospital withdrew its objections to treatment but Ms. Clark died soon anyway. In the second case, also at St. Luke's, the mother of Sun Hudson, a 6-month-old infant born with a rare and fatal form of dwarfism, wanted treatment continued. In this case the treatment was discontinued, and the infant died.

In *Medical Futility and the Evaluation of Life-Sustaining Interventions* (Cambridge University Press, 1997), Marjorie and Howard Zucker present a collection of multidisciplinary views. Also see D. L. Kasman, "When Is Medical Treatment Futile?" *Journal of General Internal Medicine* (October 2004); and M. Wreen, "Medical Futility and Physician Discretion," *Journal of Medical Ethics* (June 2004), which argues that physicians should not make decisions about nontreatment on their own. See also the American Medical Association's position in its Code of Ethics on medical futility in end-of-life care, which sets out procedural guidelines for fair decision making. It is available at: http://www.ama-assn.org/ama/pub/category/8390.html.

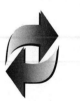

Internet References . . .

NARAL Online

This is the home page of the National Abortion and Reproductive Rights Action League (NARAL), an organization that works to promote reproductive freedom and dignity for women and their families.

http://www.naral.org

The Lindesmith Center—Drug Policy Foundation

This site offers articles concerning the issue of punishing pregnant drug users as well as articles about the case of *Cornelia Whitner v. State of South Carolina*. Search under "pregnant drug users" to access these articles.

http://www.lindesmith.org/news/

S.F.U. Students for Life

This organization run by students at Simon Fraser University in Vancouver, Canada, lists Web sites representing the diversity of pro-life views.

http://www.sfu.ca/~prolife/

Interlife

This site contains resources and information on abortion from a pro-life perspective.

http://www.interlife.org/

Choices in Reproduction

*F*ew bioethical issues could be of greater personal and social significance than questions concerning reproduction. Advances in medical technology, such as in vitro fertilization and egg donation have opened new possibilities for infertile couples, while challenging traditional notions of family. Some advances in genetic manipulation, such as cloning, are still in the experimental stage and raise complex ethical issues. Another type of technological advance, the ability to see images of the developing fetus, has enhanced our understanding of both normal growth and birth defects. This technology has provided evidence of the impact of the mother's behavior on fetal development. While many behaviors of pregnant women expose fetuses to risk, and while fathers' exposure to chemicals and other toxic substances also affect fetuses, attention has focused mainly on the mothers' use of illegal drugs. Preventing risk to fetuses raises troubling questions concerning the role of police and the courts in medical matters and the best way to assist drug-addicted women. The most polarized question remains the morality of abortion, where common ground is elusive. The issues in this section come to grips with some of the most perplexing and fundamental questions that confront medical practitioners, individual women and their partners, and society in general.

- Is Abortion Immoral?

- Should a Pregnant Woman Be Punished for Exposing Her Fetus to Risk?

ISSUE 8

Is Abortion Immoral?

YES: Patrick Lee and Robert P. George, from "The Wrong of Abortion," in Andrew Cohen and Christopher Heath Wellman, eds., *Contemporary Debates in Applied Ethics* (Blackwell, 2005)

NO: Margaret Olivia Little, from "The Morality of Abortion," in Bonnie Steinbock, John D. Arras, and Alex John London, eds., *Ethical Issues in Modern Medicine* (McGraw-Hill, 2003)

ISSUE SUMMARY

YES: Philosopher Patrick Lee and professor of jurisprudence Robert P. George assert that human embryos and fetuses are complete (though immature) human beings and that intentional abortion is unjust and objectively immoral.

NO: Philosopher Margaret Olivia Little believes that the moral status of the fetus is only one aspect of the morality of abortion. She points to gestation as an intimacy, motherhood as a relationship, and creation as a process to advance a more nuanced approach.

Abortion is the most divisive bioethical issue of our time. The issue has been a persistent one in history, but in the past 30 years or so the debate has polarized. One view—known as "pro-life"—sees abortion as the wanton slaughter of innocent life. The other view—"pro-choice"—considers abortion as an option that must be available to women if they are to control their own reproductive lives. According to the pro-life view, women who have access to "abortion on demand" put their own selfish whims ahead of an unborn child's right to life. According to the pro-choice view, women have the right to choose to have an abortion—especially if there is an overriding reason, such as preventing the birth of a child with a severe genetic defect or one conceived as a result of rape or incest.

Behind these strongly held convictions, as political scientist Mary Segers has pointed out, are widely differing views of what determines value (that is, whether value is inherent in a thing or ascribed to it by human beings), the relation between law and morality, and the use of limits of political solutions to social problems, as well as the value of scientific progress. Those who condemn abortion as immoral generally follow a classical tradition in which abortion is

124

a public matter because it involves our conception of how we should live together in an ideal society. Those who accept the idea of abortion, on the other hand, generally share the liberal, individualistic ethos of contemporary society. They believe that abortion is a private choice, and that public policy should reflect how citizens actually behave, not some unattainable ideal.

This is what we know about abortion practices in America today: Abortion has been legal since the 1973 Supreme Court decision of *Roe v. Wade* declared that a woman has a constitutional right to privacy, which includes an abortion. According to the National Center on Health Statistics, abortion at eight weeks or less gestation is seven times safer than childbirth, although there are some unknown risks—primarily the effect of repeated abortions on subsequent pregnancies. Abortion is common: In 2000 about 1.3 million abortions were performed. That is, one out of four pregnancies (and half of all unintended pregnancies) ended in abortion. According to the Alan Guttmacher Institute's 2000–2001 national survey, the overall abortion rate decreased by 11 percent between 1994 and 2000. Some of the reasons are the use of long-acting hormonal contraceptives, a lower pregnancy rate among teenagers, and growing use of emergency contraception (see Issue 20). Not all population groups showed equal decline, and abortion increased among some groups. Although the rates of teen pregnancy and abortion declined, the rate of decline was lower among black and Hispanic adolescents than among white adolescents. As a result women having abortions are increasingly those who are never-married, low-income, nonwhite and Hispanic, and have already had at least one child. The typical woman having an abortion is between the ages of 20 and 30, has never married, lives in a metropolitan area, and is Christian (42.8 percent Protestant, 27.4 percent Catholic, 7.6 percent "other," and 22.7 percent "none").

The following two selections offer thoughtful and reasoned but opposing views on abortion. Patrick Lee and Robert P. George conclude that being a mother generates a special responsibility and that the sacrifice morally required of the mother is less burdensome than the harm that would be done by expelling the child, causing his or her death, to escape that responsibility. They see abortion as objectively immoral. Margaret Olivia Little believes that if we acknowledge gestation as an intimacy, motherhood as a relationship, and creation as a process, we will be better able to appreciate the moral textures of abortion.

YES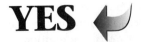

**Patrick Lee and
Robert P. George**

The Wrong of Abortion

Much of the public debate about abortion concerns the question whether deliberate feticide ought to be unlawful, at least in most circumstances. We will lay that question aside here in order to focus first on the question: is the choice to have, to perform, or to help procure an abortion morally wrong?

We shall argue that the choice of abortion is objectively immoral. By "objectively" we indicate that we are discussing the choice itself, not the (subjective) guilt or innocence of someone who carries out the choice: someone may act from an erroneous conscience, and if he is not at fault for his error, then he remains subjectively innocent, even if his choice is objectively wrongful.

The first important question to consider is: what is killed in an abortion? It is obvious that some living entity is killed in an abortion. And no one doubts that the moral status of the entity killed is a central (though not the only) question in the abortion debate. We shall approach the issue step by step, first setting forth some (though not all) of the evidence that demonstrates that what is killed in abortion—a human embryo—is indeed a human being, then examining the ethical significance of that point.

Human Embryos and Fetuses Are Complete (though Immature) Human Beings

It will be useful to begin by considering some of the facts of sexual reproduction. The standard embryology texts indicate that in the case of ordinary sexual reproduction the life of an individual human being begins with complete fertilization, which yields a genetically and functionally distinct organism, possessing the resources and active disposition for internally directed development toward human maturity.[1] In normal conception, a sex cell of the father, a sperm, unites with a sex cell of the mother, an ovum. Within the chromosomes of these sex cells are the DNA molecules which constitute the information that guides the development of the new individual brought into being when the sperm and ovum fuse. When fertilization occurs, the 23 chromosomes of the sperm unite with the 23 chromosomes of the ovum. At the end of this process there is produced an entirely new and distinct organism, originally a single cell. This organism, the human embryo, begins to grow by the normal process of cell division—it divides into 2 cells, then 4, 8, 16, and so on (the divisions are not simultaneous, so there is a 3-cell stage, and so on). This embryo gradually develops all of the organs and organ systems necessary for the full functioning of a mature human being. His or her development (sex is determined from the beginning) is very rapid in the first few weeks. For example, as early as eight or ten weeks of gestation, the fetus has a fully formed, beating heart, a complete brain (although not all of its synaptic connections are complete—nor will they be until sometime *after* the child is born), a recognizably human form, and the fetus feels pain, cries, and even sucks his or her thumb.

There are three important points we wish to make about this human embryo. First, it is from the start *distinct* from any cell of the mother or of the father. This is clear because it is growing in its own distinct direction. Its growth is internally directed to its own survival and maturation. Second, the embryo is *human:* it has the genetic makeup characteristic of human beings. Third, and most importantly, the embryo is a *complete* or *whole* organism, though immature. The human embryo, from conception onward, is fully programmed actively to develop himself or herself to the mature stage of a human being, and, *unless prevented by disease or violence, will actually do so, despite possibly significant variation in environment* (in the mother's womb). None of the changes that occur to the embryo after fertilization, for as long as he or she survives, generates a new direction of growth. Rather, *all* of the changes (for example, those involving nutrition and environment) either facilitate or retard the internally directed growth of this persisting individual.

Sometimes it is objected that if we say human embryos are human beings, on the grounds that they have the potential to become mature humans, the same will have to be said of sperm and ova. This objection is untenable. The human embryo is radically unlike the sperm and ova, the sex cells. The sex cells are manifestly not *whole* or *complete* organisms. They are not only genetically but also functionally identifiable as parts of the male or female potential parents. They clearly are destined either to combine with an ovum or sperm or die. Even when they succeed in causing fertilization, they do not survive; rather, their genetic material enters into the composition of a distinct, new organism.

Nor are human embryos comparable to somatic cells (such as skin cells or muscle cells), though some have tried to argue that they are. Like sex cells, a somatic cell is functionally only a part of a larger organism. The human embryo, by contrast, possesses from the beginning the internal resources and active disposition to develop himself or herself to full maturity; all he or she needs is a suitable environment and nutrition. The direction of his or her growth *is not extrinsically determined*, but the embryo is internally directing his or her growth toward full maturity.

So, a human embryo (or fetus) is not something distinct from a human being; he or she is not an individual of any non-human or intermediate species. Rather, an embryo (and fetus) is a human being at a certain (early) stage of development—the embryonic (or fetal) stage. In abortion, what is killed is a human being, a whole living member of the species *homo sapiens*, the same *kind* of entity as you or I, only at an earlier stage of development. . . .

The Argument That Abortion Is Justified as Non-Intentional Killing

Some "pro-choice" philosophers have attempted to justify abortion by deny-ing that all abortions are intentional killing. They have granted (at least for the sake of argument) that an unborn human being has a right to life but have then argued that this right does not entail that the child *in utero* is morally entitled to the use of the mother's body for life support. In effect, their argu-ment is that, at least in many cases, abortion is not a case of intentionally killing the child, but a choice not to provide the child with assistance, that is, a choice to expel (or "evict") the child from the womb, despite the likelihood or certainty that expulsion (or "eviction") will result in his or her death (Little, 1999; McDonagh, 1996; Thomson, 1971).

Various analogies have been proposed by people making this argument. The mother's gestating a child has been compared to allowing someone the use of one's kidneys or even to donating an organ. We are not *required* (mor-ally or as a matter of law) to allow someone to use our kidneys, or to donate organs to others, even when they would die without this assistance (and we could survive in good health despite rendering it). Analogously, the argument continues, a woman is not morally required to allow the fetus the use of her body. We shall call this "the bodily rights argument."

It may be objected that a woman has a special responsibility to the child she is carrying, whereas in the cases of withholding assistance to which abor-tion is compared there is no such special responsibility. Proponents of the bodily rights argument have replied, however, that the mother has not voluntarily assumed responsibility for the child, or a personal relationship with the child, and we have strong responsibilities to others only if we have voluntarily assumed such responsibilities (Thomson, 1971) or have consented to a personal relationship which generates such responsibilities (Little, 1999). True, the mother may have voluntarily performed an act which she knew may result in a child's conception, but that is distinct from consenting to gestate the child if a child is conceived. And so (according to this position) it is not until the woman consents to pregnancy, or perhaps not until the parents consent to care for the child by taking the baby home from the hospital or birthing center, that the full duties of parenthood accrue to the mother (and perhaps the father).

In reply to this argument we wish to make several points. We grant that in some few cases abortion is not intentional killing, but a choice to expel the child, the child's death being an unintended, albeit foreseen and (rightly or wrongly) accepted, side effect. However, these constitute a small minority of abortions. In the vast majority of cases, the death of the child *in utero* is pre-cisely the object of the abortion. In most cases the end sought is to avoid being a parent; but abortion brings that about only by bringing it about that the child dies. Indeed, the attempted abortion would be considered by the woman requesting it and the abortionist performing it to have been *unsuccess-ful* if the child survives. In most cases abortion *is* intentional killing. Thus, even if the bodily rights argument succeeded, it would justify only a small percentage of abortions.

Still, in some few cases abortion is chosen as a means precisely toward ending the condition of pregnancy, and the woman requesting the termination of her pregnancy would not object if somehow the child survived. A pregnant woman may have less or more serious reasons for seeking the termination of this condition, but if that is her objective, then the child's death resulting from his or her expulsion will be a side effect, rather than the means chosen. For example, an actress may wish not to be pregnant because the pregnancy will change her figure during a time in which she is filming scenes in which having a slender appearance is important; or a woman may dread the discomforts, pains, and difficulties involved in pregnancy. (Of course, in many abortions there may be mixed motives: the parties making the choice may intend both ending the condition of pregnancy and the death of the child.)

Nevertheless, while it is true that in some cases abortion is not intentional killing, it remains misleading to describe it simply as choosing not to provide bodily life support. Rather, it is actively expelling the human embryo or fetus from the womb. There is a significant moral difference between *not doing* something that would assist someone, and *doing* something that causes someone harm, even if that harm is an unintended (but foreseen) side effect. It is more difficult morally to justify the latter than it is the former. Abortion is the *act* of extracting the unborn human being from the womb—an extraction that usually rips him or her to pieces or does him or her violence in some other way.

It is true that in some cases causing death as a side effect is morally permissible. For example, in some cases it is morally right to use force to stop a potentially lethal attack on one's family or country, even if one foresees that the force used will also result in the assailant's death. Similarly, there are instances in which it is permissible to perform an act that one knows or believes will, as a side effect, cause the death of a child *in utero*. For example, if a pregnant woman is discovered to have a cancerous uterus, and this is a proximate danger to the mother's life, it can be morally right to remove the cancerous uterus with the baby in it, even if the child will die as a result. A similar situation can occur in ectopic pregnancies. But in such cases, not only is the child's death a side effect, but the mother's life is in proximate danger. It is worth noting also that in these cases *what is done* (the means) is the correction of a pathology (such as a cancerous uterus, or a ruptured uterine tube). Thus, in such cases, not only the child's death, but also the ending of the pregnancy, are side effects. So, such acts are what traditional casuistry referred to as *indirect* or *non-intentional*, abortions.

But it is also clear that not every case of causing death as a side effect is morally right. For example, if a man's daughter has a serious respiratory disease and the father is told that his continued smoking in her presence will cause her death, it would obviously be immoral for him to continue the smoking. Similarly, if a man works for a steel company in a city with significant levels of air pollution, and his child has a serious respiratory problem making the air pollution a danger to her life, certainly he should move to another city. He should move, we would say, even if that meant he had to resign a prestigious position or make a significant career change.

In both examples, (a) the parent has a special responsibility to his child, but (b) the act that would cause the child's death would avoid a harm to the parent but cause a significantly worse harm to his child. And so, although the harm done would be a side effect, in both cases the act that caused the death would be an *unjust* act, and morally wrongful *as such*. The special responsibility of parents to their children requires that they *at least* refrain from performing acts that cause terrible harms to their children in order to avoid significantly lesser harms to themselves.

But (a) and (b) also obtain in intentional abortions (that is, those in which the removal of the child is directly sought, rather than the correction of a life-threatening pathology) even though they are not, strictly speaking, intentional killing. First, the mother has a special responsibility to her child, in virtue of being her biological mother (as does the father in virtue of his paternal relationship). The parental relationship itself—not just the voluntary acceptance of that relationship—gives rise to a special responsibility to a child.

Proponents of the bodily rights argument deny this point. Many claim that one has full parental responsibilities only if one has voluntarily assumed them. And so the child, on this view, has a right to care from his or her mother (including gestation) only if the mother has accepted her pregnancy, or perhaps only if the mother (and/or the father?) has in some way voluntarily begun a deep personal relationship with the child (Little, 1999).

But suppose a mother takes her baby home after giving birth, but the only reason she did not get an abortion was that she could not afford one. Or suppose she lives in a society where abortion is not available (perhaps very few physicians are willing to do the grisly deed). She and her husband take the child home only because they had no alternative. Moreover, suppose that in their society people are not waiting in line to adopt a newborn baby. And so the baby is several days old before anything can be done. If they abandon the baby and the baby is found, she will simply be returned to them. In such a case the parents have not voluntarily assumed responsibility; nor have they consented to a personal relationship with the child. But it would surely be wrong for these parents to abandon their baby in the woods (perhaps the only feasible way of ensuring she is not returned), even though the baby's death would be only a side effect. Clearly, we recognize that parents do have a responsibility to make sacrifices for their children, even if they have not voluntarily assumed such responsibilities, or given their consent to the personal relationship with the child.

The bodily rights argument implicitly supposes that we have a primordial right to construct a life simply as we please, and that others have claims on us only very minimally or through our (at least tacit) consent to a certain sort of relationship with them. On the contrary, we are by nature members of communities. Our moral goodness or character consists to a large extent (though not solely) in contributing to the communities of which we are members. We ought to act for our genuine good or flourishing (we take that as a basic ethical principle), but our flourishing involves being in communion with others. And communion with others of itself—even if we find ourselves united with others because of a physical or social relationship which precedes our consent—entails duties or responsibilities. Moreover, the contribution we are morally required to make to others will likely bring each of us some discomfort and pain. This is not to say that we should simply ignore our own good, for the sake of others. Rather, since what (and who) I am is in part constituted by various relationships with others, not all of which are initiated by my will, my genuine good includes the contributions I make to the relationships in which I participate. Thus, the life we constitute by our free choices should be in large part a life of mutual reciprocity with others.

For example, I may wish to cultivate my talent to write and so I may want to spend hours each day reading and writing. Or I may wish to develop my athletic abilities and so I may want to spend hours every day on the baseball field. But if I am a father of minor children, and have an adequate paying job working (say) in a coal mine, then my clear duty is to keep that job. Similarly, if one's girlfriend finds she is pregnant and one is the father, then one might also be morally required to continue one's work in the mine (or mill, factory, warehouse, etc.).

In other words, I have a duty to do something with my life that contributes to the good of the human community, but that general duty becomes specified by my particular situation. It becomes specified by the connection or closeness to me of those who are in need. We acquire special responsibilities toward people, not only by *consenting* to contracts or relationships with them, but also by having various types of union with them. So, we have special responsibilities to those people with whom we are closely united. For example, we have special responsibilities to our parents, and brothers and sisters, even though we did not choose them.

The physical unity or continuity of children to their parents is unique. The child is brought into being out of the bodily unity and bodies of the mother and the father. The mother and the father are in a certain sense prolonged or continued in their offspring. So, there is a natural unity of the mother with her child, and a natural unity of the father with his child. Since we have special responsibilities to those with whom we are closely united, it follows that we in fact do have a special responsibility to our children anterior to our having voluntarily assumed such responsibility or consented to the relationship.[2]

The second point is this: in the types of case we are considering, the harm caused (death) is much worse than the harms avoided (the difficulties in pregnancy). Pregnancy can involve severe impositions, but it is not nearly as bad as death—which is total and irreversible. One needn't make light of the burdens of pregnancy to acknowledge that the harm that is death is in a different category altogether.

The burdens of pregnancy include physical difficulties and the pain of labor, and can include significant financial costs, psychological burdens, and interference with autonomy and the pursuit of other important goals (McDonagh, 1996: ch. 5). These costs are not inconsiderable. Partly for that reason, we owe our mothers gratitude for carrying and giving birth to us. However, where pregnancy does not place a woman's life in jeopardy or threaten grave and lasting damage to her physical health, the harm done to other goods is not total. Moreover, most of the harms involved in pregnancy are not irreversible:

pregnancy is a nine-month task—if the woman and man are not in a good position to raise the child, adoption is a possibility. So the difficulties of pregnancy, considered together, are in a different and lesser category than death. Death is not just worse in degree than the difficulties involved in pregnancy; it is worse in kind.

It has been argued, however, that pregnancy can involve a unique type of burden. It has been argued that the *intimacy* involved in pregnancy is such that if the woman must remain pregnant without her consent then there is inflicted on her a unique and serious harm. Just as sex with consent can be a desired experience but sex without consent is a violation of bodily integrity, so (the argument continues) pregnancy involves such a close physical intertwinement with the fetus that not to allow abortion is analogous to rape—it involves an enforced intimacy (Boonin, 2003: 84; Little, 1999: 300–3).

However, this argument is based on a false analogy. Where the pregnancy is unwanted, the baby's "occupying" the mother's womb may involve a harm; but the child is committing no injustice against her. The baby is not forcing himself or herself on the woman, but is simply growing and developing in a way quite natural to him or her. The baby is not performing any action that could in any way be construed as aimed at violating the mother.[3]

It is true that the fulfillment of the duty of a mother to her child (during gestation) is unique and in many cases does involve a great sacrifice. The argument we have presented, however, is that being a mother *does* generate a special responsibility, and that the sacrifice morally required of the mother is less burdensome than the harm that would be done to the child by expelling the child, causing his or her death, to escape that responsibility. Our argument equally entails responsibilities for the father of the child. His duty does not involve as direct a bodily relationship with the child as the mother's, but it may be equally or even more burdensome. In certain circumstances, his obligation to care for the child (and the child's mother), and especially his obligation to provide financial support, may severely limit his freedom and even require months or, indeed, years, of extremely burdensome physical labor. Historically, many men have rightly seen that their basic responsibility to their family (and country) has entailed risking, and in many cases, losing, their lives. Different people in different circumstances, with different talents, will have different responsibilities. It is no argument against any of these responsibilities to point out their distinctness.

So, the burden of carrying the baby, for all its distinctness, is significantly less than the harm the baby would suffer by being killed; the mother and father have a special responsibility to the child; it follows that intentional abortion (even in the few cases where the baby's death is an unintended but foreseen side effect) is unjust and therefore objectively immoral.

Notes

1. See, for example: Carlson (1994: chs. 2–4); Gilbert, (2003: 183–220, 363–90); Larson (2001: chs. 1–2); Moore and Persaud (2003: chs. 1–6); Muller (1997: chs. 1–2); O'Rahilly and Mueller (2000: chs. 3–4).

2. David Boonin claims, in reply to this argument—in an earlier and less developed form, presented by Lee (1996: 122)—that it is not clear that it is impermissible for a woman to destroy what is a part of, or a continuation of, herself. He then says that to the extent the unborn human being is united to her in that way, "it would if anything seem that her act is *easier* to justify than if this claim were not true" (2003: 230). But Boonin fails to grasp the point of the argument (perhaps understandably since it was not expressed very clearly in the earlier work he is discussing). The unity of the child to the mother is the basis for this child being related to the woman in a different way from how other children are. We ought to pursue our own good *and the good of others with whom we are united in various ways.* If that is so, then the closer someone is united to us, the deeper and more extensive our responsibility to the person will be.

3. In some sense being bodily "occupied" when one does not wish to be *is* a harm; however, just as the child does not (as explained in the text), neither does the state inflict this harm on the woman, in circumstances in which the state prohibits abortion. By prohibiting abortion the state would only prevent the woman from performing an act (forcibly detaching the child from her) that would unjustly kill this developing child, who is an innocent party.

References

Boonin, David (2003). *A Defense of Abortion.* New York: Cambridge University Press.

Carlson, Bruce (1994). *Human Embryology and Developmental Biology.* St. Louis, MO: Mosby.

Gilbert, Scott (2003). *Developmental Biology*, 7th edn. Sunderland, MA: Sinnauer Associates.

Larson, William J. (2001). *Human Embryology*, 3rd edn. New York: Churchill Livingstone.

Lee, Patrick (1996). *Abortion and Unborn Human Life.* Washington, DC: Catholic University of America Press.

Little, Margaret Olivia (1999). "Abortion, intimacy, and the duty to gestate." *Ethical Theory and Moral Practice, 2*: 295–312.

McDonagh, Eileen (1996). *Breaking the Abortion Deadlock: From Choice to Consent.* New York: Oxford University Press, 1996.

Moore, Keith, and Persaud, T. V. N. (2003). *The Developing Human, Clinically Oriented Embryology*, 7th edn. New York: W. B. Saunders.

Muller, Werner A. (1997). *Developmental Biology.* New York: Springer Verlag.

O'Rahilly, Ronan, and Mueller, Fabiola (2000). *Human Embryology and Teratology*, 3rd edn. New York: John Wiley & Sons.

Thomson, Judith Jarvis (1971). "A defense of abortion." *Philosophy and Public Affairs,* 1: 47–66; reprinted, among other places, in Feinberg (1984, pp. 173–87).

Margaret Olivia Little 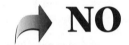 **NO**

The Morality of Abortion

Introduction

It is often noted that the public discussion of abortion's moral status is disappointingly crude. The positions staked out and the reasoning proffered seem to reflect little of the subtlety and nuance—not to mention ambivalence—that mark more private reflections on the subject. Despite attempts by various parties to find middle ground, the debate remains largely polarized—at its most dramatic, with extreme conservatives claiming abortion the moral equivalent of murder even as extreme liberals think it devoid of moral import.

To some extent, this polarization is due to the legal battle that continues to shadow moral discussions: admission of ethical nuance, it is feared, will play as concession on the deeply contested question of whether abortion should be a legally protected option for women. But to some extent, blame for the continued crudeness can be laid at the doorstep of moral theory itself.

For one thing, the ethical literature on abortion has focused its attention almost exclusively on the thinnest moral assessment—on whether and when abortion is "morally permissible." That question is, of course, a crucial one, its answer often desperately sought. But many of our deepest struggles with the morality of abortion concern much more textured questions about its placement on the scales of *decency, respectfulness,* and *responsibility.* It is one thing to decide that an abortion was permissible, quite another to decide that it was *honorable;* one thing to decide that an abortion was impermissible, quite another to decide that it was *monstrous.* It is these latter categories that determine what we might call the thick moral interpretation of the act—and, with it, the meaning the woman must live with, and the reactive attitudes such as disgust, forbearance, or admiration that she and others think the act deserves. A moral theory that moves too quickly or focuses too exclusively on moral permissibility won't address these crucial issues. . . .

To make progress on abortion's moral status, it thus turns out, requires us not just to arbitrate already familiar controversies in metaphysics and ethics, but to attend to the distinctive aspects of pregnancy that often stand at their margins. In the following, I want to argue that if we acknowledge gestation as an *intimacy,* motherhood as a *relationship,* and creation as a *process,* we will be in a far better position to appreciate the moral textures of abortion. I explore these textures, in the first half on stipulation that the fetus is a person, in the second half under supposition that early human life has an important value worthy of respect.

Fetal Personhood: From Wrongful Interference to Positive Responsibilities

If fetuses are persons, then abortion is surely an enormously serious matter: What is at stake is nothing less than the life of a creature with full moral standing. To say that the stakes are high, though, is not to say that moral analysis is obvious (which is why elsewhere in moral theory, conversation usually starts, not stops, once we realize people's lives are at issue). I think the most widely held objection to abortion is badly misguided; more importantly, it obscures the deeper ethical question at issue.

On the usual view, it is perfectly obvious what to say about abortion on supposition of fetal personhood: if fetuses are persons, then abortion is murder. Persons, after all, have a fundamental right to life, and abortion, it would seem, counts as its gross violation. On this view, we can assess the status of abortion quite cleanly. In particular, we needn't delve too deeply into the burdens that continued gestation might present for women—not because their lives don't matter or because we don't sympathize with their plight, but because we don't take hardship as justification for murder.

In fact, though, abortion's assimilation to murder will seem clear-cut only if we have already ignored key features of gestation. While certain metaphors depict gestation as passive carriage—as though the fetus were simply occupying a room until it is born—the truth is of course far different. One who is gestating is providing the fetus with sustenance—donating nourishment, creating blood, delivering oxygen, providing hormonal triggers for development—without which it could not live. For a fetus, to live *is* to be receiving aid. And whether the assistance is delivered by way of intentional activity (as when the woman eats or takes her prenatal vitamins) or by way of biological mechanism, assistance it plainly is. But this has crucial implications for abortion's alleged status as murder. To put it simply, the right to life, as Judith Thomson famously put it, does not include the right to have all assistance needed to maintain that life (Thomson, 1971). Ending gestation will, at early stages at least, certainly lead to the fetus's demise, but that does not mean that doing so would constitute murder. . . .

Even if the fetus is a person, then, abortion would not be murder. More broadly put, abortion, whatever its rights and wrongs, isn't a species of *wrongful interference*.

None of this, though, is to say that abortion under such supposition is therefore unproblematic. It is to argue, instead, that the crucial moral issue needs to be re-located. Wrongful interference is a central concern in morality, but it isn't the only one. We are also concerned with notions of *neglect, abandonment* and *disregard*. These are issues that involve abrogations of positive responsibilities to help others, not injunctions against interfering with them. If fetuses are persons, the question we really need to decide is what positive responsibilities, if any, do pregnant women have to continue gestational assistance? This is a question that takes us into far richer, and far more interesting, territory than that occupied by discussions of murder.

One issue it raises is: what do pregnant women owe to the fetuses they carry as a matter of *general beneficence?* Philosophers, of course, familiarly divide over the ambitions of beneficence, generically construed; but abortion raises distinct difficulties of its own. On the one hand, the beneficence called for here is of a particularly urgent kind: the stakes are life and death, and the pregnant woman is the *only* one who can render the assistance needed. It's a rare (and, many of us will think, dreadful) moral theory that will think she faces no responsibilities to assist here: passing a drowning person for mere convenience when no one else is within shouting distance is a very good example of moral indecency. On the other hand, gestation is not just any activity. It involves sharing one's very body. It brings with it an emotional intertwinement that can reshape one's entire life. It brings another person into one's family. Being asked to gestate another person, that is, isn't like being asked to write a check to support an impoverished child; it's like being asked to adopt the child. Doing so is a caring, compassionate act; it is also an enormous undertaking that has reverberations for an entire lifetime. Deciding whether, and if so when, such action is obligatory rather than admirable is no light matter.

I don't think moral theory has begun to address the rich questions at issue here. When are intimate actions owed to generic others? How do we weigh the sacrifice morality requires of us when it is measured, not in terms of risk, but of intertwinement? What should we think of such obligations if the required acts would be performed under conditions of profound self-alienation? The *type* of issue paradigmatically represented by gestation—an assistance that combines life and death stakes with deep intimacy—is virtually nowhere discussed in ethical theory. (We aren't called upon in the usual course of events to save people's lives by, say, having sexual intercourse with them.) By ignoring these issues, mainstream moral theory has ended up deeply under-selling the moral complexity of abortion.

Difficult as these questions are, though, it is actually a second issue, I suspect, that is responsible for much of the passion that surrounds abortion on supposition of fetal personhood. On reflection, many will say, the issues confronting the pregnant woman aren't about generic beneficence at all. The considerations she faces are not just those that would face someone uniquely well placed to serve as Good Samaritan to some stranger—as when one passes the drowning person: for the pregnant woman and fetus, crucially, aren't strangers. If the fetus is a person, many will say, it is *her child;* and for this reason she has special responsibilities to meet its needs. In the end, I believe, much of the animating concern with abortion is not about what we owe to generic others; it's about what parents owe their children.

But if it's parenthood that is carrying normative weight, then we need an ethics of parenthood—a theory of what makes someone a parent in this thickly normative sense and what the contours of its responsibilities really are. This should raise something of a warning flag. Philosophers, it must be said, have by and large done a rather poor job when it comes to parenthood—

variously avoiding it, romanticizing it, or assimilating it to categories, like contractual relations, to which it stands in paradigmatic contrast. This general shortcoming is evident in discussions of abortion, where two remarkably unhelpful models dominate.

One position, advocated by Judith Thomson and some of the most recent treatments of abortion, is a classically liberal one. It agrees that special responsibilities attach to parenthood but argues that parenthood is thereby a status that is entered into only by consent. That consent is usually tacit, to be sure—taking the baby home from the hospital qualifies; nonetheless, special responsibilities to a child accrue only when one voluntarily assumes them.

Such a model is surely an odd one. The model yields the plausible view that the rape victim does not face the very same set of duties as many other pregnant women, but it does so by implying that a man who fathers a child during a one-night stand has no special responsibilities toward that child unless he decides he does. Perhaps most strikingly, such a view has no resources for acknowledging that there may be moral reasons why one *should* consent to the status. Those who sustain a biological connection may have a tendency to enter the role of parent, but on this scheme it's a mere psychological proclivity that rides atop nothing normative.

Another position is classically conservative. According to this view, the special responsibilities of parenthood are grounded in biological progenitor-ship. It is blood ties, to use the old-fashioned vernacular—"passing on one's genes," in more current translation—that makes one a parent and grounds heightened responsibilities. This view has its own blind spot. It has the resources for agreeing that a man who fathers a child from a one-night stand faces special responsibilities for the child whether he likes it or not, but none for distinguishing between the responsibilities of someone who has served as the special steward for a child—who has engaged for years in the *activity* of parenting—and the responsibilities of someone who bears literally no con-nection beyond a genetic or causal contribution to existence. On this view, a sperm donor faces all the responsibilities of a social father.

What both positions have in common is the supposition that parenthood is an all or nothing affair. Applied to pregnancy, the gestating woman either owes everything we imagine we owe to the children we love and rear or she owes nothing beyond general beneficence unless she decides she does. But parenthood—like all familial relations—is surely a more complicated moral notion than this. Parenthood, and its attendant responsibilities, admit of *layers*. It has a crucial existence as a social *role*—something with institutionally defined entrances, exits, and expectations that can attach to us quite indepen-dently of what our self-conceptions might say. It also has a crucial existence as a *relationship*—an emotional connection, a shared history, an intertwinement of lives. It is because of that intertwinement that parents' motivation to sacrifice is so often immediate. But it is also because of that relationship that even especially ambitious sacrifices are legitimately expected, and why failure to undertake them would be so problematic: absent unusual circumstances, it becomes a betrayal of the relationship itself. In short, parenthood is not monolithic: some of the responsibilities we paradigmatically associate as parental attach, not to the role, but to the relationship that so often accompanies it.

These layers matter especially when we get to gestation, for the pregnant woman stands precisely at their intersection. If a fetus is a person, then there is surely an important sense in which she is its mother: to regard her as just a passing stranger uniquely able to help it would grossly distort the situation. But she is not yet a mother most thickly described—a mother in standing relationship with a child, with the responsibilities born of shared history and the enterprise of caretaking.

These demarcations are integral, I think, to understanding the distinctive sorts of conflicts that pregnancy can represent—including, most notably, the conflicts it can bring *within* the mantle of motherhood. Women sometimes decide to abort even though they regard the fetus they carry as their child, because they realize, grimly, that bringing this child into the world will leave too little room to care adequately for the children they are already raising. This is a conflict we cannot even name, much less arbitrate, on standard views—if the fetus is her child, how could she possibly choose to sacrifice its life unless the stakes are literally equivalent for the others? But this is to ignore the layers of parenthood. She occupies the *role* of mother to the fetus, but with the other children, she is, by dint of time, interaction, and intertwinement, in a *relationship* of motherhood. The fetus is her baby, then,—not just some passing stranger she alone can help—which is why this conflict brings the kind of agony it does. But if it is her child in the role sense only, she does not yet owe all that she owes to her other children. Depending on the circumstances, other family members with whom she is already in relationship may, tragically, come first.

None of this is to make light to the responsibilities pregnant women face on supposition of fetal personhood. If fetuses are persons, such responsibilities are surely profound. It is, rather, to insist that they admit of layer and degree, and that these distinctions, while delicate, are crucial to capturing the *types* of tragedy—and the types of moral compromise—abortion can here represent.

The Sanctity of Life: Respect Revisited

. . . For many women who contemplate abortion, the desire to end pregnancy is not, or not centrally, a desire to avoid the nine months of pregnancy; it is to avoid what lies on the far side of those months—namely, motherhood. If gestation were simply a matter of rendering, say, somewhat risky assistance to help a burgeoning human life they've come across—if they could somehow render that assistance without thereby adding a member to their family—the decision faced would be a far different one. But gestation doesn't just allow cells to become a person; it turns one into a mother.

One of the most common reasons women give for wanting to abort is that they do not want to become a mother—now, ever, again, with this partner, or no reliable partner, with these few resources, or these many that are now, after so many years of mothering, slated finally to another cause. Nor does adoption represent a universal solution. To give up a child would be for some a life-long trauma; others occupy fortunate circumstances that would, by their own lights, make it unjustified to give over a child for others to rear. Or again—and most frequently—she doesn't want to raise a child just now but knows that if she *does* carry the pregnancy to term, she won't *want* to give up the child for adoption. Gestation, she knows, is likely to reshape her heart and soul, transforming her into a mother emotionally, not just officially; and it is precisely that transformation she does not want to undergo. It is because continuing pregnancy brings with it this new identity and, likely, relationship, then, that many feel it legitimate to decline.

But pregnancy's connection to motherhood also enters the phenomenology of abortion in just the opposite direction. For some women, that it would be her child is precisely why she feels she must continue the pregnancy—even if motherhood is not what she desired. To be pregnant is to have one's potential child knocking at one's door; to abort is to turn one's back on it, a decision, many women say, that would haunt them forever. On this view, the desire to avoid motherhood, so compelling as a reason to contracept, is uneasy grounds to abort: for once an embryo is on the scene, it isn't about rejecting motherhood, it's about rejecting one's *child.* Not literally, of course, since there is no child yet extant to stand as the object of rejection. But the stance one should take to pregnancy, sought or not, is one of *acceptance:* when a potential family member is knocking at the door, one should move over, make room, and welcome her in.

These two intuitive stances represent just profoundly different ways of gestalting the situation of ending pregnancy. On the first view, abortion is closer to contraception—hardly equivalent, because it means the demise of something of value. But the desire to avoid the enterprise and identity of motherhood is an understandable and honorable basis for deciding to end a pregnancy. Given that there is no child yet on the scene, one does not owe special openness to the relationship that stands at the end of pregnancy's trajectory. On the second view, abortion is closer to exiting a parental relationship—hardly equivalent, for one of the key relata is not yet fully present. But one's decision about whether to continue the pregnancy already feels specially constrained: that one would be related to the resulting person exerts now some moral force. It would take especially grave reasons to refuse assistance here, for the norms of parenthood already have a toehold. Assessing the moral status of abortion, it turns out, then, is not just about assessing the contours of generic respect owed to burgeoning human life, it's about assessing the salience of *impending relationship.* And this is an issue that functions in different ways for different women—and, sometimes, in one and the same woman.

In my own view, until the fetus is a person, we should recognize a moral prerogative to decline parenthood and end the pregnancy. Not because motherhood is necessarily a burden (though it can be); but because it so thoroughly changes what we might call one's fundamental practical identity. The enterprise of mothering restructures the self—changing the shape of one's heart, the primary commitments by which one lives one's life, the terms by which one judges one's life a success or a failure. If the enterprise is eschewed and one decides to give the child over to another, the identity of mother still changes the normative facts that are true of one, as there is now someone by whom one does well or poorly. And either way—whether one rears the child or lets it go—to continue a pregnancy means that a piece of one's heart, as the saying goes, will forever walk outside one's body. As profound as the respect we should have for burgeoning human life, we should acknowledge moral prerogatives over identity-constituting commitments and enterprises as profound as motherhood.

But I also don't think this is the whole of the moral story. If women find themselves with different ways of gestalting the prospective relationship involved in pregnancy, it is in part because they have different identities, commitments, and ideals that such a prospect intersects with—commitments which, while permissibly idiosyncratic, are morally authoritative for *them*. If a woman feels already duty-bound by the norms of parenthood to nurture this creature, it may be for the very good reason that, in an important personal sense, she already *is* its mother. She finds herself—perhaps to her surprise, happy or otherwise—with a maternal commitment to this creature. As philosophers forget but women and men have long known, something can be your child even if it is not yet a person. But taking on the identity of mother towards something just *is* to take on certain imperatives about its well-being as categorical. Her job is thus clear—it's to help this creature reach its fullest potential. For other women, the identity is still something that can be assessed—tried on, perhaps accepted, but perhaps declined: in which case respect is owed, but is saved, or confirmed, for others—other relationships, other projects, other passions.

And again, if a woman feels she owes a stance of welcome to burgeoning human life that comes her way, it may be, not because she thinks such a stance authoritative for all, but because of the virtues around which her practical identity is now oriented: receptivity to life's agenda, for instance, or responsiveness to that which is most vulnerable. For another woman, the executive virtues to be exercised tug in just the other direction: loyalty to treasured life plans, a commitment that it be she, not the chances of biology, that should determine her life's course, bolstering self-direction after a life too long ruled by serendipity and fate.

Deciding when it is morally decent to end a pregnancy, it turns out, is an admixture of settling impersonally or universally authoritative moral requirements, and of discovering and arbitrating—sometimes after agonizing deliberation, sometimes in a decision no less deep for its immediacy—one's own commitments, identity, and defining virtues.

A similarly complex story appears when we turn to the second theme. Another thread that appears in many women's stories in the face of unsought pregnancy is respect for the weighty responsibility involved in creating human life. Once again, it is a theme that pulls and tugs in different directions.

In its most familiar direction, it shows up in many stories of why an unsought pregnancy is continued. Many people believe that one's responsibility to nurture new life is importantly amplified if one is responsible for bringing about its existence in the first place. Just what it takes to count as responsible here is a point on which individuals diverge (whether voluntary but contracepted intercourse is different from intercourse without use of birth control, and again from intentionally deciding to become pregnant at the IVF clinic). But triggering the relevant standard of responsibility for creation, it is felt, brings with it a heightened responsibility to nurture: it is disrespectful to create human life only to allow it to wither. Put more rigorously, one who is responsible for bringing about a creature that has intrinsic value in virtue of its potential to become a person has a special responsibility to enable it to reach that end state.

But the idea of respect for creation is also, if less frequently acknowledged, sometimes the reason why women are moved to *end* pregnancies. As Barbara Katz Rothman (1985) puts it, decisions to abort often represent, not a decision to destroy, but a refusal to create. Many people have deeply felt convictions about the circumstances under which they feel it right for them to bring a child into the world—can it be brought into a decent world, an intact family, a society that can minimally respect its agency? These considerations may persist even after conception has taken place; for while the *embryo* has already been created, a person has not. Some women decide to abort, that is, not because they do not *want* the resulting child—indeed, they may yearn for nothing more, and desperately wish that their circumstances were otherwise—but because they do not think bringing a child into the world the right thing for them to do.

These are abortions marked by moral language. A woman wants to abort because she knows she couldn't give up a child for adoption but feels she couldn't give the child the sort of life, or be the sort of parent, she thinks a child *deserves;* a woman who would have to give up the child thinks it would be *unfair* to bring a child into existence already burdened by rejection, however well grounded its reasons; a woman living in a country marked by poverty and gender apartheid wants to abort because she decides it would be *wrong* for her to bear a daughter whose life, like hers, would be filled with so much injustice and hardship.

Some have thought that such decisions betray a simple fallacy: unless the child's life were literally going to be worse than non-existence, how can one abort out of concern for the future child? But the worry here isn't that one would be imposing a *harm* on the child by bringing it into existence (as though children who are in the situations mentioned have lives that aren't worth living). The claim is that bringing about a person's life in these circumstances would do violence to her ideals of creating and parenthood. She does not want to bring into existence a daughter she cannot love and care for, she does not want to bring into existence a person whose life will be marked by disrespect or rejection.

Nor does the claim imply judgment on women who *do* continue pregnancies in similar circumstances—as though there were here an obligation to abort. For the norms in question, once again, need not be impersonally authoritative moral chums. Like ideals of good parenting, they mark out considerations all should be sensitive to, perhaps, but equally reasonable people may adhere to different variations and weightings. Still, they are normative for those who do have them; far from expressing mere matters of taste, the ideals one does accept carry an important kind of categoricity, issuing imperatives whose authority is not reducible to mere desire. These are, at root, issues about *integrity,* and the importance of maintaining integrity over one's participation in this enterprise precisely because it is so normatively weighty.

What is usually emphasized in the morality of abortion is the ethics of destruction; but there is a balancing ethics of creation. And for many people, conflict about abortion is a conflict *within* that ethics. On the one had, we now have on hand an entity that has a measure of sanctity: that it has begun is reason to help it continue—perhaps especially if one had a role in its procreation—which is why even early abortion is not normatively equivalent to contraception. On the other hand, not to end a pregnancy *is* to do something else, namely, to continue creating a person, and for some women, pregnancy strikes in circumstances in which they cannot countenance that enterprise. For some, the sanctity of developing human life will be strong enough to tip the balance towards continuing the pregnancy; for others, their norms of respectful creation will hold sway. For those who believe that the norms governing creation of a person are mild relative to the normative telos of embryonic life, being a responsible creator means continuing to gestate, and doing the best one can to bring about the conditions under which that creation will be more respectful. For others, though, the normativity of fetal telos is mild and their standards of respectful creation high, and the lesson goes in just the other direction: it is a sign of respect not to continue creating when certain background conditions, such as a loving family or adequate resources, are not in place.

However one thinks these issues settle out, they will not be resolved by austere contemplation of the value of human life. They require wrestling with the rich meanings of creation, responsibility, and kinship. And these issues, I have suggested, are just as much issues about one's integrity as they are about what is impersonally obligatory. On many treatments of abortion, considerations about whether or not to continue a pregnancy are exhausted by preferences, on the one hand, and universally authoritative moral demands, on the other; but some of the most important terrain lies in between.

References

Rothman, B. K. (1989). *Recreating motherhood: ideology and technology in a patriarchal society.* New York: Norton.

Thomson, J. J. (1971). A defense of abortion. *Philosophy and Public Affairs, 1,* 47–66.

POSTSCRIPT

Is Abortion Immoral?

According to the Centers for Disease Control and Prevention, more than half of all abortions in the United States are performed during the first eight weeks of pregnancy, and 88 percent before the twelfth week. Though uncommon, abortions performed in the second trimester of pregnancy are very controversial. Most often the reasons are fetal abnormalities, illness in the mother, or late diagnosis of pregnancy in a teenager. The procedure, which involves delivering a dead but intact fetus, is particularly troubling. The technical term is intact dilatation and extraction (D&X), but the more commonly used (and emotionally loaded) term is "partial-birth abortion."

In June 2000, the U.S. Supreme Court struck down a Nebraska law making it a crime to perform a partial-birth abortion. The five-to-four vote was the first abortion rights ruling in 8 years. Congress twice passed a bill banning partial-birth abortions, and President Bill Clinton twice vetoed it. President George W. Bush, however, signed the Partial-Birth Abortion Act of 2003. In June 2004, a federal judge in San Francisco struck down the bill, ruling that the law jeopardizes other legal forms of abortion and threatens the health of women. The federal government appealed, and the case of *Gonzales v. Carhart* went to the U.S. Supreme Court in 2006. Oral arguments were presented in November, and a decision is expected in the spring of 2007. For an article describing Dr. Leroy Carhart's clinic in Nebraska, see Alexi A. Wright and Ingrid T. Katz, "*Roe* versus Reality—Abortion and Women's Health," *New England Journal of Medicine,* July 6, 2006.

While most attention focuses on federal challenges to *Roe v. Wade,* state legislatures have been very active in this arena. In November 2006 South Dakota voters overturned a law enacted earlier in the year that would have banned almost all abortions, including those resulting from rape or incest. Some states have tried to restrict access through laws requiring parental consent for a minor seeking an abortion, for example, or special building restrictions not applied to other medical facilities. Other states have restricted protests at abortion clinics. See www.stateline.org for information on abortion regulations in specific states.

For a history of the political and ethical issues surrounding abortion in the United States, see Eva R. Rubin's *The Abortion Controversy: A Documentary History* (Greenwood, 1994). Also see Robert M. Baird and Stuart E. Rosenbaum, *The Ethics of Abortion: Pro-Life vs. Pro-Choice*, 3rd ed. (Prometheus Books, 2001).

ISSUE 9

Should a Pregnant Woman Be Punished for Exposing Her Fetus to Risk?

YES: Jean Toal, from Majority Opinion, *Cornelia Whitner, Respondent, v. State of South Carolina, Petitioner* (July 15, 1997)

NO: Lynn M. Paltrow, from "Punishment and Prejudice: Judging Drug-Using Pregnant Women," in Julia E. Hanigsberg and Sara Ruddick, eds., *Mother Troubles: Rethinking Contemporary Maternal Dilemmas* (Beacon Press, 1999)

ISSUE SUMMARY

YES: In a case involving a pregnant woman's use of crack cocaine, a majority of the supreme court of South Carolina ruled that a state legislature may impose additional criminal penalties on pregnant drug-using women without violating their constitutional right of privacy.

NO: Attorney Lynn Paltrow argues that treating drug-using pregnant women as criminals targets poor, African American women while ignoring other drug usage and fails to provide the resources to assist them in recovery.

At first glance, Cornelia Whitner and Bobbi McCaughey have absolutely nothing in common. Cornelia Whitner gave birth to a baby after using crack cocaine in the last trimester of pregnancy. She was arrested and convicted of child neglect. Bobbi McCaughey gave birth to seven babies in November 1997 to public acclaim and an avalanche of gifts and community support. Yet she too placed her babies at risk, simply by the use of fertility drugs and her decision to continue the multiple pregnancy. Through laws and public attitudes, society views the risks taken by Whitner and McCaughey very differently and punishes or rewards women accordingly.

In 1989, fueled by the specter of an epidemic of drug use resulting in the birth of thousands of "crack babies," the Medical University of South Carolina established a program that required drug-using pregnant women to seek treatment and prenatal care or face criminal prosecution. This program applied only to patients attending the university's obstetric clinic, primarily poor black women, and not to private patients. Patients enrolled in the clinic saw a video and were given written information about the harmful effects of substance abuse during pregnancy. The information warned that the Charleston, South Carolina, police, the court system, and child protective services might become involved if illegal drug use were detected.

Women who met certain criteria were required to undergo periodic urine screening for drugs. A patient who had a positive urine test or who failed to keep scheduled appointments for therapy or prenatal care could be arrested and placed in custody. If a woman delivered a baby who tested positive for drugs, she would be arrested immediately after her medical release and her newborn taken into protective custody. If the drug use was detected within the first 27 weeks of gestation, the patient was charged with possession of an illegal substance; after that date, the charge was possession and distribution of an illegal substance to a minor. If the drug use were detected during delivery, the woman would be charged with unlawful neglect of a child.

This stringent policy was developed as a result of clinicians' concern about the harmful effects of drug use on fetal development and prosecutors' desires to take a strong public stand condemning drug use. Although the stated goal was to get women into treatment, there were few places that women could receive treatment and the necessary support, such as transportation and child care. At the time there was no women-only residential treatment center for substance-abusing pregnant women anywhere in the state.

The program ended because the federal Office of Protection from Research Risks determined that it constituted human experimentation conducted without required institutional review board approval. This determination was based on a published report comparing the outcomes before and after the program. The university's approval as a site that could receive federal funds was placed in jeopardy.

By the time the policy was discontinued in September 1994 as the result of a settlement with the Civil Rights Division of the federal Department of Health and Human Services, 42 pregnant women had been arrested. One of those women was Cornelia Whitner, whose baby was born with cocaine metabolites in his system. Whitner admitted to using crack cocaine during her pregnancy. Charged with criminal child neglect, she pled guilty and was sentenced to eight years in prison. She appealed the decision on the grounds that the law covered children, not fetuses, and her case went to the supreme court of South Carolina.

The court's majority decision, written by Justice Jean Toal, found that the state's statute includes a fetus within its definition of "child" and ruled that the state was not violating Whitner's constitutional right of privacy by punishing her for endangering her child through an already illegal activity. This ruling was appealed to the U.S. Supreme Court. Lynn Paltrow believes that criminalization of drug use is a punitive response that denies the humanity of the women who are denied treatment and support for recovering from their addiction.

YES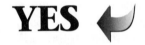

Jean Toal

Majority Opinion

Whitner *v.* South Carolina . . . ,

This case concerns the scope of the child abuse and endangerment statute in the South Carolina Children's Code. We hold the word "child" as used in that statute includes viable fetuses.

Facts

On April 20, 1992, Cornelia Whitner (Whitner) pled guilty to criminal child neglect, S.C.Code Ann. § 20-7-50 (1985), for causing her baby to be born with cocaine metabolites in its system by reason of Whitner's ingestion of crack cocaine during the third trimester of her pregnancy. The circuit court judge sentenced Whitner to eight years in prison. Whitner did not appeal her conviction.

Thereafter, Whitner filed a petition for Post Conviction Relief (PCR), pleading the circuit court's lack of subject matter jurisdiction to accept her guilty plea as well as ineffective assistance of counsel. Her claim of ineffective assistance of counsel was based upon her lawyer's failure to advise her the statute under which she was being prosecuted might not apply to prenatal drug use. The petition was granted on both grounds. The State appeals.

Law/Analysis

. . . South Carolina law has long recognized that viable fetuses are persons holding certain legal rights and privileges. In 1960, this Court decided Hall v. Murphy, 236 S.C. 257, 113 S.E.2d 790 (1960). That case concerned the application of South Carolina's wrongful death statute to an infant who died four hours after her birth as a result of injuries sustained prenatally during viability. The Appellants argued that a viable fetus was not a person within the purview of the wrongful death statute, because, inter alia, a fetus is thought to have no separate being apart from the mother.

We found such a reason for exclusion from recovery "unsound, illogical and unjust," and concluded there was "no medical or other basis" for the "assumed identity" of mother and viable unborn child. In light of that conclusion, this Court unanimously held: "We have no difficulty in concluding

Whitner v. State, 328 S.C. 1, 492 S.E.2d 777 (1997).

that a fetus having reached that period of prenatal maturity where it is capable of independent life apart from its mother is a person."

Four years later, in Fowler v. Woodward, 244 S.C. 608, 138 S.E.2d 42 (1964), we interpreted Hall as supporting a finding that a viable fetus injured while still in the womb need not be born alive for another to maintain an action for the wrongful death of the fetus.

> Since a viable child is a person before separation from the body of its mother and since prenatal injuries tortiously inflicted on such a child are actionable, it is apparent that the complaint alleges such an "act, neglect or default" by the defendant, to the injury of the child. . . .
>
> Once the concept of the unborn, viable child as a person is accepted, we have no difficulty in holding that a cause of action for tortious injury to such a child arises immediately upon the infliction of the injury. . . .

More recently, [in State v. Horne,] we held the word "person" as used in a criminal statute includes viable fetuses. . . . The defendant in that case stabbed his wife, who was nine months' pregnant, in the neck, arms, and abdomen. Although doctors performed an emergency caesarean section to deliver the child, the child died while still in the womb. The defendant was convicted of voluntary manslaughter and appealed his conviction on the ground South Carolina did not recognize the crime of feticide.

This Court disagreed. In a unanimous decision, we held it would be "grossly inconsistent . . . to construe a viable fetus as a 'person' for the purposes of imposing civil liability while refusing to give it a similar classification in the criminal context." Accordingly, the Court recognized the crime of feticide with respect to viable fetuses.

Similarly, we do not see any rational basis for finding a viable fetus is not a "person" in the present context. Indeed, it would be absurd to recognize the viable fetus as a person for purposes of homicide laws and wrongful death statutes but not for purposes of statutes proscribing child abuse. Our holding in Hall that a viable fetus is a person rested primarily on the plain meaning of the word "person" in light of existing medical knowledge concerning fetal development. We do not believe that the plain and ordinary meaning of the word "person" has changed in any way that would now deny viable fetuses status as persons.

The policies enunciated in the Children's Code also support our plain meaning reading of "person." S.C. Code Ann. § 20-7-20(C) (1985), which describes South Carolina's policy concerning children, expressly states: "It shall be the policy of this State to concentrate on the prevention of children's problems as the most important strategy which can be planned and implemented on behalf of children and their families." . . . The abuse or neglect of a child at any time during childhood can exact a profound toll on the child herself as well as on society as a whole. However, the consequences of abuse or neglect which takes place after birth often pale in comparison to those resulting from abuse suffered by the viable fetus before birth. This policy of prevention supports a reading of the word "person" to include viable fetuses. Furthermore, the scope of the Children's Code is quite broad. It applies "to all children who have need of services." . . . When coupled with the comprehensive remedial purposes of the Code, this language supports the inference that the legislature intended to include viable fetuses within the scope of the Code's protection.

Whitner advances several arguments against an interpretation of "person" as used in the Children's Code to include viable fetuses. We shall address each of Whitner's major arguments in turn.

Whitner's first argument concerns the number of bills introduced in the South Carolina General Assembly in the past five years addressing substance abuse by pregnant women. Some of these bills would have criminalized substance abuse by pregnant women; others would have addressed the issue through mandatory reporting, treatment, or intervention by social service agencies. Whitner suggests that the introduction of several bills touching the specific issue at hand evinces a belief by legislators that prior legislation had not addressed the issue. Whitner argues the introduction of the bills proves that section 20-7-50 was not intended to encompass abuse or neglect of a viable fetus.

We disagree with Whitner's conclusion about the significance of the proposed legislation. Generally, the legislature's subsequent acts "cast no light on the intent of the legislature which enacted the statute being construed." . . . Rather, this Court will look first to the language of the statute to discern legislative intent, because the language itself is the best guide to legislative intent. . . . Here, we see no reason to look beyond the statutory language. . . . Additionally, our existing case law strongly supports our conclusion about the meaning of the statute's language.

Whitner also argues an interpretation of the statute that includes viable fetuses would lead to absurd results obviously not intended by the legislature. Specifically, she claims if we interpret "child" to include viable fetuses, every action by a pregnant woman that endangers or is likely to endanger a fetus, whether otherwise legal or illegal, would constitute unlawful neglect under the statute. For example, a woman might be prosecuted under section 20-7-50 for smoking or drinking during pregnancy. Whitner asserts these "absurd" results could not have been intended by the legislature and, therefore, the statute should not be construed to include viable fetuses.

We disagree for a number of reasons. First, the same arguments against the statute can be made whether or not the child has been born. After the birth of a child, a parent can be prosecuted under section 20-7-50 for an action that is likely to endanger the child without regard to whether the action is illegal in itself. For example, a parent who drinks excessively could, under certain circumstances, be guilty of child neglect or endangerment even though the underlying act—consuming alcoholic beverages—is itself legal. Obviously, the legislature did not think it "absurd" to allow prosecution of parents for such otherwise legal acts when the acts actually or potentially endanger the "life, health or comfort" of the parents' born children. We see no reason such a result should be rendered absurd by the mere fact the child at issue is a viable fetus.

Moreover, we need not address this potential parade of horribles advanced by Whitner. In this case, which is the only case we are called upon to decide here, certain facts are clear. Whitner admits to having ingested crack cocaine during the third trimester of her pregnancy, which caused her child to be born with cocaine in its system. Although the precise effects of maternal crack use during pregnancy are somewhat unclear, it is well documented and within the realm of public knowledge that such use can cause serious harm to the viable unborn child. . . . There can be no question here Whitner endangered the life, health, and comfort of her child. We need not decide any cases other than the one before us.

We are well aware of the many decisions from other states' courts throughout the country holding maternal conduct before the birth of the child does not give rise to criminal prosecution under state child abuse/ endangerment or drug distribution statutes. . . . Many of these cases were prosecuted under statutes forbidding delivery or distribution of illicit substances and depended on statutory construction of the terms "delivery" and "distribution." . . . Obviously, such cases are inapplicable to the present situation. The cases concerning child endangerment statutes or construing the terms "child" and "person" are also distinguishable, because the states in which these cases were decided have entirely different bodies of case law from South Carolina. . . .

Massachusetts, however, has a body of case law substantially similar to South Carolina's, yet a Massachusetts trial court [in Commonwealth v. Pellegrini,] has held that a mother pregnant with a viable fetus is not criminally liable for transmission of cocaine to the fetus. . . . Specifically, Massachusetts law allows wrongful death actions on behalf of viable fetuses injured in utero who are not subsequently born alive. Mone v. Greyhound Lines, Inc., 368 Mass. 354, 331 N.E.2d 916 (1975). Similarly, Massachusetts law permits homicide prosecutions of third parties who kill viable fetuses. See Commonwealth v. Cass, 392 Mass. 799, 467 **783 N.E.2d 1324 (1984) (ruling a viable fetus is a person for purposes of vehicular homicide statute); Commonwealth v. Lawrence, 404 Mass. 378, 536 N.E.2d 571 (1989) (viable fetus is a person for purposes of common law crime of murder). Because of the similarity of the case law in Massachusetts to ours, the Pellegrini decision merits examination.

In Pellegrini, the Massachusetts Superior Court found that state's distribution statute does not apply to the distribution of an illegal substance to a viable fetus. The statute at issue forbade distribution of cocaine to persons under the age of eighteen. Rather than construing the word "distribution," however, the superior court found that a viable fetus is not a "person under the age of eighteen" within the meaning of the statute. In so finding, the court had to distinguish [Commonwealth v.] Lawrence and [Commonwealth v.] Cass, both of which held viable fetuses are "persons" for purposes of criminal laws in Massachusetts.

The Massachusetts trial court found Lawrence and Cass "accord legal rights to the unborn only where the mother's or parents' interest in the potentiality of life, not the state's interest, are sought to be vindicated." In other words, a viable fetus should only be accorded the rights of a person for the sake of its mother or both its parents. Under this rationale, the viable fetus lacks rights of its own that deserve vindication. Whitner suggests we should interpret our decisions in Hall, Fowler, and Horne to accord rights to the viable fetus only when doing so protects the special parent-child relationship rather than any individual rights of the fetus or any State interest in potential life. We do not think Hall, Fowler, and Horne can be interpreted so narrowly.

If the Pellegrini decision accurately characterizes the rationale underlying Mone, Lawrence, and Cass, then the reasoning of those cases differs substantially from our reasoning in Hall, Fowler, and Horne. First, Hall, Fowler, and Horne were decided primarily on the basis of the meaning of "person" as understood in the light of existing medical knowledge, rather than based on any policy of protecting the relationship between mother and child. As a homicide case, Horne also rested on the State's—not the mother's—interest in vindicating the life of the viable fetus. Moreover, the United States Supreme Court has repeatedly held that the states have a compelling interest in the life of a viable fetus. . . . If, as Whitner suggests we should, we read Horne only as a vindication of the mother's interest in the life of her unborn child, there would be no basis for prosecuting a mother who kills her viable fetus by stabbing it, by shooting it, or by other such means, yet a third party could be prosecuted for the very same acts. We decline to read Horne in a way that insulates the mother from all culpability for harm to her viable child. Because the rationale underlying our body of law—protection of the viable fetus—is radically different from that underlying the law of Massachusetts, we decline to follow the decision of the Massachusetts Superior Court in Pellegrini. . . .

Right to Privacy

Whitner argues that prosecuting her for using crack cocaine after her fetus attains viability unconstitutionally burdens her right of privacy, or, more specifically, her right to carry her pregnancy to term. We disagree.

Whitner argues that section 20-7-50 burdens her right of privacy, a right long recognized by the United States Supreme Court. . . . She cites Cleveland Board of Education v. LaFleur, 414 U.S. 632, 94 S.Ct. 791, 39 L.Ed.2d 52 (1974), as standing for the proposition that the Constitution protects women from measures penalizing them for choosing to carry their pregnancies to term.

In LaFleur, two junior high school teachers challenged their school systems' maternity leave policies. The policies required "every pregnant school teacher to take maternity leave without pay, beginning [four or] five months before the expected birth of her child." A teacher on maternity leave could not return to work "until the beginning of the next regular school semester which follows the date when her child attains the age of three months." The two teachers, both of whom had become pregnant and were required against their wills to comply with the school system's policies, argued that the policies were unconstitutional.

The United States Supreme Court agreed. It found that "[b]y acting to penalize the pregnant teacher for deciding to bear a child, overly restrictive maternity leave regulations can constitute a heavy burden on the exercise of these protected freedoms." The Court then scrutinized the policies to determine whether "the interests advanced in support of" the policy could "justify the particular procedures [the School Boards] ha[d] adopted." Although it found that the purported justification for the policy—continuity of instruction—was a "significant and legitimate educational goal," the Court concluded that the "absolute requirement[s] of termination at the end of the fourth or fifth month of pregnancy" was not a rational means for achieving continuity of instruction and that such a requirement "may serve to hinder attainment of the very continuity objectives that they are purportedly designed to promote." Finding no rational relationship between the purpose of the maternity leave policy and the means crafted to achieve that end, the Court concluded the policy violated the Due Process Clause of the Fourteenth Amendment.

Whitner argues that the alleged violation here is far more egregious than that in LaFleur. She first suggests that imprisonment is a far greater burden on her exercise of her freedom to carry the fetus to term than was the unpaid maternity leave in LaFleur. Although she is, of course, correct that imprisonment is more severe than unpaid maternity leave, Whitner misapprehends the fundamentally different nature of her own interests and those of the government in this case as compared to those at issue in LaFleur.

First, the State's interest in protecting the life and health of the viable fetus is not merely legitimate. It is compelling. . . .

Even more importantly, however, we do not think any fundamental right of Whitner's—or any right at all, for that matter—is implicated under the present scenario. It strains belief for Whitner to argue that using crack cocaine during pregnancy is encompassed within the constitutionally recognized right of privacy. Use of crack cocaine is illegal, period. No one here argues that laws criminalizing the use of crack cocaine are themselves unconstitutional. If the State wishes to impose additional criminal penalties on pregnant women who engage in this already illegal conduct because of the effect the conduct has on the viable fetus, it may do so. We do not see how the fact of pregnancy elevates the use of crack cocaine to the lofty status of a fundamental right.

Moreover, as a practical matter, we do not see how our interpretation of section 20-7-50 imposes a burden on Whitner's right to carry her child to term. In LaFleur, the Supreme Court found that the mandatory maternity leave policies burdened women's rights to carry their pregnancies to term because the policies prevented pregnant teachers from exercising a freedom they would have enjoyed but for their pregnancies. In contrast, during her pregnancy after the fetus attained viability, Whitner enjoyed the same freedom to use cocaine that she enjoyed earlier in and predating her pregnancy—none whatsoever. Simply put, South Carolina's child abuse and endangerment statute as applied to this case does not restrict Whitner's freedom in any way that it was not already restricted. The State's imposition of an additional penalty when a pregnant woman with a viable fetus engages in the already proscribed behavior does not burden a woman's right to carry her pregnancy to term; rather, the additional penalty simply recognizes that a third party (the viable fetus or newborn child) is harmed by the behavior.

Section 20-7-50 does not burden Whitner's right to carry her pregnancy to term or any other privacy right. Accordingly, we find no violation of the Due Process Clause of the Fourteenth Amendment.

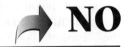

Punishment and Prejudice: Judging Drug-Using Pregnant Women

The Villain Cocaine

In the late 1980s and into the 1990s newspapers, magazines, and television were full of stories documenting the devastating effects of cocaine and predicting a lost generation irredeemably damaged by the effects of their mothers' cocaine use. For example, in 1991 *Time* magazine ran a cover story on the subject.[1] Bold yellow letters read "Crack Kids" followed by the headline: "Their mothers used drugs, and now it's the children who suffer." The face of a tearful child filled the page beneath the words. . . .

The same year the *New York Times* ran a front page story entitled "Born on Crack and Coping with Kindergarten."[2] The story is accompanied by a photograph of a school teacher surrounded by young children. Underneath the caption reads: "I can't say for sure it's crack, said Ina R. Weisberg, a kindergarten teacher at P.S. 48 in the Bronx, but I can say that in all my years of teaching I've never seen so many functioning at low levels."

Throughout these years medical and popular journals, public school teachers and judges alike were willing to assume that if a child had a health or emotional problem and he or she had been exposed prenatally to cocaine, then cocaine and cocaine alone was the cause of the perceived medical or emotional problem. Rather than wait for careful research and evaluation of the drug's effect there was, as several researchers later criticized, a "rush to judgment" that blamed cocaine for a host of problems that the research simply has not borne out.[3]

Indeed, an article in the medical journal *Lancet* in 1989 found that scientific studies that concluded that exposure to cocaine prenatally had adverse effects on the fetus had a significantly higher chance of being published than more careful research finding no adverse effects.[4] The published articles, delineating the harmful effects on infants prenatally exposed to cocaine, reported brain damage, genito-urinary malformations, and fetal demise as just a few of the dire results of a pregnant woman's cocaine use. Infants that survived the exposure were described as inconsolable, unable to make eye contact, emitting a strange high-pitched piercing wail, rigid and jittery. These early studies, however, had numerous methodologic flaws that made generalization from them

From *Mother Troubles: Rethinking Contemporary Maternal Dilemmas Trouble,* ed. by Julia E. Hanigsberg, Sara Ruddick, 1999. Copyright © 1999 by Beacon Press. Reprinted by permission.

completely inappropriate. For example, these studies were based on individual case reports or on very small samples of women who used more than one drug. Researchers often failed to control for the other drugs and problems the mother might have, and/or failed to follow up on the child's health.[5] The articles describing these studies were nevertheless relied upon to show that cocaine alone was the cause of an array of severe and costly health problems.

Like alcohol and cigarettes, using cocaine during pregnancy can pose risks to the woman and the fetus. More carefully controlled studies, however, are finding that cocaine is not uniquely or even inevitably harmful. For example, unlike the devastating and permanent effects of fetal alcohol syndrome, which causes permanent mental retardation, cocaine seems to act more like cigarettes and marijuana, increasing certain risks like low birth weight but only as one contributing factor and only in some pregnancies.[6] Epidemiological studies find that statistically speaking many more children are at risk of harm from prenatal exposure to cigarettes and alcohol. In fact, one recent publication on women and substance abuse has created the label "Fetal Tobacco Syndrome" to draw attention to the extraordinarily high miscarriage and morbidity rates associated with prenatal exposure to cigarette smoke.[7]

By the late 1980s it was already becoming clear to researchers in the field that the labels "crack babies" and "crack kids" were dangerous and counterproductive.[8] If one read far enough in the *Time* article—past the pictures of premature infants and deranged children—the story reported that

> [a]n increasing number of medical experts, however, vehemently challenge the notion that most crack kids are doomed. In fact, they detest the term crack kids, charging that it unfairly brands the children and puts them all into a single dismal category. From this point of view, crack has become a convenient explanation for problems that are mainly caused by a bad environment. When a kindergartner from a broken home in the impoverished neighborhood misbehaves or seems slow, teachers may wrongly assume that crack is the chief reason, when other factors, like poor nutrition, are far more important.

Even the *New York Times* article about crack-exposed children in kindergarten eventually revealed that researchers "after extensive interviews [found] the problems in many cases were traced not to drug exposure but to some other traumatic event, death in the family, homelessness, or abuse, for example."[9] And despite the fact that school administrators "rarely know who the children are who have been exposed to crack . . . and the effects of crack are difficult to diagnose because they may mirror and be mixed up with symptoms of malnutrition, low birth-weight, lead poisoning, child abuse and many other ills that frequently afflict poor children," the article resorts to crack as the only reasonable explanation for an otherwise seemingly inexplicable phenomenon. . . .

The Public Responds

The public response to the media and medical journal reports was largely one of outrage. The harshest reaction was the call for the arrest of the pregnant women and new mothers who used drugs. Numerous states considered legislation to make it a crime for a woman to be pregnant and addicted.[10] Although not a single state legislature passed a new law creating the crime of fetal abuse, individual prosecutors in more than thirty states arrested women whose infants tested positive for cocaine, heroin, or alcohol. Many of these women were arrested for child abuse, newly interpreted as "fetal" abuse. Others, like Jennifer Johnson in Florida, were charged with delivery of drugs to a minor.[11] In that case, the prosecutor argued that the drug delivery occurred through the umbilical cord after the baby was born but before the umbilical cord was cut. Still other women were charged with assault with a deadly weapon (the weapon being cocaine), or feticide (if the woman suffered a miscarriage), or homicide (if the infant, once born, died). Some women were charged with contributing to the delinquency of a minor.

While arrests were almost always the result of the action of an individual prosecutor, in the state of South Carolina there was unprecedented coordination between health care providers, the prosecutor's office, and the police.

In 1989, the city of Charleston, South Carolina, established a collaborative effort among the police department, the prosecutor's office, and a state hospital, the Medical University of South Carolina (MUSC), to punish pregnant women and new mothers who tested positive for cocaine. Under the policy, the hospital tested certain pregnant women for the presence of cocaine. Women were tested for the presence of cocaine to further criminal investigations, but the women never consented to these searches and search warrants were never obtained.

While the hospital refused to create a drug treatment program designed to meet the needs of pregnant addicts, or to put even a single trained drug counselor on its obstetrics staff, it did create a program for drug-testing certain patients, their in-hospital arrest, and removal to jail (where there was neither drug treatment nor prenatal care); the ongoing provision of medical information to the police and prosecutor's office; and tracking for purposes of ensuring their arrest. Some women were taken to jail while still bleeding from having given birth. They were handcuffed and shackled while hospital staff watched with approval. All but one of the women arrested were African American. The program itself had been designed by and entrusted to a white nurse who admitted that she believed that the "mixing of races was against God's will."[12] She noted in the medical records of the one white woman arrested that she lived "with her boyfriend who is a Negro."[13] . . .

Who Are These Mothers?

As a report from the Southern Regional Project on Infant Mortality observed:

> Newspaper reports in the 1980s sensationalized the use of crack cocaine and created a new picture of the "typical" female addict; young, poor, black, urban, on welfare, the mother of many children and addicted to crack. In interviewing nearly 200 women for this study, a very different picture of the "typical" chemically dependent woman emerges. She is most likely white, divorced or never married, age 31, a high school graduate, on public assistance, the mother of two or three children, and addicted

to alcohol and one other drug. It is clear from the women we interviewed that substance abuse among women is not a problem confined to those who are poor, black, or urban, but crosses racial, class, economic and geographic boundaries.[14]

African American women have been disproportionately targeted for arrest and punishment, not because they use more drugs or are worse mothers, but because, as Dorothy Roberts explains, "[t]hey are the least likely to obtain adequate prenatal care, the most vulnerable to government monitoring, and the least able to conform to the white middle-class standard of motherhood. They are therefore the primary targets of government control."[15]

Beyond the stock images and prejudicial stereotypes, the media has given the public little opportunity to meet or get to know the pregnant women on drugs. If we never learn who they are it is inevitable that their drug use will seem inexplicably selfish and irresponsible. Yet, if we could meet them and learn their history, we might be able to begin to understand them and the problems that need to be addressed.

Let me give an example. In the popular television show *NYPD Blue* we get to know the irascible Detective Sipowicz. While he is neither handsome nor charming, we come to care for him. We learn that he is an alcoholic who is able to stop drinking and improve his life. When he has a massive relapse and behaves outrageously, effectively abandoning his new wife and their newborn son, committing crimes of violence and countless violations of his responsibilities as a police officer, we nevertheless want to forgive him and give him another chance.

We are able to sympathize, at least in part because we have been given the information about why he has relapsed. His first son, whom he has finally reconnected with, is murdered, and Sipowicz, who can't handle it emotionally, turns back to the numbing, relief-giving effects of alcohol.

Sipowicz, in the end, is supported by his police colleagues who cover up for him and give him yet another chance. By contrast, when the same program did an episode involving a heroin-addicted pregnant woman, whose drug habit leads her two older sons to a life of crime, we never get to know why she has turned to drugs. We do not know as we did with Sipowicz what could have driven her to this behavior. The viewer can only assume that her drug use is purely selfish, stemming from a thoughtless hedonism. Thus, she is not entitled to understanding, sympathy, or the many second chances Sipowicz's character routinely gets.

But like Sipowicz, pregnant women who use drugs also have histories and complex lives that affect their behavior and their chances of recovery. We know that substance abuse in pregnancy is highly correlated with a history of violent sexual abuse.[16] In one study 70 percent of the pregnant addicted women were found to be in violent battering relationships. A hugely disproportionate number, compared to a control group, were raped as children. Drugs appear to be used as a means to numb the pain of a violent childhood and adulthood. Like Vietnam veterans who self-medicated with drugs for their post-traumatic stress disorders, at least some pregnant women also use drugs to numb the pain of violent and traumatic life experiences.[17]

Are their difficult childhoods or their experiences with violence an excuse for drug use? No. But the information begins to provide some idea of root causes that might need to be taken into consideration when trying to imagine the appropriate societal reaction. Will the threat of jail remove the trauma and pain that in many instances prompted the drug use and stands in the way of recovery? It is not that a woman who uses drugs is not responsible, but rather that we have to hold her responsible in a context that takes into account the obstacles, internal and external, that stand in the way of recovery. . . .

All pregnant women, not just poor ones, are routinely denied access to the limited drug treatment that exists in this country. In a landmark study in 1990, Dr. Wendy Chavkin surveyed drug treatment programs in New York City. She found that 54 percent flat out refused to take pregnant women.[18] Sixty-seven percent refused to take women who relied on Medicaid for payment, and 84 percent refused to take crack-addicted pregnant women.

One hospital in New York was sued for excluding women from drug treatment. The program argued that its exclusion of all women was justified and no different from its medical judgment to exclude all psychotics.[19] While New York State courts found that such exclusion violated state law, this did not automatically increase needed services. . . .

Other barriers also exist. [In the case of Jennifer Johnson, a pregnant Florida woman,] Judge Eaton ruled that "the defendant also made a choice to become pregnant and to allow those pregnancies to come to term." The prosecutor argued that "[w]hen she delivered that baby she broke the law." By saying this, the judge makes clear that it was having a child that was against the law. If Ms. Johnson had had an abortion she would not have been arrested—even for possessing drugs.[20] But this statement not only reveals a willingness to punish certain women for becoming mothers, it also reflects a host of widely held beliefs and assumptions about access to reproductive health services for women.

For example, implicit in this statement is the assumption that Ms. Johnson had sex and became pregnant voluntarily. Given the pervasiveness of rape in our society, assuming voluntary sexual relations may not be justified. Perhaps, though, the judge, like many others, simply thought that addicts have no business becoming pregnant in the first place. A South Carolina judge put it bluntly: "I'm sick and tired of these girls having these bastard babies on crack cocaine." Apparently concerned about his candor, he later explained: "They say you're not supposed to call them that but that's what they are . . . when I was a little boy, that's what they called them."[21]

On call-in radio talk shows someone inevitably asks why these mothers can't just be sterilized or injected with Depo Provera until they can overcome their drug problems and, while they are at it, their low socioeconomic status. The consistency of this view should not be surprising given our country's history of eugenics and sterilization abuse. Indeed, the U.S. Supreme Court has declared sterilization of men unconstitutional, but has never overturned its decision upholding the sterilization of women perceived to be a threat to society.[22]

The suggestion of sterilization, however, is particularly attractive if there is no explanation about why a pregnant woman with a drug problem would want to become pregnant or to have a child in the first place. But drug-using pregnant women become pregnant and carry to term for the same range of reasons all women do. Because contraception failed. Because they fell in love again and hoped this time they could make their family work. Because they are "prolife" and would never have an abortion. Because when they found out the beloved father of the baby was really already married, they thought it was too late to get a legal abortion. Because they do not know what their options might be. Because they have been abused and battered for so long they no longer believe they can really control any aspect of their lives including their reproductive lives. Because they wanted a child. Because their neighbors and friends, despite their drug use, had healthy babies and they believed theirs would be healthy too.

The threat of sterilization is just another punitive response that denies the humanity of the women themselves. Although Judge Eaton did not propose sterilization as part of the sentence he imposed on Ms. Johnson, as some judges in related cases have,[23] he undoubtedly assumed that Ms. Johnson could decide, once pregnant, whether or not to continue that pregnancy to term. Since 1976, however, the United States government has refused to pay for poor women's abortions and few states have picked up the costs.[24] In Florida, like most other states, the "choice" Judge Eaton spoke of does not exist for low-income women. . . .

Lack of access to abortion services is only one of the many barriers that exist for a drug-addicted pregnant woman who attempts to make responsible "choices." There are many other barriers that make it extremely difficult for pregnant women on drugs to get the kind of help and support they need. Access to services for drug-addicted women who are physically abused is also limited. For example, many battered women's shelters are set up to deal with women who have experienced violence, but are not equipped to support a woman who has become addicted to drugs as a way to numb the pain of the abuse.[25] Other barriers include lack of housing, employment, and access to prenatal care. As one of the few news stories to discuss these women's dilemmas explains:

> Soon after she learned she was pregnant, [Kimberly] Hardy [who was eventually prosecuted for delivery of drugs to a minor], convinced she had to get away from her crowd of crack users as well as her crumbling relationship with her [boyfriend] Ronald, took the kids home to Mississippi for the duration of her pregnancy. But by moving, she lost her welfare benefits, including Medicaid. Unable to pay for clinic visits, she had to go without prenatal care.[26]

And what about the men in their lives? Their contributions to the problem, physiologically and socially, are ignored or deliberately erased. Rarely in the media do we know what has happened to the potential fathers. Their drug use, abandonment, and battering somehow miraculously disappear from view.

Nevertheless, men often do play a significant role. For example, in California Pamela Rae Stewart was arrested after her newborn died. One of her alleged crimes contributing to the child's ultimate demise was having sex with her husband on the morning of the day of the delivery. Her husband, with whom she had had intercourse, was never arrested for fetal abuse. Indeed, the prosecutor's court papers argued that Ms. Stewart had "subjected herself to the rigors of intercourse," thereby totally nullifying the man's involvement or culpability.[27]

Prosecutors in South Carolina have also managed to ignore male culpability, even when it is the father who is supplying the pregnant woman with cocaine or other potentially harmful substances. Many women arrested in this state were not identified as substance addicted until after they had given birth, a point at which their drug use could not even arguably have a biological impact on the baby. Prosecutors argued that arrest was still justified because evidence of a woman's drug use during pregnancy is predictive of an inability to parent effectively. But fathers identified as drug users are not automatically presumed to be incapable of parenting. Indeed, when a man who happens to be a father is arrested for drunk driving, a crime that entails a serious lack of judgment and the use of a drug, he is not automatically presumed to be incapable of parenting and reported to the child welfare authorities. Prosecutors nevertheless rely on biological differences between mothers and fathers, arguing that a man's drug use could not have hurt the developing baby in the first place. However, studies indicate that male drug use can affect birth outcome: Studies on male alcohol use have demonstrated a relationship between male drinking and low birth weight in their children and a study of cocaine and men suggests that male drug use can also affect birth outcome.[28]

We continue to live in a society with double standards and extremely different expectations for men and women. Drug use by men is still glorified, while drug use by women is shameful, and by pregnant women a crime. This could not have been better demonstrated than by an advertising campaign by Absolut vodka. On Father's Day, as a promotional gimmick, Absolut sent 250,000 free ties to recipients of the *New York Times* Sunday edition. Scores of little sperm in the shape of Absolut vodka bottles swim happily on the tie's blue background. So while many call for arrest when a pregnant woman uses drugs or alcohol, fathers who drink are celebrated and, in effect, urged to "tie one on."

Of course, none of these arguments is made to suggest that women are not responsible for their actions or that they are unable to make choices that reflect free will. Rather, it is to say that popular expectations of what acting responsibly looks like and notions of "choice" have to be modified by an understanding of addiction as a chronic relapsing disease, of the degree to which our country has abandoned programs for poor women and children, and of the time, strength, and courage it takes for a drug-addicted woman to confront her history of drug use, violence, and abandonment. Compassion and significantly more access to coordinated and appropriate services will not guarantee that all of our mothers and children are healthy. But medical experts and both children's and women's rights advocates agree that such an approach is far more likely to improve health than are punishment and blame. . . .

The problem with treating the fetus as a person is that women will not simply continue to be less than equal, they will become nonpersons under the law. [To oppose the recognition of fetal personhood as a matter of law is not to deny the value and importance of potential life as a matter of religious belief, emotional conviction, or personal experience. Rather, by opposing such a new legal construct, we can avoid devastating consequences to women's health, prenatal health care, and women's hope for legal equality.— L.P.] No matter how much value we place on a fetus's potential life, it is still inside the woman's body. To pretend that the pregnant woman is separate is to reduce her to nothing more than, as one radio talk show host asserted, a "delivery system" for drugs to the fetus.

Notes

1. *Time Magazine* (13 May 1991).

2. Suzanne Dale, "Born on Crack and Coping with Kindergarten," *New York Times* (7 February 1991), A1.

3. Linda C. Mayes, R. H. Granger, M. H. Bornstein, and B. Zuckerman, "The Problem of Cocaine Exposure, A Rush to Judgment," *Journal of the American Medical Association* 267 (1992): 406.

4. Gideon Koren, Karen Graham, Heather Shear, and Tom Einarson, "Bias Against the Null Hypothesis: The Reproductive Hazards of Cocaine," *Lancet* (1989): 1, 1440–1442.

5. Mayes, "The Problem of Cocaine Exposure"; B. Lutiger, K. Graham, T. R. Einarson, and G. Koren, "Relationship Between Gestational Cocaine Use and Pregnancy Outcome: A Meta-Analysis," *Teratology* (1991): 44, 405–414.

6. Barry Zuckerman et al., "Effect of Maternal Marijuana and Cocaine Use on Fetal Growth," *New England Journal of Medicine* 320, no. 12 (23 March 1990): 762–768; Deborah A. Frank and Barry S. Zuckerman, "Children Exposed to Cocaine Prenatally: Pieces of the Puzzle," *Neurotoxicology and Teratology* 15 (1993): 298–300; Deborah A. Frank, Karen Breshahn, and Barry Zuckerman, "Maternal Cocaine Use: Impact on Child Health and Development," *Advances in Pediatrics* 40 (1993): 65–99.

7. Center on Addiction and Substance Abuse at Columbia University, *Substance Abuse and the American Woman* (1997); Joseph R. DiFranza and Robert A. Lew, "Effect of Maternal Cigarette Smoking on Pregnancy Complications and Sudden Death Syndrome," *Journal of Family Practice* 40 (1995): 385. Cigarette smoking has been linked to as many as 141,000 miscarriages and 4,800 deaths resulting from perinatal disorders, as well as 2,200 deaths from sudden infant death syndrome, nationwide.

8. American Academy of Pediatrics, Committee on Substance Abuse. Drug Exposed Infants, *Pediatrics* 86 (1990): 639.

9. Dale, "Born on Crack."

10. Allison Marshall, 1992, 1993, 1994 Legislative Update, in *National Association for Families and Addiction Research and Education Update* (Chicago, 1993, 1994, 1995).

11. *Johnson v. State,* 602 So.2d 1288 (Fla. 1992).

12. Brown Trial Transcript, *Ferguson et al. v. City of Charleston et al.,* U.S. District Court for the District of South Carolina, Charleston Division, C/A No. 2:93-2624-1 at 5:18–21 (Dec. 10, 1996).

13. Plaintiffs' Exhibit 119, *Ferguson et al. v. City of Charleston et al.,* U.S. District Court for the District of South Carolina, Charleston Division, C/A No. 2:93-2624-1.

14. Shelley Geshan, "A Step Toward Recovery, Improving Access to Substance Abuse Treatment for Pregnant and Parenting Women," *Southern Regional Project on Infant Mortality* (1993): 1.

15. Dorothy Roberts, "Punishing Drug Addicts Who Have Babies: Women of Color, Equality, and the Right of Privacy," *Harvard Law Review* 104, no. 7 (1991): 1419, 1422.

16. Dianne O. Regan, Saundra M. Ehrlich, and Loretta P. Finnegan. "Infants of Drug Addicts: At Risk for Child Abuse, Neglect, and Placement in Foster Care," *Neurotoxicology and Teratology* 9 (1987): 315–319.

17. Sheigla Murphy and Marsha Rosenbaum, *Pregnant Women on Drugs: Combating Stereotypes and Stigma* (New Brunswick, N.J.: Rutgers University Press, forthcoming).

18. Wendy Chavkin, "Drug Addiction and Pregnancy: Policy Crossroads," *American Journal of Public Health* 80, no. 4 (April 1990): 483–487.

19. *Elaine W. v. Joint Diseases North General Hospital Inc.,* 613 N.E.2d 523 (N.Y. 1993).

20. Lynn M. Paltrow, "When Becoming Pregnant Is a Crime," *Criminal Justice Ethics* 9, no. 1 (Winter–Spring 1990): 41–47.

21. *State v. Crawley,* Transcript of Record (Ct. Gen. Sess. Anderson Cnty., S.C., Oct. 17, 1994).

22. *Skinner v. Oklahoma,* 316 U.S. 535 (1942); *Buck v. Bell,* 274 U.S. 200 (1927); Stephen J. Gould, "Carrie Buck's Daughter," *Natural History* (July 1984).

23. *People v. Johnson,* No. 29390 (Cal.Super.Ct. Jan. 2, 1991).

24. *Harris v. McRae,* 448 U.S. 297 (1980).

25. Amy Hill, "Applying Harm Reduction to Services for Substance Using Women in Violent Relationships," *Harm Reduction Coalition* 6 (Spring 1998): 7–8.

26. Jan Hoffman, "Pregnant, Addicted and Guilty?" *New York Times Magazine* (19 August 1990): 53.

POSTSCRIPT

Should a Pregnant Woman Be Punished for Exposing Her Fetus to Risk?

In March 2001 the U.S. Supreme court ruled in the case of *Ferguson v. City of Charleston* (121 S.C. 1281) that the Medical University of South Carolina's policy was unconstitutional. In a six-to-three decision, the Court reversed the decision of the lower Fourth Circuit Court of Appeals and sent the case back to the circuit court for a factual determination of whether the women had actually consented to the search that led to their arrest and imprisonment. The circuit court had ruled that the searches were reasonable under the Fourth Amendment to the Constitution (which prohibits "unreasonable" searches) because of the "special need" to protect women and children from the consequences of cocaine use in pregnant women.

The Supreme Court, however, rejected this claim, arguing that it did not meet the same standard as, for example, the purpose of testing railway workers, customs employees, and high school athletes. Because the Court's decision rested on an interpretation of the Fourth Amendment, it did not settle the public policy and ethical challenges that remain concerning drug use and pregnant women.

For more on this decision, see George Annas, "Testing Poor Pregnant Women for Cocaine: Physicians as Police Investigators," *The New England Journal of Medicine* (May 31, 2001) and Lawrence O. Gostin, "The Rights of Pregnant Women: The Supreme Court and Drug Use," *Hastings Center Report* (September–October, 2001).

In Talbot County, Maryland, two women were convicted of child endangerment for continuing to take illegal drugs while pregnant. In August 2006 the state's highest court, the Court of Appeals, overturned the convictions on the grounds that the state did not intend the law prohibiting reckless endangerment of children to apply to women in relationship to their own pregnancies. If interpreted in this way, it could be used to apply to an array of activities, such as exercising too much or too little, or almost any potentially injury-inducing activity.

See also Drew Humphries, *Crack Mothers: Pregnancy, Drugs, and the Media* (Ohio State University Press, 1999).

Internet References . . .

Society for Adolescent Medicine

The Society for Adolescent Medicine is composed of professionals committed to improving the physical and psychosocial health of adolescents. This Web site provides many resources on the topic of adolescent health.

http://www.adolescenthealth.org

Center for Adolescent Health and the Law

This site has extensive material about minors' right to consent to medical treatment and access to health care.

http://www.cahl.org

Jehovah's Witnesses and Blood

The Watchtower Web site contains the official view of Jehovah's Witnesses on blood. The Web site of the Associated Jehovah's Witnesses for Reform on Blood interprets the ban differently.

http://www.watchtower.org/medical_care_and_blood.htm

http://ajwrb.org

Children and Bioethics

*C*hildren are often the subjects of controversies in biomedical ethics. Too young to make fully autonomous decisions, vulnerable to the pressures and interests of adults (including parents and health care providers), children are nonetheless persons in their own right with clear interests and a need for guidance and protection. Unless proven otherwise, parents are presumed to be the primary decision makers for their children. The common belief is that parents know and love their children, have a family history of values and choices, and can make informed choices about the best interests of their children. Yet this ideal does not always hold true, and in many cases what parents find acceptable, physicians or public health officials see as medical negligence. This section presents some of the most vexing dilemmas in medical ethics.

- Should Adolescents Make Their Own Life-and-Death Decisions?

- Do Parents Harm Their Children When They Refuse Medical Treatment on Religious Grounds?

ISSUE 10

Should Adolescents Be Allowed to Make Their Own Life-and-Death Decisions?

YES: Robert F. Weir and Charles Peters, from "Affirming the Decisions Adolescents Make About Life and Death," *Hastings Center Report* (November–December 1997)

NO: Lainie Friedman Ross, from "Health Care Decisionmaking by Children: Is It in Their Best Interest?" *Hastings Center Report* (November–December 1997)

ISSUE SUMMARY

YES: Ethicist Robert F. Weir and pediatrician Charles Peters assert that adolescents with normal cognitive and developmental skills have the capacity to make decisions about their own health care. Advance directives, if used appropriately, can give older pediatric patients a voice in their care.

NO: Pediatrician Lainie Friedman Ross counters that parents should be responsible for making their child's health care decisions. Children need to develop virtues, such as self-control, that will enhance their long-term, not just immediate, autonomy.

A patient is brought to the emergency room after an accident. The physicians believe that he will die if he does not receive a blood transfusion, but the patient says that he is a Jehovah's Witness and will not accept blood. A cancer patient has undergone months of debilitating therapy with discouraging results; she says that she does not want any more treatment. These patients have the right to refuse treatment because they are adults. What if they were 15 or 16 years old? Would they have the same rights or could their wishes be overruled?

If there is one Golden Rule of contemporary bioethics, it is that competent adults are legally and ethically empowered to make health care decisions for themselves. Competent in this context means able to understand the choices and the consequences of decisions made. People base these decisions on values and preferences, personal experiences, religious beliefs, the availability of alternatives, level of pain and suffering, economic consequences, or any combination of these and other factors.

Except in unusual situations, parents are presumed to be in the best position to make these decisions for their children. Children, especially young children, are assumed to have neither the cognitive skills nor the mature judgment to make complex choices that may have far-reaching health consequences. Parents share the consequences of the decision so they make it with the best interests of their children and themselves in mind.

But adolescents are neither children nor fully mature adults. Where do they fit in this scheme? There are differences of opinion of how to define adolescence. Depending on the definition, adolescence may begin as young as 10 and end as late as 21. Legally the age of 18 defines the end of adolescence. However, that may not be an appropriate boundary for health care decision making. Those who support the idea that young people of a certain age should make their own health care decisions tend to call them "adolescents"; those who are critical of this view tend to call them "children" or "minors." In general adolescents have achieved a degree of emotional and intellectual maturity that surpasses that of young children. Still, they may be unable to appreciate long-term consequences of their actions.

In making health care decisions for children and adolescents, an alliance among the patient, parents, and physicians sometimes develops. Together they choose among alternative plans for treatment or, in the case of terminal illness, palliative care instead of aggressive treatment. However, parents, adolescents, and physicians do not always agree.

The selections that follow present two opposing views on whether adolescents should make their own life-and-death decisions. Robert F. Weir and Charles Peters argue for adolescent capacity and autonomy. They summarize an expanding body of professional literature to indicate that, with a few exceptions, adolescents are capable of making major health decisions and giving informed consent. Lainie Friedman Ross argues against the 1995 American Academy of Pediatrics recommendations that give children a greater voice in their care. She contends that it is the parents' right and responsibility to make decisions that enhance their children's long-term autonomy.

165

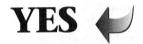

YES

**Robert F. Weir and
Charles Peters**

Affirming the Decisions Adolescents
Make About Life and Death

Some Illustrative Cases

Scott Rose was a talented adolescent who loved poetry, music, writing, and acting. Unfortunately, he had Nezelof syndrome, a cellular immunodeficiency disease similar to the condition of the famous "bubble boy" in Houston. Scott refused to remain in a similar enclosure, preferring to live as normal a life as his condition permitted. At the age of fourteen, with his lungs deteriorating and his suffering increasing, Scott decided that he could accept no more life-sustaining treatment. Against his physician's wishes but with tacit approval from his family, Scott died by disconnecting himself from the ventilator that was keeping him alive in a community hospital in Oklahoma.

C.G. was a fifteen-year-old with end-stage cystic fibrosis. During the last year of his life, he was hospitalized four times in a critical care unit for pneumonia and respiratory distress. He repeatedly expressed fear that his life would end in a slow, agonizing death. He realized that he was dying and stated that he did not want to "smother" or die on a ventilator. On his last admission, he experienced increasing respiratory distress and became disoriented as his carbon dioxide rose. However, his parents were adamant, insisting to the attending physician that "everything possible" be done to keep C.G. alive, including prolonged intubation and mechanical ventilation.

Benito Agrela was born with an enlarged liver and spleen. He received a liver transplant when he was eight years old, had a second liver transplant when he was fourteen, and then stopped taking his medication several months after the second transplant because he could not tolerate its side effects. When the Florida Department of Social Services discovered that he was not taking his antirejection medications, they forcibly removed him from his parents' home and admitted him to a transplant floor of a Miami hospital. After he refused further treatment, his case was taken to court; the circuit court judge spent several hours with Benito and his physicians, then ruled that Benito had a legal right to refuse the medications and return home. Before his death at the age of fifteen, Benito said: "I should have the right to make my own decision. I know the consequences, I know the problems."

M.C. was ten years old when she was diagnosed with acute lymphoblastic leukemia. During two years of chemotherapy, she maintained excellent grades, joined a swim team, and demonstrated, according to her teachers, "a particularly mature and far-reaching perspective on her life." Then the leukemia relapsed. Following discussions with a health care team and her parents, she decided that a partially matched, related donor bone marrow transplant was her best chance for continued life. Before she received the transplant, at the age of thirteen, she told her parents and others that she did not want to "grow up to be a vegetable," did not want to be supported on "a lot of machines," and did not want to be a psychological or financial burden on the family. Two months after the transplant, she was diagnosed as having an Epstein Barr virus-associated lymphoproliferative disorder. Despite aggressive treatment efforts in a pediatric ICU, her condition did not improve. Four days later the ventilator sustaining her life was withdrawn, at the request of her family and in keeping with her previously expressed wishes.

B.C. was a sixteen-year-old adolescent who was diagnosed with cystic fibrosis shortly after birth. Over the years, both his medical condition and his relationship with his parents deteriorated. He watched several friends with cystic fibrosis die, and mentioned on several occasions that he did not want to be placed on a ventilator. Nevertheless, even as his pulmonary tests deteriorated rapidly, his parents refused to discuss death with him, or any decisions that might need to be made about limiting life-sustaining treatment, the possibility of do-not-resuscitate status, or his preferences about treatment options. When he was soon thereafter admitted, unresponsive, following an unsuccessful suicide attempt, his parents requested that no life-sustaining measures be employed. They forbade the medical staff from discussing this matter with B.C., even when he became sufficiently alert to communicate.

Our reason for presenting these cases is simple. Every day, in hospitals throughout this country, adolescent patients cope with chronic conditions, struggle to survive with life-threatening illnesses, and think about the burdens of continued existence compared with the prospect of death. Sometimes, as indicated by Scott Rose and Benito Agrela, these adolescent patients conclude that death is preferable to the suffering they are experiencing, decide to refuse further life-sustaining interventions, and carry out that decision in spite of opposition from physicians and/or parents. Other times, as in the case of M.C., parents and physicians carry out the decision to abate life-sustaining treatment, knowing it to be consistent with the adolescent patient's wishes. Yet other times, as in the cases of C.G. and B.C., parents request, and physicians carry out, a plan of care that has not been discussed with the adolescent patient and may be completely contrary to his or her expressed wishes.

Such cases reflect the considerable uncertainty that sometimes surrounds the medical management of these patients. Do most adolescents have the capacity to make major decisions about their lives and health, even when they are hospitalized? Do only *some* adolescents have this decisionmaking capacity and, if so, what kinds of lines need to be drawn in terms of adolescent decisional abilities? Do adolescents have the right not only to *assent,* but also to *consent*—and to refuse to consent—to recommended medical treatment or participation in research studies? . . .

Adolescents as Capable Decisionmakers

An expanding body of professional literature indicates that adolescents, with some exceptions, are capable of making major health decisions and giving informed consent, whether in a clinical or research setting. An increasing number of professionals in developmental psychology, pediatrics, biomedical ethics, and health law agree that a fundamental reorientation toward adolescents—in clinical medicine, in research settings, and in the law—is necessary to increase adult acceptance of the important decisions that many adolescents now seem capable of making for themselves.

Numerous studies can be cited to make the basic point. Almost twenty years ago, a comprehensive analysis of the literature in developmental psychology by Thomas Grisso and Linda Vierling indicated that "generally minors below the ages of 11–13 do not possess many of the cognitive capacities one would associate with the psychological elements of 'intelligent' consent."[1] By contrast, the authors stated that there "is little evidence that minors of age 15 and above as a group are any less competent to provide consent than are adults." On the basis of their literature analysis, they concluded that "minors are entitled to have some form of consent or dissent regarding the things that happen to them in the name of assessment, treatment, or other professional activities that have generally been determined unilaterally by adults in the minor's interest." Similar conclusions came from an empirical study reported by Lois Weithron and Susan Campbell.[2]

In the pediatric literature, Sanford Leikin surveyed the findings of developmental psychologists, mainly those of Jean Piaget, and applied them to the issue of minors' assent or dissent to medical treatment. He observed that while cognitive development cannot always be equated with chronological age, good evidence exists "that, by age 14 years, many minors attain the cognitive developmental stage associated with the psychological elements of rational consent." As to other adolescent ages, he concluded that "minors between 11 and 14 years of age appear to be in a transition period . . . [and] there appear to be no psychological grounds for the general assumption that minors 15 years of age or older cannot provide competent consent."[3]

In a subsequent publication Leikin addressed the question of how parents and physicians should respond to the decisions made by adolescents to withhold or withdraw life-sustaining treatment. In large part, he argued, it depends on the psychological development of the adolescent in question and that person's ability to make "authentic choices" guided by logical thought patterns, a physiologic understanding of illness, and a willingness to make decisions independent of authority figures (a willingness, he pointed out, not usually found in adolescents less than fourteen or fifteen years of age).[4] Other writers agree.[5] . . .

Legal Developments

Even if most adolescents between age fourteen and seventeen increasingly are regarded as having the capacity to make health decisions for themselves, and even if leading pediatric groups have for over twenty years called for an expansion of adolescent rights in health care settings, important questions about the law remain. . . .

Traditionally, state laws reflected the view that adolescents and other legal minors under the age of twenty-one were incapable of understanding, deliberating about, and making decisions regarding important health care choices. The power to make such decisions was vested in parents, legal guardians, or someone standing in *loco parentis* to a child. Any physician who might have provided nonemergency medical care to a legal minor without parental consent risked being charged with civil battery (performing treatment without consent), even if there was no charge of malpractice.[6]

Legal minors and personal health decisions. During the past three decades, this view of legal minors has changed in a number of ways. One important change involves the age of majority. Until 1971, the standard age of majority was twenty-one, with a perennial debate focusing on the differences in age required for voting compared with the age required for being drafted into the military. That debate stopped with the passage of the 26th amendment to the Constitution in 1971, thereby permitting persons aged between eighteen and twenty to vote in federal elections. Most state legislatures subsequently lowered the age of majority to eighteen, thus granting legal adulthood to millions of persons who previously could not vote, make contractual obligations, or consent to medical treatment apart from their parents.[7]

Another change in the law involves the creation of exceptional legal categories for some adolescents to make personal health decisions. Two such categories are common among the states. Some adolescents, depending on the state, are legally recognized as *emancipated minors* on the basis of marriage, parenthood, military service, consent of parents (for example, adolescents who are "thrown away" by parents after family conflicts), judicial order of emancipation, or financial independence. Some state statutes (such as in Arizona, Idaho, Massachusetts, Montana, Nevada, North Carolina, Oregon, and Texas) specifically grant emancipated minors the right to consent to medical treatment.

Other adolescents are legally recognized in some jurisdictions as *mature minors* for the purpose of making health decisions because of their individual ability to understand the nature and purposes of recommended medical treatment. The "mature minor rule" recognizes that some adolescents are sufficiently mature to make their own decisions about recommended medical treatment and, when necessary, to go against their parents' views regarding the treatment. Physicians who carry out these decisions seem to run little legal risk, since there are no reported judicial decisions over the past twenty-five years in which parents have recovered damages for the medical treatment of an adolescent over the age of fifteen without parental consent.[8]

A third change in the law pertains to *minor treatment statutes* according to which states permit legal minors to consent to certain types of medical care. These statutes usually specify certain health problems for which legal minors can seek medical treatment without parental consent, precisely because the nature of the health problems is such that some adolescents would probably choose to go without medical treatment rather than seek their parents' consent for the treatment. Such statutes are typically limited to treatment for sexually transmitted diseases, pregnancy and pregnancy prevention (including abortion in some states, but not sterilization), alcohol and other drug abuse, and in some states, psychiatric problems.

Legal minors, end-of-life decisions, and state legislatures.   Despite these changes, most state legislatures have not addressed the issue of treatment refusal by adolescents, especially in circumstances in which a refusal of life-sustaining treatment is likely to result in the adolescent's death. Thus, even though forty-seven states have living will statutes (the exceptions are Massachusetts, Michigan, and New York) and forty-eight states have surrogate decisionmaking statutes that include end-of-life decisions (the exceptions are Alabama and Alaska), the legislative statutes in thirty-eight states and the District of Columbia do not specifically address end-of-life decisions made by legal minors.[9]

Most state legislatures seem to think that adolescents either do not die in clinical settings, or are incapable of making informed consent or informed refusal decisions about treatment options, must be protected from their own lack of judgment, or simply should not be permitted to give legally binding advance directions regarding life-sustaining treatments and surrogate decisionmakers. If a given adolescent does not qualify for emancipation under state law, does not live in one of the three states (Alaska, Arkansas, and Mississippi) having a mature-minor statute, and is unable or unwilling for some reason to go through a judicial hearing to be designated a mature minor, he or she is left with only three options: (1) persuading parents and physicians to act according to the adolescent's expressed views on life-sustaining treatment, (2) persuading parents to execute an advance directive on the patient's behalf (in the seven states having this legal option), or (3) acquiescing to the views of legal adults (namely, parents and physicians) regarding the medical circumstances under which the remaining portion of life is to be lived. . . .

Advance Directives and Moral Persuasion

Most adolescents who want to participate in the decisionmaking process connected with their medical conditions, especially in regard to decisions about life-sustaining medical interventions, have chronic conditions that often deteriorate over time: certain kinds of cancer, cystic fibrosis, AIDS, complicated types of heart disease, and so on. Having experienced years of physical and psychological suffering, gone through multiple hospitalizations and numerous treatments, probably experienced depression, and probably observed the suffering and dying of several hospitalized friends with similar medical problems, these adolescent patients are frequently mature beyond their chronological years. They have had, at the very least, multiple opportunities to think about the inescapable suffering that characterizes their lives, the features of life that make it worth continuing, the benefits and burdens that accompany medical treatment, and the prospect of death. At least some of these adolescents want to give voice to their values, provide directions for parents, physicians, and nurses regarding end-of-life care, and be assured that their wishes and preferences will be respected and carried out should their medical conditions deteriorate to the point that they will no longer be able to communicate their deeply felt views.

How parents, physicians, nurses, and other health professionals respond to these adolescents' desires for control and self-determination at the end of life is vitally important. These adults, individually and collectively, may simply *choose not to* listen. Alternatively, parents, physicians, and other adults involved in these cases may think that these personal life-and-death decisions are *primarily matters of law,* quite apart from the wishes and preferences expressed by individual patients. If so, the attending physician will likely check with hospital legal counsel, who will report on relevant statutory and case law and give legal advice that, understandably, will be protective of the hospital's legal interests. . . .

There is a third alternative. Parents, physicians, and other adults involved in these cases may regard the thoughtful comments, the verbalized reflections on the meaning of life and death, and the communicated choices regarding treatment options by *at least some* (perhaps most) adolescents with life-threatening conditions as *efforts of moral persuasion,* quite apart from what the law may or may not say.[10] Parents may reluctantly conclude that their son or daughter has suffered enough, seen enough, and communicated enough to convince them that however much they may want their child to live, he or she has the moral right to make end-of-life decisions that, when carried out, will result in death. Physicians, nurses, and other health care professionals also may be convinced.

Advance directives can help meet this goal, especially if the use of such directives becomes an acceptable part of the informed consent process in pediatric medicine. Enabling at least some adolescent patients—patients with chronic, life-threatening conditions—to communicate their decisions about treatment options through oral or written advance directives would also provide a measure of legal protection for physicians. Pediatricians, family practice physicians, and other physicians having such cases would be more able to document the specific end-of-life treatment decisions made by these patients, the maturity and decisionmaking capacity of individual patients, and the conversations about consenting to or refusing life-sustaining treatment that had taken place with the patients and their parents.

References

1. Thomas Grisso and Linda Vierling, "Minors' Consent to Treatment: A Developmental Perspective," *Professional Psychology* 9 (August 1978): 412–427, at 420.

2. Lois A. Weithorn and Susan B. Campbell, "The Competency of Children and Adolescents to Make Informed Treatment Decisions," *Child Development* 53 (1982): 1589–98.

3. Sanford L. Leikin, "Minors' Assent or Dissent to Medical Treatment," *Journal of Pediatrics* 102 (1983): 173.

4. Sanford L. Leikin, "A Proposal Concerning Decisions to Forgo Life-Sustaining Treatment for Young People," *Journal of Pediatrics* 108 (1989): 17–22, at 20; Leikin, "The Role of Adolescents in Decisions Concerning Their Cancer Therapy," *Cancer Supplement* 71 (15 May 1993): 3342–46.

5. For example, C. E. Lewis, "A Comparison of Minors' and Adults' Pregnancy Decisions," *American Journal of Orthopsychiatry* 50 (1980): 446–53; Richard H. Nicholson, ed., *Medical Research with Children* (Oxford: Oxford University Press, 1986), p. 140–52; Angela Holder, *Legal Issues in Pediatrics and Adolescent Medicine,* 2d ed. (New Haven: Yale University Press, 1985), p. 133.

6. Sarah D. Cohn, "The Evolving Law of Adolescent Health Care," *Clinical Issues* 2 (1991): 201–7, at 201; Angela R. Holder, "Disclosure and Consent Problems in Pediatrics," *Law, Medicine & Health Care* 16 (1988): 219–28; Steven M. Selbst, "Treating Minors Without Their Parents," *Pediatric Emergency Care* 1 (1985): 168–73.

7. Richard A. Leiter, ed., *National Survey of State Laws* (Detroit: Gale Research Inc., 1993), pp. 279–91.

8. Angela R. Holder, "Children and Adolescents: Their Right to Decide about Their Own Health Care," in *Children and Health Care: Moral and Social Issues,* ed. Loretta Kopelman and John C. Moskop (Boston: Kluwer Academic Publishers, 1989), p. 163.

9. Information from Choice in Dying, New York, 1995.

10. Robert F. Weir, "Advance Directives as Instruments of Moral Persuasion," in *Medicine Unbound,* ed. Robert H. Blank and Andrea L. Bonnicksen (New York: Columbia University Press, 1994), pp. 171–87.

Lainie Friedman Ross 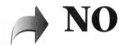 **NO**

Health Care Decisionmaking by Children

In pediatrics, the doctor-patient relationship traditionally has included three parties: the physician, the child, and his or her parents. Parents were not merely surrogate decisionmakers on the grounds of child incompetence, but rather, parents were believed to have both a right and a responsibility to partake in their child's medical decisions.[1] In this [selection] I will examine the evolving position regarding the role of the child in the decisionmaking process as advocated by the American Academy of Pediatrics (AAP). I will offer both moral and pragmatic arguments why I believe this position is misguided.

Recommendations of the American Academy of Pediatrics

In 1995, the AAP published its recommendations for the role of children in health care decisionmaking. The AAP recommended that the child's voice be given greater weight as the child matured. The AAP categorized children as (1) those who lack decisionmaking capacity; (2) those with a developing capacity; and (3) those who have decisionmaking capacity for health care decisions.[2]

For children who lack decisionmaking capacity, the AAP recommended that their parents should make decisions unless their decisions are abusive or neglectful. When children have developing decisionmaking capacity, the physician should seek parental permission and the child's assent. In many cases, the child's dissent should be binding, or at minimum, the physician should seek third-party mediation for parent-child disagreement. Although the child who dissents to life-saving care can be overruled, attempts should be made to persuade the child to assent for "coercion in diagnosis or treatment is a last resort." When children have decisionmaking capacity, the AAP concluded that the children should give informed consent for themselves and their parents should be viewed as consultants.

A major problem with the AAP recommendations is that it assumes decisionmaking capacity can be defined and measured, although the AAP offers no guidance as to what this definition is or how to test for it. Instead, the AAP

From *Hastings Center Report,* November–December 1997, pp. 41–45. Copyright © 1997 by Hastings Center Report. Reprinted by permission.

recommends individual assessment of decisionmaking capacity in each case. However, since there are no criteria on which to base maturity or decision-making capacity, the decision of whether to respect a child's decision is dependent upon the judgment of the particular pediatrician—a judgment he or she has no training to make.

My main concern with the AAP recommendations, however, is what should be done when parents and children disagree on health care decisions: according to the AAP, if there is parental-child disagreement and the child is judged to have decisionmaking authority, the child's decision should be binding. If the child has developing capacity, various mechanisms to resolve the conflict should be attempted. They propose:

> short term counseling or psychiatric consultation for patient and/or family, "case management" or similar multidisciplinary conference(s), and/or consultation with individuals trained in clinical ethics or a hospital based ethics committee. In rare cases of refractory disagreement, formal legal adjudication may be necessary.

I will ignore the difficulties in determining whether a minor has decisionmaking capacity and assume that some minors are competent to make at least some health care decisions. If autonomy is based solely on competency, then competent children should have decisionmaking autonomy in the health care setting. It is my view, however, that even if children are competent, there is a morally significant difference between competent minors and adults. Competency is a necessary but not a sufficient condition on which to base respect for a minor's health care decisionmaking autonomy.

Competency of Children

The psychological literature divides the process of giving informed consent into three components: the patient's consent is informed (made knowingly), is competent (made intelligently), and is voluntary.[3] Although a survey of the literature reveals scant empirical data, existing data suggest that most health care decisions made by adults and children do not fulfill these three components.[4] The data also suggest that adults and older children do not significantly differ in their consent skills.[5] If competency is the only criterion on which respect for autonomy in health care is based, then this difference in treatment cannot be justified.

No test has been developed that uniformly distinguishes all competent individuals from incompetent individuals. Given that competency is context-specific, it is doubtful whether such a test could be developed. And even if a nonculturally biased, objective test could be devised, individual testing of every potential patient would exact a high price in terms of efficiency, privacy, and respect for autonomy. Instead, adults have traditionally been presumed competent and children have been presumed incompetent. That is, respect for autonomy in health care uses both a threshold concept of competency and an age-standard.

To some extent the age-standard is arbitrary as there are individuals above the line (older than the legal age of emancipation) who are incompetent and individuals below the line (younger than the legal age of emancipation) who are competent. But the statutes are not capricious: in general, individuals above the line are more likely to be competent than individuals below it.

Autonomy of Children

One reason to limit the child's present-day autonomy is based on the argument that parents and other authorities need to promote the child's life-time autonomy. Given the value that is placed on self-determination, it makes sense to grant adults autonomy provided that they have some threshold level of competency. Respect is shown by respecting their present project pursuits. But respect for a threshold of competency in children places the emphasis on present-day autonomy rather than on a child's life-time autonomy. Children need a protected period in which to develop "enabling virtues"—habits, including the habit of self-control, which advance their life-time autonomy and opportunities. Although many adults would also benefit from developing their potentials and improving their skills and self-control, at some point (and it is reasonable to use the age of emancipation as the proper cut-off), the advantages of self-determination outweigh the benefits of further guidance and its potential to improve life-time autonomy.

A second reason to limit the child's present-day autonomy is the fact that the child's decisions are based on limited world experience and so her decisions are not part of a well-conceived life plan. Again, many adults have limited world experience, but children have a greater potential for improving their knowledge base and for improving their skills of critical reflection and self-control. . . . By protecting the child from his own impetuosity, his parents help him obtain the background knowledge of the world and the capacities that will allow him to make decisions that better promote his life plans. His parents' attempt to help him flourish may not be achieved, but that does not invalidate their attempt.

A third reason childhood competency should not necessarily entail respect for a child's autonomy is the significant role that intimate families play in our lives. Elsewhere, I have argued that when the family is intimate, parents should have wide discretion in pursuing family goals, goals which may compete and conflict with the goals of particular members.[6] In general, parental autonomy promotes the interests and goals of both children and parents. It serves the needs and interests of the child to have autonomous parents who will help him become an autonomous individual capable of devising and implementing his own life plan. It serves the adults' interest in having and raising a family according to their own vision of the good life. These interests do not abruptly cease when the child becomes competent. If anything, now parents have the opportunity to inculcate their beliefs through rational discourse, instead of through example, bribery, or force.

There are also pragmatic reasons to permit parents to override the present-day autonomy of competent children. First, one can argue for a determination of competency that allows unusually mature children to be emancipated. The problem, as I have already mentioned, is that no such test exists. Second, one can acknowledge that it is best if parents recognize their child's maturity and treat them accordingly, but deny that this justifies granting competent children legal emancipation. Many parents respect their mature child's decisions voluntarily. Laura Purdy remarks: "It is plausible to think that children's maturity is not completely unrelated to parental good sense."[7] Child liberationists may object because a voluntary approach only encourages parents to respect their children's autonomy, but it does not legally enforce it. However, the voluntary approach is more consistent with a policy to limit the state's role in intrafamilial decisions, which is important for the family's ability to flourish.

Health Care Rights in Context

A final argument against respecting the health care decisions of minors is based on placing the notion of health care rights in context. Most individuals who support health care decisionmaking for children view it as an exception and do not seek to emancipate children in other spheres. But why should a child who is competent to make major health care decisions not have the right to make other types of decisions? That is, if a fourteen-year-old is competent to make life-and-death decisions, then why can't this fourteen-year-old buy and smoke cigarettes? Participate in interscholastic football without his parents' consent? Or even drop out of school? . . .

What would it mean to endorse equal rights for children? It is a radical proposal with wide repercussions.[8] It would mean that children could make binding contracts, and that there would be the dissolution of child labor laws, mandatory education, statutory rape laws, and child neglect statutes. As such, it would give children rights for which they are ill-prepared and deny them the protection they need from predatory adults. It would leave children even more vulnerable than they presently are.

Endorsement of child liberation would make a child's membership in a family voluntary. For example, Howard Cohen argues that children should be allowed to change families, either because the child's parents are abusive, or because a neighbor or wealthy stranger offers him a better deal.[9] Such freedom ignores the important role that continuity and permanence play in the parent-child relationship—a significance the child may not yet appreciate.[10] . . .

The Family as the Locus of Decisionmaking

One of my major concerns with the AAP's recommendations is their willingness to involve third-parties in the decisionmaking process. My concern is that these decisions undermine the family. Physicians provide only for the child's transient medical needs; his parents provide for all of his needs and are responsible for raising the child in such a way that he becomes an autonomous responsible adult. Goldstein and colleagues at Yale University's Child Study Center expressed their concern that health care professionals sometimes forget where their professional responsibilities end, and described the harm that we do when we think we can replace parents.[11] By deciding that the child's decision should be respected over the parents' decision, physicians are replacing the parents' judgment that the decision should be overridden with their judgment that the child's decision should be respected. To do so makes this less an issue of respecting the child's autonomy, and more about deciding who knows what is best for the child. In general, parents are the better judge as they have a more vested interest in their child's well-being and are responsible for the day-to-day decisions of child-rearing. It behooves physicians to be humble as they are neither able nor willing to take over this daily function.

I do not mean to suggest that children, particularly mature children, should be ignored in the decisionmaking process. Diagnostic tests and treatment plans should be explained to children to help them understand what is being done to them and to garner, when possible, their cooperation. Parents should include their children in the decisionmaking process both to get their active support and to help them learn how to make such decisions. However, when there is parental-child disagreement, the child's decision should not be decisive nor should health care providers, as I have argued, seek third-party mediation. Rather, as I have already argued, there are both moral and pragmatic reasons why the parents should have final decisionmaking authority.

References

1. Allen Buchanan and Dan Brock, *Deciding for Others: The Ethics of Surrogate Decision Making* (New York: Cambridge University Press, 1989).

2. American Academy of Pediatrics, Committee on Bioethics, "Informed Consent, Parental Permission, and Assent in Pediatric Practice," *Pediatrics* 95 (1995): 314–17.

3. Thomas Grisso and Linda Vierling, "Minor's Consent to Treatment: A Developmental Perspective," *Professional Psychology* 9, no. 3 (1978): 412-27.

4. Paul S. Appelbaum, Charles W. Lidz, and Alan Meisel, *Informed Consent: Legal Theory and Clinical Practice* (New York: Oxford University Press, 1987); Stanley Milgram, *Obedience to Authority: An Experimental View* (New York: Harper and Row, 1974).

5. Grisso and Vierling, "Minor's Consent to Treatment."

6. Lainie Friedman Ross, *Health Care Decision Making for Children*, unpublished manuscript, 1996.

7. Laura M. Purdy, *In Their Best Interest? The Case Against Equal Rights for Children* (New York: Cornell University Press, 1992).

8. Richard Farson, "A Child's Bill of Rights," in *Justice: Selected Readings,* ed. Joel Feinberg and Hyman Gross (Belmont, Calif.: Dickenson Publishing Co. 1977).

9. Howard Cohen, *Equal Rights for Children* (Totowa, N.J.: Rowman and Littlefield, 1980); John Harris, "The Political Status of Children," in *Contemporary Political Philosophy,* ed. Keith Graham (Cambridge, Mass.: Cambridge University Press, 1982), pp. 35–55.

10. Joseph Goldstein, Anna Freud, and Albert J. Solnit, *Before the Best Interests of the Child* (New York: The Free Press, 1979).

11. Joseph Goldstein et al., *In the Best Interest of the Child* (New York: The Free Press, 1986).

POSTSCRIPT

Should Adolescents Be Allowed to Make Their Own Life-and-Death Decisions?

In August 2006, Starchild Abraham Cherrix, a 16-year-old Virginia adolescent with Hodgkin's disease, a form of cancer, was granted the right to pursue a course of Hoxsey therapy instead of chemotherapy. Hoxsey therapy is an alternative form of herbal therapy that is illegal in the United States but is available in Mexico. The case was settled out of court at the start of what was to be a two-day hearing. In this case starchild Abraham's parents supported his decision to forego the second round of chemotherapy that his doctors recommended.

Three earlier cases are discussed in Isabel Traugott and Ann Alpers, "In Their Own Hands: Adolescents' Refusals of Medical Treatment," *Archives of Pediatric and Adolescent Medicine* (September 1, 1997). Although published in 1985, *Legal Issues in Pediatrics and Adolescent Medicine* by Angela Roddey Holder (Yale University Press) is still a classic text. She supports the right of competent adolescents to make treatment decisions. Other documents supporting this position are the 1995 statement of the American Academy of Pediatrics (cited in the selection by Ross) and "Health Care Decision Making Guidelines for Minors," (Midwest Bioethics Center, 1995). Hillary Rodham Clinton also supports children's rights in several articles, including "Children's Rights: A Legal Perspective," *Children's Rights: Contemporary Perspectives*, edited by Patricia A. Vardin and Ilene N. Brody (Teachers College Press, 1979). Among those critical of the movement to grant children and adolescents more decision-making authority is Laura M. Purdy, *In Their Best Interests? The Case Against Equal Rights for Children* (Cornell University Press, 1992). In "Minor Rights and Wrongs," *Journal of Law, Medicine & Ethics* (Summer 1996), Michelle Oberman urges particular concern about cases in which adolescents refuse life-sustaining treatment.

In *The Adolescent "Alone": Decision Making in Health Care in the United States* (Cambridge University Press, 1999), Jeffrey Blustein, Nancy N. Dubler, and Carol Levine present a series of papers and case studies concerning adolescents who do not have a parent or surrogate in their lives to help them make health care decisions.

ISSUE 11

Do Parents Harm Their Children When They Refuse Medical Treatment on Religious Grounds?

YES: Massachusetts Citizens for Children, from "Death by Religious Exemption," http://www.masskids.org/dbre/dbre_1.html (January 1992)

NO: Mark Sheldon, from "Ethical Issues in the Forced Transfusion of Jehovah's Witness Children," *The Journal of Emergency Medicine* (vol. 14, no. 2, 1996)

ISSUE SUMMARY

YES: Massachusetts Citizens for Children, an advocacy organization, asserts that laws exempting parents from responsibility to provide medical care for their seriously ill children, on the basis of religious beliefs, result in needless deaths and mislead parents about their legal responsibilities.

NO: Professor of philosophy Mark Sheldon assesses the case of Jehovah's Witness parents who refuse to allow their children to undergo blood transfusions and concludes that they cannot be said to be truly harming or neglecting their children. Rather, they are placing their children's spiritual interests above worldly ones.

On May 6, 1989, an 11-year-old Minnesota boy named Ian Lundman complained of stomach pains. Acting in accordance with her beliefs as a lifelong Christian Scientist, his mother, Katherine McKown, prayed for Ian but did not call a doctor. When the boy had not improved the following day, Ms. McKown sought the healing prayers of two Christian Science practitioners. Three days later, Ian was dead.

Christian Scientists believe that healing through prayer is scientific and effective and that if a patient dies, it is because the prayers had not been strong enough. Based on a state law that allows parents to rely on spiritual treatment for their children, Minnesota courts dismissed manslaughter charges against Ian's mother, stepfather, and the Christian Science practitioners. In 1993 Ian's father, Douglass Lundman, filed a civil suit against the four people who were involved in his son's death. A doctor testified that Ian had diabetes that could easily have been treated with insulin, while representatives of the First Church of Christ, Scientist (the official name of the church) testified that many people have been healed through prayer. The jury awarded Mr. Lundman $1.5 million in damages and assessed the Christian Science Church $9 million. An appeals court upheld the judgment against the four defendants but dismissed the punitive damages against the church. In January 1996 the U.S. Supreme Court turned down a petition to restore the punitive damages, leaving the $1.5 million award intact.

Although few such cases reach the Supreme Court, they occur with troubling frequency and place some of the most cherished values in American society into conflict. Religious freedom and family privacy are pitted against society's obligation, through the medical profession and the courts, to protect the health and welfare of all children. In the most extreme cases, such as Ian's, honoring one value inevitably means violating the other.

Some of the debate turns on what constitutes child abuse and neglect. The legal picture is neither clear nor consistent. The federal Child Abuse Prevention and Treatment Act of 1974 defines abuse and neglect as "the physical and mental injury, negligent treatment, or maltreatment of a child under the age of 18 by a person who is responsible for the child's welfare under circumstances which indicate that the child's health and welfare is harmed or threatened thereby." However, state interpretations of the federal definition vary.

Cultural and religious differences clearly influence the interpretation of abuse and neglect statutes, especially where medical neglect is involved. Christian Scientists have been leaders in convincing many state legislatures to exclude religiously based refusals of medical treatment from child abuse and neglect statutes, and more than 40 states have passed laws recognizing spiritual treatment as an acceptable form of health care for children. In the past decade, however, some states have revoked these laws.

In general, the perspective of Jehovah's Witnesses differs from those of Christian Science and other religions that offer alternatives to modern medical care. Jehovah's Witnesses refuse only one intervention: the transfusion of whole blood and blood products. This refusal reflects a core belief in their religion. Jehovah's Witnesses take biblical bans on "eating" blood literally. Blood transfusion is held to violate this ban, and those who accept blood in this manner face loss of eternal life. Because blood transfusion is a common procedure in surgery and in the treatment of some diseases, cases involving refusal by Jehovah's Witnesses arise relatively frequently.

The following selections probe these dilemmas. Massachusetts Citizens for Children argues that parents harm children when they deny them the benefits of medical care because of religious beliefs. Laws that exempt parents not only result in preventable deaths but still leave parents open to prosecution. Mark Sheldon asserts that the concept of harm is not appropriately applied to cases involving Jehovah's Witnesses because parents are sincerely acting in what they believe to be the child's higher interests—protecting the possibility of eternal life.

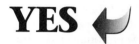
Death By Religious Exemption

Religious Exemption Laws Lead to Cruel Deaths, Mislead Parents

Religious Exemption Laws Lead to the Cruel and Unnecessary Deaths of Helpless Children; These Laws also Falsely Mislead Parents Regarding Their Legal Duty to Provide Necessary Medical Care for Their Seriously Ill Children

The deadly consequences of religious exemption laws are apparent nationwide: over the past 25 years there have been over 150 reported deaths of children whose parents chose to rely on faith healing rather than medicine.

There are at least 20 different sects and religious groups in the U.S. whose teachings deny the use of medical care. These groups include: Faith Assembly, Christian Science, The Believer's Fellowship, Faith Tabernacle, Church of the First Born, Church of God of the Union Assembly, Church of God Chapel, Faith Temple Doctoral Church of Christ in God, Jesus through John and Judy, Christ Miracle Healing Center, NE Kingdom Community Church, Christ Assembly, The Source, True Followers of Christ, "No Name" Fellowship, End Time Ministries, Faith Cathedral Fellowship, Living Word Assembly of God, Traveling Ministries Everyday Church.

Christian Science is the largest and most prominent of these groupings. Church membership is estimated at 100,000–200,000 persons. The church estimates it has 1,800 churches and societies active in all parts of the United States. Since the 1970's there have been at least 18 deaths of Christian Science children; these deaths occurred when the parents denied their children medical care in favor of purely "spiritual healing." Of these deaths: three were from juvenile onset diabetes, an illness which can be controlled by insulin but which is otherwise invariably fatal; four from bacterial meningitis, a deadly illness which, with proper administration of antibiotics, is 90 percent curable; one from a ruptured appendix; one from pneumonia, and one from diphtheria (due to lack of vaccination).

Forty-four states have had religious exemption laws in force since the mid-1970's. (In 1990 South Dakota became the first state to repeal its religious exemptions from health care requirements for sick children.) Furthermore, the above deaths are only those that have come to public attention. Certainly there are other known and unknown cases of death, injury, prolonged suffering, and permanent disability of children whose parents have refused effective medical treatment.

In 1988, the national office of the American Civil Liberties Union made the following statement regarding state religious exemption laws:

> *Children have rights too, and parents have certain rights which end when they intrude too far into a child's right to live . . . the parent's right to bring up the child in the way the parent thinks best—an important right . . . ends at the point at which the parents' actions endanger the lives of kids . . . there cannot be in our view a religious exemption no matter how sincere a parent's belief. . .*

Prior to 1982, "For nearly seven years after religious immunity was put under federal mandate, no charges of child abuse, neglect, or manslaughter were filed in any cases of religiously-based medical neglect. Beginning in 1982, though, prosecutors filed charges in some deaths of children due to religious beliefs against medical care. From 1982 through 1989, criminal charges were filed in 29 such cases. To date there have been 21 convictions, 5 acquittals . . . of the 29 cases, 7 involved Christian Scientists, with a result of 5 convictions for manslaughter and child endangerment." (Swan, The Law's Response When Religious Beliefs Against Medical Care Impact on Children, 1990).

How is it that parents can be prosecuted in the deaths of their children when states have legislated religious exemption? Prosecutors and courts have determined that the state religious exemption laws do not necessarily exempt parents from responsibility from obtaining medical care if a child is seriously ill or if the illness results in the child's death. In 1988, the California Supreme Court (*People v. Walker*) determined that the state's religious exemption law applies only to the neglect statute and does not carry over to the state's manslaughter statute. The Twitchells in Boston were convicted under a similar interpretation of the Massachusetts religious exemption law.

Not only do the religious exemption laws leave children vulnerable to death and disability, the laws can mislead (and be used by their churches to mislead) parents into believing that the state allows the substitution of prayer for medical care. Only when it is too late, after the agony of a child's death, do parents come to realize they are accountable under the law. In effect, religious exemption laws are punitive rather then preventative.

> *It would be better, however, to make a parent's legal duty clear before a child dies. Many parents would be relieved to obey the law if the state would make its standards clear. They do not comprehend the risks they are taking with their child when the state seems to endorse the withholding of medical care.*

Rita Swan, "Barriers to Medical Care for Children: How You Can Help," The Exchange, Jan.–Feb., 1988.

Swan, in the same article, further went on to state:

No one is trying to outlaw prayer. Doctors are willing for people of any denomination to pray for their patient. Religious exemptions appear to make prayer a legal substitute for the medical care needed by a sick child.

Prayer cannot be a substitute for medicine in serious childhood illnesses in which medical treatment has proven its effectiveness over decades or when medicine is expected to have some reasonable likelihood of success.

Faith and reason may both have their place in healing, but not the same place. The state must remain neutral between religions, defending everyone's right to believe. But that does not mean it must remain neutral between "treatment," as if spiritual healing and science were equal options for curing a bowel obstruction.

Ellen Goodman, "Healing: Faith vs. Reason,"
Boston Globe, July 12, 1990

But where the issue is beyond real scientific dispute—as for example, with an operable malignant tumor, a case of acute appendicitis or treatable condition like juvenile diabetes—the state must have the power to compel parents to treat their children medically until they become adults.

Alan Dershowitz, "Let's Not Sacrifice Kids to Religion,"
Boston Herald, April 16, 1990

Religious exemption laws are unconscionable because they deprive a group of children of the basic rights and protections of life and health guaranteed by law to all other children. In effect religious exemption to medical care constitutes an apparent state sanction of child abuse/neglect.

The conviction that led to a sentence of 10 years' probation for David and Ginger Twitchell ought to alert Americans to a legal double standard that subjects the children of Christian Scientists to risks that are not tolerated for any other child. In ordinary circumstances, parental failure to safeguard a child's health, including seeking medical care for a grave illness, constitute child neglect or abuse and is subject to prosecution. But 43 states, including Massachusetts . . . provide an exemption for Christian Scientists, whose faith rejects medical care in favor of "spiritual healing." Given modern scientific knowledge, the legal exemptions can't be excused. Society has a duty to say that Christian Science parents may take whatever personal hazards they choose on practicing their religion—but they may not expose their children to the risk of death and disability by refusing medical treatment. Editorial, Chicago Tribune, July 8, 1990.

Lawrence Tribe, a leading constitutional lawyer at Harvard, stated in a Boston Herald article on July 7, 1990: There should be a very clear duty on the part of all parents to take children to the doctor when a certain threshold is reached. Repealing the religious exemption would make it clear in the future that people like the Twitchells have to call in a doctor.

⌘

Why Reporting System and Court Orders Are Not Sufficient

Why the Abuse Reporting System and Court Orders Are Not Sufficient to Protect the Life and Health of Children Whose Parents Rely on Spiritual Healing to the Exclusion of Medicine

The Christian Science Church and other proponents of religious exemption laws claim that the preservation of the religious exemption to the parental duty to provide children with necessary medical care does not unduly threaten the life of children. Supporters of religious exemptions argue that, under the Chapter 119 child abuse and neglect reporting system, a Massachusetts court can order necessary medical care for a seriously ill child through a temporary custody proceeding.

Why deprive parents of their right to practice their religion when, if it is absolutely necessary, a court can order necessary medical care?

The dangerous fallacy in this argument is that very often, seriously ill Christian Science children and children in other sects never come to the attention of a reporting authority until it is too late to prevent permanent disability or death.

Serious illness in Christian Science children often occurs *completely outside the reporting system*; unlike Jehovah's Witnesses who will use doctors and hospitals, Christian Science parents, in many cases, deny the effectiveness of medicine and will not take their children to doctors. A doctor or a hospital cannot request a court order for a child they are unaware of.

Christian Science utilizes its own organization of "spiritual healers" and (non-medical) "nurses" to treat childhood illnesses, including serious and life-threatening illnesses. These practitioners are *not* mandated reporters under the Massachusetts abuse and neglect reporting law. And in states where they are, practitioners may not report because they may not believe the child to be in danger. Christian Science healers and nurses have no training in medical diagnosis and treatment. In order to be accredited by the church, the spiritual healer must complete only a two-week class in non-physical, spiritual healing.

In fact, Christian Science healers believe that illness does not result from physical causes, but rather occurs because of lack of spiritual closeness to God. They believe that medical care can be an obstacle to health because it mistakenly treats the body rather than the spirit. The sole method of treatment is prayer and most often this treatment is conducted at a distance by telephone. Moreover,

> The Christian Science Church tells its health care providers not to report contagious diseases to the state. It dissuades them from reporting cases of sick children deprived of medical care to protective services agencies.

Rita Swan, "The Law's Response When Religious Beliefs
Against Medical Care Impact on Children," 1990

Because Christian Science healers and nurses cannot be expected to either identify or report serious childhood illness, Christian Science children are often insulated from the reporting system.

Additionally, school teachers and other public authorities cannot be counted on to make the reporting system work for seriously ill Christian Science children. The following is a direct quotation from the "Legal Rights and Obligation Handbook of Christian Science Parents in Massachusetts" published by the church in 1983: (This book was taken out of circulation only after it was criticized by the Twitchell Inquest judge.)

> *But it should be recognized that care of children is given special importance under Massachusetts laws relating to the protection and care of children, to the extent that the right of the parent can be usurped by court order . . . Thus, if a child is being given Christian Science treatment for an illness, inquiries made by school or other public officials as to care of the child should be answered with assurance that such child is being given good care and is having treatment for the illness. Otherwise, such official may incorrectly conclude that the child is a neglected child. In talking with such officials, a parent should stay clear of statements such as "belief of illness" or "claim of sickness" which may result in the official thinking that the illness is being ignored . . .*

In other words, the Church is not encouraging its parents to help the reporting system work.

Massachusetts cannot place life and health of Christian Science children or the children of other religious sects exclusively in the hands of the reporting system. The tragic fact is that the reporting systems in Massachusetts and other states have been unable to prevent the deaths of Christian Science children and the children of other faith-healing sects. No doctor or court ever knew that Robyn Twitchell lay dying in his own home. In Florida, in 1986, six-year-old Amy Hermanson died of juvenile onset diabetes. Amy deteriorated over a six week period; a report was made to Child Protective Services only shortly before her death and a hearing was concluded the hour before she died. Abuse reporting systems did not intervene to prevent the deaths of three Christian Science children in 1984 of bacterial meningitis in California.

The combination of the religious exemption law and the Massachusetts Chapter 119 reporting system seriously exacerbates the threat to the lives and health of children whose parents choose to rely exclusively on spiritual healing. Because the religious exemption appears to allow parents to rely solely on prayer, parents may try to shield an ill child from the reporting system so that they may continue to avoid medical care.

The religious exemption creates an incentive for parents to keep a child's illness hidden, thereby avoiding necessary medical assessment. This contradiction fails to meet a proper moral and practical standard for guiding responsible parental behavior and ensuring protection.

The Massachusetts religious exemption law must be repealed so that parents who utilize spiritual healing will have the same legal duty as all other parents to provide their seriously ill children with necessary medical care. Children's lives cannot be left totally dependent on Protective Services action. Parents have the legal custody of children and, therefore, have 24-hour a day responsibility for them. As such, they have far more awareness of their children's illnesses than do mandatory reporters. The state cannot and should not be in the position of having to continually monitor the health of Christian Science children or the children of other faith-healing sects.

Mark Sheldon 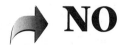 **NO**

Ethical Issues in the Forced Transfusion of Jehovah's Witness Children

Beliefs of Jehovah's Witnesses

Jehovah's Witnesses are Christians who believe the Bible is the Word of God in its entirety. Their name is taken from a statement that appears in the book of Isaiah: "Ye are my witnesses, saith Jehovah" (Isa. 43:10). . . . Presently, there are estimated to be approximately 2.2 million Jehovah's Witnesses in more than 200 countries around the world, with about 554,000 Witnesses in the United States (1).

As a group, Jehovah's Witnesses have faced numerous challenges. In the 1930s and 1940s, when their right to make home visitations was challenged, the courts affirmed their right to freedom of speech. Jehovah's Witnesses comply with most modern medical and surgical procedures, and a number of Witnesses are physicians and surgeons (2). They do not smoke, use recreational drugs, or have abortions. They view life as sacred. Why, then, do Witnesses appear to contradict this commitment to the idea that life is sacred, and reject blood transfusions at critical moments when it is a matter of life and death? In their pamphlet, *Jehovah's Witnesses and the Question of Blood* (3), they make the following statement:

> The issues of blood for Jehovah's Witnesses . . . involves the most fundamental principles on which they as Christians base their lives. Their relationship with their creator and God is at stake.

The seriousness of the question of blood for Witnesses can be compared to the seriousness of idolatry for Jews. . . .

It is the Acts of Apostles, in particular, which serves most centrally as the basis for the rejection of blood transfusions. After listing those things from which believers should abstain, it reads: ". . . from which if ye keep yourselves, ye shall do well" (Acts 15:28 29).

Therefore, Jehovah's Witnesses take literally the numerous passages which proscribe the consumption of blood. They believe that the violation of

From *The Journal of Emergency Medicine,* vol. 14, no. 2, 1996, pp. 251 257. Copyright © 1996 by American Academy of Emergency Medicine. Reprinted by permission of Elsevier Science, Inc.

this proscription will result in loss of eternal life. Witnesses do not reject this world. To the contrary, they value and seek bodily health. Still, they do not think "physical life is limited to this present, temporal existence" (4). They believe that it is wrong to contrast "physical life" with "eternal life." Rather, Witnesses believe that God will, in the future, destroy life on earth, ending both personal life and conscious spiritual life. Eventually, they believe, God will resurrect the bodies of the faithful, and a limited number "will reign with God in heaven, while the remainder will live a life without end on a renewed earth" (4). They believe that life in the future, therefore, will be physical, earthly, and eternal. . . .

The Legal Framework

. . . When adults are concerned, the courts generally have determined that the competent adult Jehovah's Witness, who has no dependent minor children, has a right to refuse blood transfusion (5). When children are concerned, however, the situation is very different. Interestingly enough, the decision that appears to have set the major precedent, *Prince v. Massachusetts* (1944), was not a case dealing with medical treatment, but with child labor laws (5). An aunt, who was the legal custodian of a 9-year-old, had the child on the street with her selling Jehovah's Witness magazines. Although this was in violation of child labor laws, the defense claimed that Jehovah's Witnesses were required by their religion to spread the gospel. The little girl indicated that she wanted to sell the magazines to avoid eternal damnation. Defense, therefore, claimed that this was a violation of her right to freedom of religious belief. In response, the Supreme Court ruled that the state has authority as *parens patriae* to act in the interest of the child's well being, and that, on this basis, parental control can be restricted. While this particular decision had nothing to do with transfusion, the court (6) reached this conclusion:

> Neither the rights of religion nor the rights of parenthood are beyond limitation. . . . Parents may be free to make martyrs of themselves, but they are not free to make martyrs of their children before they have reached the age when they can make that choice for themselves.

A series of court decisions followed upholding *Prince,* but also dealing with the legitimacy of state intervention in matters that do or do not involve life-or-death situations. Again, it is interesting to note that *Prince* did not involve a life-and-death situation (5).

Witnesses' Views Regarding Children

In their pamphlet, *Jehovah's Witnesses and the Question of Blood* (3), the Witnesses make the following statement:

> Jehovah's Witnesses are sure that obeying the directions from their Creator is for their lasting good. . . .

The Witnesses then make the point that their refusal of blood transfusion cannot rightfully be construed either as suicide or as an exercise of the right to die, but it must be seen as respect for God's word (3).

In addressing the issue of children, Witnesses (3) make the following argument:

> Likely the aspect of this matter that is most highly charged with emotion involves the treating of children. All of us realize that children need care and protection. God-fearing parents particularly appreciate this. They deeply love their children and keenly feel their God-given responsibility to care for them and make decisions for their lasting welfare.—Ephesians 6:14.
>
> Society, too, recognizes parental responsibility, acknowledging that parents are the ones primarily authorized to provide for and decide for their children. Logically, religious beliefs in the family have a bearing on this. Children are certainly benefited if their parents' religion stresses the need to care for them. That is so with Jehovah's Witnesses, who in no way want to neglect their children. They recognize it as their God-given obligation to provide food, clothing, shelter and health care for them. Moreover, a genuine appreciation of the need to provide for one's children also requires inculcating in them morality and regard for what is right. . . .
>
> Parents who are Jehovah's Witnesses show great love for their children as well as their God by using the Bible to become moral persons. Thus, when these children are old enough to know what the Bible says about blood, they themselves support their parents decision to abstain from blood.—Acts 15:29.

. . . Witnesses indicate that they are fully aware of the significance of their refusal of blood transfusion for their children. However, they state that they do this out of devotion to God and out of love for their children. They claim that they cherish their children and are concerned for their children's future welfare. They do not believe that their actions should be construed as neglect. Rather, they believe that they probably are better parents than many parents in the larger society. They point to society's toleration for loose parenting, which leads to children growing up without respect for life, morality, or themselves. They hold up as examples the early Christian families who died at the hands of the Romans as models. Further, Witnesses claim to have evidence that as their children grow, they made the same choices that their parents previously made for them.

The aspect of the quote that should be emphasized is that Jehovah's Witness parents perceive themselves as acting in their children's best interest. They do not want their children to be "cut off" from the possibility of obtaining eternal life. They do not believe that it is in any way appropriate to describe their actions as involving neglect or disregard for their children. It is true, of course, that their belief that they may be better parents than others does not provide support for their right to deny blood transfusion to their children. Also, it is not clear what evidence they have to support their claim that their children will, when grown, reach the same decision as they have. But it seems clear that to describe their actions as neglectful is problematic. . . .

The Ethics Literature

Uniformly, the ethics literature expresses the view that it is right for the state to take temporary custody of a child to force it to undergo a blood transfusion in cases 1) when the lack of transfusion will lead to the child's death and 2) when the child is too young to give assent. However, I also believe that the basis upon which the state takes such action is not well defended in the existing ethics literature. This section consists of a review of representative arguments supporting state intervention, along with criticism of these arguments.

In 1977, Ruth Macklin (7) wrote, in an article still much referred to and often anthologized, the following:

> It might be argued that Jehovah's Witness parents, in refusing permission for blood to be given to their child, are acting in accordance with their perceived duty to God, as dictated by their religion, and that this duty to God overrides whatever secular duties they may have to preserve the life and health of their child.

Macklin (7) criticized this belief:

> Here it can only be replied that when an action done in accordance with perceived duties to God results in the likelihood of harm or death to another person (whether child or adult), then the duties to preserve life here on earth take precedence. The duties of a physician are to preserve and prolong life and to alleviate suffering. . . . Freedom of religion does not include the right to act in a manner that will result in harm or death to another.

A few points in response to Macklin's argument are in order. The first and fundamental question is: from whose perspective is "harm" being defined? Second, she identifies "harm" with "death." These are not necessarily the same. She (7) states:

> If the parents refuse to grant permission for blood to be given to their child when failure to give blood will result in death or severe harm . . . , their prima facie right to retain control over their child no longer exists. . . . the case [at this point] sufficiently resembles that of child neglect [in respect to harm to the child]. . . . in the absence of fulfillment of their duties, it is morally justifiable to take control of the child away from the parent.

From Macklin's point of view, the act "sufficiently resembles child neglect." However, on what basis is this determined to be child neglect? This is only possible to claim if the religious perspective of the parents is set aside. What makes this move acceptable? The vague comment "sufficiently resembles child neglect" does not seem to provide such a basis.

Another interesting discussion of this issue appears in a 1983 article (8) that appeared in *Hospital Progress*. The article states: "The basic ethical principle involved is beneficence: One is obliged to do whatever good one reasonably can for another person" (8). The argument is different from Macklin's in that duty is seen positively (doing good) rather than negatively (avoiding harm). The article indicates a certain concern for the family and recognizes that it is "especially dangerous today, when society tends increasingly to allow the state to take over parents' functions" (8). However, it makes the following point (8):

> When the person is a minor, the obligation of beneficence falls primarily on the parents. When the parents for whatever reasons, even sincerely held religious beliefs, fail in this regard, then society, usually through its legal processes, must step in and provide for the child's good. Certain members of society, such as physicians or hospital administrators, are in a position to detect parental failure in these matters and therefore have a moral obligation to call the child's plight to civil authorities attention.

Two comments are necessary. The first is that the use of the language "parental failure" is heavily condemnatory, and not clearly appropriate. Second, while there may not be a problem, as there was above, in defining "harm," there is the problem of defining "good."

Another document that addresses the issue of state intervention is "Religious Exemptions From Child Abuse Statutes," produced by the Committee on Bioethics of the American Academy of Pediatrics in 1988 (9). This document is essentially a recommendation to change child abuse and neglect statutes that exempt parents on the basis of religious freedom. . . .

Again, as in the Macklin article, the problem exists concerning the fact that whether harm is present depends on the perspective from which it is identified. Also, what truly constitutes the "welfare" of the child is a matter of perspective.

Another representative approach in the ethics literature appears in an article by Gary Benfield, MD, published in *Legal Aspects of Medical Practice* (10). He attempts, he points out, to address the human side of the issue, and he does, one can argue, make a sincere effort to try to understand the feelings of the Jehovah's Witness parents. He describes one of his cases that involved a young Rh-positive mother who gave birth to an Rh-positive male. He quotes (10) the mother:

> Three days after the birth of our son, we were told that on the very day of his birth he was taken from us, by a simple dial of the phone, and given blood. . . . You have touched the very depth of my being. The pain I felt is the same pain had I been told of my son's death. . . . I realize it is difficult to understand how two people claiming to love their child are willing to let that child die. We as Jehovah's Witnesses believe in that promised kingdom of God's as a real ruling power, and when that kingdom that we all pray for does come to this earth, our son will be given back to us. We would just have to wait a little longer to watch him grow and to give him all the love we stored up for him in our hearts over the last few months. . . . Jehovah's Witnesses do not reject blood for their children due to lack of love. . . . If we violate God's law on blood and the child dies, we have endangered his opportunity for everlasting life in God's new world.

Benfield's comments, in response to the mother's statement, are interesting and revealing. He remarks that after he considered all the options, he chose the one that "would best benefit my innocent patient" (10), a description which seems to impute something negative and possibly exploitative to the mother's relationship with the child. Second, he explains the basis for his choice. This consists of him asking himself, "Can I live with this decision?" (10). His answer is, "Yes." One can argue, however, that there is a problem in resolving an ethical dilemma on this basis. Such a criterion allows for anything that human beings "can live with." It is probably the case that Benfield is a sensitive and caring person, but this is a dangerous way to proceed. Presumably (this comment is not meant to reflect on Benfield but on the methodology he employs to resolve ethical dilemmas), Nazi doctors could "live with" their decisions.

Benfield (10) continues:

> The parents felt that, by giving blood, I would compromise their son's chances for everlasting life. I disagreed. I felt that Jehovah, a loving God, would welcome their child in "God's new world" were he to die having received blood or not. Who was right?

In this passage, Benfield ventures beyond the basis justifying intervention expressed in the ethics literature quoted above. He does not focus on the issue of "harm" or "good" or "welfare." Instead, he is engaged in theological debate. This, of course, prompts a question concerning the expertise a physician must have in order to engage in such commentary, to make a judgment concerning the validity of another's religious belief. The question is not what Benfield does, but why. What legitimately entitles him to force a transfusion on the child? A claim to possess a more valid religious insight than the mother is not available to him simply by virtue of being a physician. Nothing about being a physician provides a basis for his conviction that he understands better than the mother does how God works. In addition, she does not make a decision on the basis of what she "can live with." She acts on the basis of scripture. For her, this is not a matter of speculation or theological debate. She acts in a way that is prescribed for her by her religious tradition.

Observations and Conclusions

The following observations and conclusions should be viewed as preliminary thoughts in response to the issues raised in this article. They are preliminary in the sense that more discussion is warranted. . . .

- The criticism of the ethics literature, contained in this paper, does not imply that there is no basis for the existence of statutes concerned with child abuse and neglect. This is a different question. The state, on this issue, appropriately takes guidance from scientists (psychiatrists and psychologists) who do studies, determine consequences, and measure pain and adverse reaction related to abuse and neglect. The state can develop expertise in this area and can claim knowledge of what constitutes child welfare, benefit, best interest, and harm. But where the issue is ultimately spiritual and where obtaining eternal life is the objective, it is clear that the state can make no claim to any sort of knowledge. Undergoing a blood transfusion may, in fact, cut off one from obtaining eternal life, and the state simply does not have the expertise and knowledge that would enable it to judge the merits of such a claim.

- Given this lack of expertise in such ultimate questions, the state, it seems to me, must accede that all talk of harm, benefit, best interest, and martyrdom amounts to what appears to be rhetoric and not argument. Jehovah's Witness parents, in refusing blood transfusion, cannot be said to be truly harming or neglecting their children. It is simply not the case that knowledge, which would make such a judgment legitimate, is available. That refusing a transfusion is harmful can certainly be believed, and one can argue that such is the case, but it cannot be known. Therefore, the state, in taking temporary guardianship to transfuse the child, cannot be said, with certainty, to be doing this for the child's welfare. It is simply not known whether this is the case.

What, therefore, makes it legitimate to order transfusions for the children of Jehovah's Witness? The most defensible argument is that the state's weakness is also its strength. That is, while the state does not know truly what is in the child's best interest, neither does anyone else. What the parents believe is in the child's best interest may be mistaken. Given that no one knows what is in the child's best interest, the role of the state is to ensure that children ultimately become adults, able to decide, independently, what is in their own best interest. It is not even that the state assumes that it knows it to be in the child's best interest to become an adult. It may not be. It is simply that no one knows what is in the child's best interest, and the responsibility of the state is to make certain that persons who make decisions which are irrevocable do so when they are competent. A source of disquiet is that many people believe, with good reason, that parents know what is in their child's best interest. This is a belief that is not easily dismissed. And, in fact, it is not dismissed here. Ideally, the family is a very significant moral institution. More than any other institution in society, the family, properly focused, values human beings simply because they *are,* not because of any use to which they can be put. And, for this reason, it is probably in a child's best interest (and society's best interest, as well) that the family be maintained to the extent that it is, as a unit, consistent with this objective of such nurturance.

References

1. Mead FS. Handbook of denominations in the United States. Nashville: Abingdon Press; 1980:148.

2. Dixon JL, Smalley MG. Jehovah's Witnesses: the surgical/ethical challenge. JAMA. 1981;246(27): 2471-2.

3. Jehovah's Witnesses and the question of blood. Brooklyn, NY: Watchtower Bible and Tract Society; 1977.

4. Studdard PA, Greene JY. Jehovah's Witnesses and blood transfusion: toward the resolution of a conflict of conscience. Ala J Med Sci. 1986;23(4):455.

5. Hirsh HL, Phifer H. The interface of medicine, religion, and the law: religious objections to medical treatment. Med Law. 1985;4(2):121–39.

6. Prince v. Massachusetts.

7. Macklin R. Consent, coercion and conflict of rights. Perspect Biol Med. 1977;20(365):365–6.

8. Editorial. May a Catholic hospital allow bloodless surgery for children? Hosp Prog. 1983;64(9): 58, 60.

9. Committee on Bioethics of the American Academy of Pediatrics. Religious exemptions from child abuse statutes. Pediatrics. 1988;81(1): 169–71.

10. Benfield DG. Giving blood to the critically ill newborn of Jehovah's Witness parents: the human side of the issue. Leg Aspects Med Pract. 1978;6(6):19–22.

POSTSCRIPT

Do Parents Harm Their Children When They Refuse Medical Treatment on Religious Grounds?

One solution to the problem posed by the refusal of Jehovah's Witnesses to undergo blood transfusions is to use alternative treatment methods, such as nonblood replacement fluids and surgical techniques that reduce the need for blood. Under many circumstances, these management alternatives allow even major surgery to be performed without additional risk. Another way to circumvent the religious prohibition is to choose medical, rather than surgical, treatment. In "Accommodating Jehovah's Witnesses' Choice of Nonblood Management," *Perspectives in Health Care Management* (Winter 1990), Donald Ridley, an attorney, argues that the sometimes inappropriate or unproven use of blood transfusions—as well as the lingering danger of transfusion-related infectious diseases, such as hepatitis—means that it may be reasonable to view Jehovah's Witnesses as "people making an informed choice between alternative courses of management." See also J. K. Vinicky et al., "The Jehovah's Witness and Blood: New Perspectives on an Old Dilemma," *Journal of Clinical Ethics* (Spring 1990).

Some of the most difficult situations arise when the patient is an adolescent. Determining whether or not an adolescent has the capacity to refuse blood transfusions is fraught with hazards. Some states have a provision for declaring an adolescent a "mature minor," that is, a person under the legal age of consent who has the capacity to make medical and other decisions.

Courts have ruled in different ways in these cases. In "My God, My Choice: The Mature Minor Doctrine and Adolescent Refusal of Life-Saving of Sustaining Medical Treatment Based upon Religious Beliefs," attorney Jonathan F. Will reviews statutory and case law on mature minors (*Journal of Contemporary Health Law and Plolicy,* Spring 2006). He concludes that when adolescents "refuse life-saving or sustaining medical treatment based upon religious belief, they must show by clear and convincing evidence that they both have understanding of the medical aspects of the decision, and also that the religious beliefs . . . are deeply rooted and central to their life plan."

Internet References . . .

Human Genome Project Information

This site contains information on the ethics, legal, and social issues related to advances in genetics.

http://www.ornl.gov/sci/techresources/Human_Genome/elsi.shtml

President's Council on Bioethics

This site has all the reports on cloning and stem cell research of this council, as well as those of prior commissions.

http://www.bioethics.gov

Council for Responsible Genetics

This organization has a newsletter and articles on the political, medical, consumer, and scientific aspects of genetics.

http://www.gene-watch.org

Genetics

*T*he explosion of technology for unraveling the mysteries of human genetics has created enormous possibilities for the future in terms of understanding heredity and its influence on disease, of identifying people who are at risk for genetic diseases, and eventually of treating at-risk people. All scientific and technical breakthroughs bring unresolved problems. The ability to replicate basic genetic material raises fundamental questions about the ethics of creating and using human embryos and what limits should be set on use of genetic material, even in the advance of scientific knowledge that might be used to treat devastating diseases or to enhance existing characteristics. Earlier abuses of genetic information (much of it misinformation) haunt efforts today to use this information wisely and compassionately. What impact will this knowledge have on individuals' lives and futures? And on the lives and futures of their children? These are some of the challenging issues raised in this section.

- Is the Ban on Federal Funding of Human Stem Cell Research Justifiable?

- Is Genetic Enhancement an Unacceptable Use of Technology?

ISSUE 12

Is the Ban on Federal Funding of Human Stem Cell Research Justifiable?

YES: **The President's Council on Bioethics,** from *Monitoring Stem Cell Research: A Report of the President's Council on Bioethics* (January 2004)

NO: **Jerome Groopman,** from "Forward, Medicine! Science, Morality, and Embryonic Stem Cells," *New Republic* (November 1, 2004)

ISSUE SUMMARY

YES: The President's Council on Bioethics supports the current ban on federal funding of embryonic stem cell research based on the law and its underlying principle, and the significance of federal funding.

NO: Jerome Groopman, professor of medicine at Harvard, says that the policy fails on scientific and moral accounts and is essentially a political choice.

$\mathbf{F}$ew bioethical issues have become so controversial in recent years as stem cell research. Perhaps only abortion, to which this issue is related, seems to evoke such passionate advocacy on both sides. To understand the ethical dimensions of this question, it is important to understand the scientific basis for the research.

Every human has stem cells of different kinds. Some stem cells exist to repair some of the everyday wear and tear of the body's blood, skin, and other organs. Others have more differentiated functions; that is, when they divide, their successors mature into specific types of cells, such as heart, muscle, blood, or brain cells. While all stem cells are capable of constant renewal, the most fundamental and versatile stem cells are found in the early (four-to-five-day) embryo, called the blastocyst. These embryonic stem cells have the special ability to develop into nearly any cell type, unlike the more differentiated or other cell types. Embryonic germ cells originate in the basic reproductive cells of the developing fetus and have properties similar to but not exactly like embryonic stem cells.

Because these special stem cells are so adaptable, they could possibly be used to develop new cells that would replace cells damaged by injuries or neurological diseases, such as Alzheimer's or Parkinson's, or common ailments like heart disease or kidney failure. They could also be used to develop new drugs for these and other diseases.

Although researchers have been working for more than 20 years with animal models, a breakthrough came in 1998 when James Thomson of the University of Wisconsin–Madison and John Gearhart at Johns Hopkins University, in different privately funded laboratories, were able to isolate and culture human embryonic stem cell lines. Other scientists have since developed other cell lines using different approaches, and research on adult stem cells is also continuing to determine both similarities and differences.

If this type of research is to continue, more stem cell lines would have to be developed. Where would these stem cells come from? Here is the crux of the problem. The potential sources are human fetal tissue following elective abortion; human embryos created by in vitro fertilization, which are not going to be implanted; human embryos created solely for this purpose; or, potentially, human or hybrid embryos created by cloning techniques. All these potential sources raise, to differing degrees, questions about the moral status of the human embryo and whether or not it is ethical to destroy an embryo in the pursuit of scientific knowledge, even for humanitarian purposes. Much of the debate focuses on whether or not federal funds should be used to support this research, even if it is not illegal.

In 1998, in response to the research developments of Thomson and Gearhart, President Bill Clinton asked the National Bioethics Advisory Commission to study the questions around stem cell research. The commission's report, issued in 1999, recommended that federal sponsorship of research that involves the derivation and use of human embryonic stem and germ cells should be limited in two ways. First, federally sponsored research should be limited to using aborted fetal tissue and embryos remaining after infertility treatments. Second, there should be an open and appropriate system of national oversight and review. Late in 2000 the National Institutes of Health (NIH) issued guidelines following the commission's suggestions.

The controversy did not end, however. The following selections crystallize the debate. The President's Council on Bioethics supports the Bush administration's ban on federal funding by citing the moral concerns raised by the new frontiers of science. Jerome Groopman calls the current policy a political decision, not one supported by science or moral values.

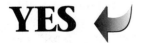

YES

Monitoring Stem Cell Research

Current Federal Law and Policy

The Significance of Federal Funding

The national debate over human embryonic stem cell research often raises the most fundamental questions about the moral status of human embryos and the legitimacy of research that destroys such embryos. Yet, looking over this debate, it is easy to forget that the question at issue is not whether research using embryos should be allowed, but rather whether it should be financed with the federal taxpayer's dollars.

The difference between *prohibiting* embryo research and *refraining from funding* it has often been blurred by both sides to the debate. Ignored in the battles over embryo research itself, the ethical-political question regarding funding is rarely taken up in full.

That question arises because modern governments do more than legislate and enforce prohibitions and limits. In the age of the welfare state, the government, besides being an enforcer of laws and a keeper of order, is also a major provider of resources. Political questions today, therefore, reach beyond what ought and ought not be allowed. They include questions of what ought and ought not be encouraged, supported, and made possible by taxpayer funding. The decision to fund an activity is more than an offer of resources. It is also a declaration of official national support and endorsement, a positive assertion that the activity in question is deemed by the nation as a whole, through its government, to be good and worthy. When something is done with public funding, it is done, so to speak, in the name of the country, with its blessing and encouragement.

To offer such encouragement and support is therefore no small matter. The federal government is not required to provide such material support, even for activities protected by the Constitution, let alone for those permitted but not guaranteed.[1] "The affording of most federal funding is entirely optional, and the choice to make such an offer is therefore laden with moral and political meaning, well beyond its material importance. In the age of government funding, the political system is sometimes called upon to decide not only the lowest standards of conduct, but also the highest standards of legitimacy and importance. When the nation decides an activity is worth its public money, it declares that the activity is valued, desired, and favored.

From Monitoring Stem Cell Research: A Report of the President's Council on Bioethics, January 2004, pp. Ch. 2, Section IV, VI, Footnotes, Endnotes.

The United States has long held the scientific enterprise in such high regard. Since the middle of the twentieth century, the federal government, with the strong support of the American people, has funded scientific research to the tune of many hundreds of billions of dollars. The American taxpayer is by far the greatest benefactor of science in the world, and the American public greatly values the contributions of science to human knowledge, human health, and human happiness. And we Americans have overwhelmingly been boosters of medical science and medical progress, deeming them worthy of support for moral as well as material reasons.

But this enthusiasm for medical science is not without its limits. As already noted, we attach restrictions to federally funded research, for instance to protect human subjects. In fact at times we even use funding to *place* restrictions on research that might otherwise not be constrained. Indeed, federal funding sometimes serves as a means by which *private* research can be subjected to critical standards, since institutions that receive federal funds are often inclined (and given strong administrative incentives) to abide by the prescribed ethical standards throughout all of their activities, not only those directly receiving public dollars. Some supporters of funding therefore argue that extending public money to research is the most effective means of making certain that nearly all researchers, public and private, adhere to basic standards of ethics and safety. Public funding also requires researchers to make their work available to the public and for critical review by their peers, and it may encourage some degree of responsibility not necessarily encouraged by commercial endeavors.[2]

In addition to conditions attached to government funding of research, law sometimes erects specific limits on certain practices that might be medically beneficial. For example, we put limits on some practices that might offer life-saving benefits, such as the buying and selling of organs for transplantation, currently prohibited under the National Organ Transplant Act. Also, as in the present case, many Americans and their congressional representatives have moral reasons for opposing certain lines of research or clinical practice, for example those that involve the exploitation and destruction of human fetuses and embryos.

The two sides of the embryo research debate tend to differ sharply on the fundamental moral significance of the activity in question. One side believes that what is involved is morally abhorrent in the extreme, while the other believes embryo research is noble or even morally obligatory and worthy of praise and support. It would be very difficult for the government to find a middle ground between these two positions, since the two sides differ not only on what should or should not be done, but also on the moral premises from which the activity should be approached.

To this point, the federal government has pursued a policy whereby it does not explicitly prohibit embryo research but also does not officially condone it, encourage it, or support it with public funds (though state governments have often taken more active roles in both directions . . .). This approach, again, combines prudential demands with moral concerns. It has allowed the political system to avoid banning embryo research against the wishes of those who believe it serves an important purpose, while not compelling those citizens who oppose it to fund it with their tax money. This approach is also based, at least in part, on the conviction that debates over the federal budget are not the place to take up the anguished question of the moral status of human embryos.

But the position is not only a compromise between those who would have the government bless and those who would have the government curse this activity. It is also a statement of a certain principle: namely, that public sanction makes a serious difference and ought not to be conferred lightly. While embryo destruction may be something that some Americans support and engage in, it is not something that America as a nation has officially supported or engaged in.[3]

Of course, if the funding issue were merely a proxy for the larger dispute over the moral status of human embryos, then the present arrangement might appeal only to those who would protect human embryos, and it would succeed only as long as they were able to enact it. The argument might end there, with a vote-count on the question of the moral status or standing of human embryos. But some proponents of the present law suggest that the particulars and contours of the embryo research debate offer an additional rationale for that arrangement. Here again, it is important to remember that the issue in question is public funding, not permissibility. Opponents of embryo research have in most cases acquiesced (likely owing to various prudential and moral factors) in narrowing the debate at the federal level to the question of funding. They do not argue for a wholesale prohibition of embryo research by national legislation, even though many of them see such work as an abomination and even a form of homicide. In return, proponents of the Dickey Amendment argue that it would be appropriate for supporters of research to agree to do without federal funding in this particular field.

On the other hand, it might reasonably be argued that part of living under majority rule is living with the consequences of sometimes being in the minority. Were the Congress to overturn the current policy of withholding public funds from the destruction of embryos, opponents of funding for embryo research would not be alone in being compelled to pay for activities they abhor. We all see our government do things, in our name, with which we disagree. Some of these might even involve life and death questions of principle, for instance in waging wars that some citizens deeply oppose. The existence of strong moral opposition to some policy is not in itself a decisive argument against proceeding with that policy.

These concerns give the question of funding its own crucial ethical significance, even apart from the more fundamental question of the legitimacy and propriety of the act being funded. This matter of funding broadly understood, together with the moral and prudential aims apparently motivating the administration's policy, as well as the legal context created by the Dickey Amendment, are the essential prerequisites for thinking about the underlying logic of the current policy. The combination of these elements gives form not only to the specific rules set forth in the administration's funding policy, but also to the implementation of that policy. . . .

Conclusion

The administration's policy on the funding of embryonic stem cell research rests on several moral and ethical-legal principles, set upon the reality of existing law:

1. *The law:* The Dickey Amendment, which the President is required to enforce.
2. *The principle underlying the law:* The conviction, voiced by the administration, a majority of the Congress, and some portion of the public, that federal taxpayer dollars should not be used to encourage the exploitation or destruction of nascent human life, even if scientific and medical benefits might come from such acts.
3. *The principle underlying the desire to offer funding:* That efforts to heal the sick and the injured are of great national importance and should be vigorously supported, provided that they respect important moral boundaries.
4. *The significance of federal funding:* That federal funding constitutes a meaningful positive statement of national approval and encouragement, which should be awarded only with care, particularly in cases where the activity in question arouses significant public moral opposition.

The significance of the policy is best understood in light of these key elements. Its soundness is most reasonably measured against them and against the policy's implementation by the National Institutes of Health.

Though the prudential and principled considerations raised in this chapter governed the formulation of the policy, or at least defined its articulation by its advocates and authors, these are not the only terms by which federal funding policy might be conceived or measured. In the next chapter we present an overview of the ethical and policy debates that have raged for the past two years around both the wisdom of the present policy and the fundamental issues at stake in human embryonic stem cell research.

Notes

1. This question has been addressed by the Supreme Court on a number of occasions, in which the Court found that even activities protected as rights under the Constitution are not thereby inherently worthy of financial support from the federal government. See, for instance, *Maher v. Roe* 432 U.S. 464 (1977); *Harris v. McRae* 448 U.S. 297 (1980); and *Rust v. Sullivan* 500 U.S. 173 (1991). Also see Berkowitz, P. "The Meaning of Federal Funding," a paper commissioned by the Council and included in Appendix F of this report.
2. Indeed, some even argue that the terms and conditions set for federal funding of research could be defined in such a way as not only to subject private research to general standards but also to help influence the eventual distribution of the products of that research to all those in need, or to serve other goods deemed publicly worthy.
3. The repeated reenactment of the Dickey Amendment by the Congress may be taken as evidence of some support for this assertion.

Jerome Groopman

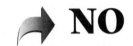 **NO**

Forward, Medicine! Science, Morality, and Embryonic Stem Cells

The President's Council for Bioethics has produced several reports detailing the reasons for its opposition to federal support for less restrictive human embryonic-stem-cell research. There are, in essence, three arguments made in these documents. The first is that embryonic-stem-cell research is a slippery slope that will lead society into a moral abyss. The second is that the manipulation of early embryos for purposes of research and development of therapeutics ignores the innate humanness of these embryos. The third argument, which is mostly a whisper from the council but is in fact the major cause of much of the public debate, is rooted in religious dogma.

The slippery-slope argument applies, of course, to every scientific advance. References to literature are frequently made by council members to heighten concern about inadvertently skidding into catastrophe: Hawthorne, for example, famously imagined a scientist obsessed with perfect beauty who gives a cleansing but fatal potion to his wife in order to erase an innocuous birthmark. The trouble with these cautionary tales is that scientific researchers rarely resemble their caricatures in fiction. The scientists I know who are laboring on stem-cell research are intent on erasing deadly pediatric diseases and debilitating maladies such as ALS and Parkinson's. Skin blemishes are not on their research agenda. Nor is anyone trying to create Superman—so-called "human enhancement." There is a great gulf between fixing a genetic lesion in an embryo that would lead to the birth of a child with Fanconi's anemia or muscular dystrophy, and meddling in the DNA to try to produce a baby who will one day have perfect SATs or win an Olympic medal.

The slippery-slope argument is made also about the scenario of an industry for body parts. Poor women may be paid to donate their eggs for IVF, and then the embryonic stem cells will be subverted for less than salubrious purposes, such as a market for replacement organs to prevent aging among the rich. These fears about exploitation for "human enhancement" are legitimate, and they need to be discussed. But they are certainly not dispositive: they can be securely guarded against by means of legislation.

All of these dystopian anxieties put one in mind of the furious public debates that occurred when recombinant DNA technology was developed in the 1970s and when IVF with "test-tube babies" succeeded in 1978. Decades later, the nightmare arguments about the slippery slope (then they came from the left) have proved to be wrong. The moratorium on recombinant DNA work sponsored by the far left was in force for nearly a year in Cambridge, Massachusetts, and it did nothing more than cause some scientists to migrate to California and others to be retarded in their work. Instead of Frankenstein or an Andromeda strain, recombinant DNA technology has yielded a plethora of desperately needed therapies, including human insulin, the blood cell growth factors erythropoietin and CSF used in cancer therapy and bone marrow transplantation, and cytokine inhibitors for rheumatoid arthritis and Crohn's disease. The lives of hundreds of thousands of patients have been made immeasurably better by the application of cloning genes.

Slippery-slope arguments shut down serious thought. They are essentially appeals to fear. No monsters and no plagues have been unleashed by the cloning of genes. Similarly, hundreds of thousands of children conceived by IVF now fill families that were previously empty. And there are no IVF factories for body parts. Fringe scientists who share the fantasies of Mary Shelley or Michael Crichton are vigorously condemned in the scientific community, and they could be criminally prosecuted with the right legislation. Fences could readily be constructed by Congress around such awful prospects, as they have been in the United Kingdom, Israel, South Korea, and Singapore. All these states have outlawed so-called "reproductive cloning," meaning producing a human being or body parts from a manipulated embryonic stem cell. All permit work with IVF discards to create new treatments for incurable diseases.

The President's Council largely avoided invoking theology as the primary rationale for limiting stem-cell research. This is unfortunate, because it is theology that is the real motive behind most of the political opposition to embryonic-stem-cell research. But not all theology: the various monotheistic traditions do not have the same analysis of conception and the origins of life. The Catholic and evangelical Protestant churches firmly reject embryo research because it amounts to murder. The soul, they believe, enters the body at the moment of conception; their opposition is in concert with their stance on abortion. But several other traditions, including Judaism, Islam, and liberal branches of Protestantism, do not posit that human life occurs at such an early stage.

The exegesis of verses from Genesis and the Prophets has led to different religious opinions. Because God breathed into a lump of earth to form Adam, Judaism and Islam generally view life arriving when organs such as the lungs appear, many weeks after conception. The Talmud states that before forty days what is in the uterus is akin to water. Jewish thinkers point out, moreover, that the potential for life is not the same as life itself. Since IVF occurs outside the uterus, rabbinical opinion holds that it is permitted, and that the excess fertilized eggs can be discarded without moral qualms. Catholic and evangelical Protestant thinkers, by contrast, draw their conclusion that life begins at the moment the egg and sperm fuse, extrapolating in part from the verse in the beginning of Jeremiah where God says, "I knew you before you were formed in the womb."

The important fact is that this is all theology. From a scientific point of view, no one can know when ensoulment occurs, or if it occurs. It is a metaphysical question that cannot be empirically answered. In this matter, no data can be sought from experimentation. And so aspects of our humanness are considered by scientists as surrogates for the soul, most notably whether the embryo is sentient at such an early stage—that is, whether it has sufficient neural development to perceive pain or to react to noxious stimuli. And the empirical truth is that it does not do so at day five or six, when stem cells are taken from the blastocyst.

Some moral philosophers and bioethicists look not to biology but to cultural norms to try to assess the humanness of a five-day-old IVF embryo composed of some two hundred cells. . . . Such fertilized embryos are routinely discarded. These discarded blastocysts, the philosophers argue, are not mourned or afforded a funeral. Absent such rituals, they should be considered less than truly human. To my mind, these are weaker arguments for the right conclusion. Such cultural inferences are too relative to decide the case. Vivisection, for example, was banned for centuries as a desecration of the body. And slavery was condoned with biblical references.

On October 8, [2004], in *The Washington Post*, Leon R. Kass, the chairman of the President's Council on Bioethics, published an illuminating article called "Playing Politics with the Sick." . . .

Kass argues that the Bush policy is a Solomonic compromise:

> Wise public policy concerning embryonic-stem-cell research must attend to three important—sometimes competing—responsibilities: to seek scientific knowledge and cures for terrible diseases, to protect human life in all its vulnerable stages, and to respect the diverse yet deeply held moral views of the American people. The president's policy on funding this research offers a prudent means of doing all three. It provides an effective way to vigorously promote embryonic stem cell research and seek cures for disease without violating respect for nascent human life, and without conferring the nation's official blessing, through the awarding of federal taxpayer dollars, on practices many Americans find morally reprehensible.

In fact, the policy falls short on all accounts, scientific and moral. It fails to "vigorously promote embryonic stem cell research," to put it mildly. Stem-cell lines available through federal programs tightly constrict the scope of scientific research and its potential therapeutic applications. Kass argues that expansion of this scope should be done without the use of taxpayers' money. But it is federal money that has brought America a level of science unparalleled in the world. No other country has made more contributions to the health and the welfare of humankind than the United States. This American glory is owed to the structure and the support of the NIH and other federal funding agencies.

Kass refers to efforts at universities such as Harvard, Stanford, and Johns Hopkins to set up stem-cell institutes with donations from wealthy individuals and foundations; but such initiatives are born of desperation rather than desire. They are a throwback to the days when scientists sought wealthy patrons to underwrite their efforts. Although philanthropy is often a powerful catalyst to initiate scientific projects, in almost every case it has been taxpayer money that has brought such work to fruition. Should creative and energetic scientists who could make important contributions to stem-cell research be frustrated or penalized if they are unable to secure a rich patron? Will patients with juvenile diabetes or Parkinson's disease or ALS have to be uprooted from their communities to enter into clinical trials using embryonic stem cells created after August 2001 that are available only in Baltimore or Boston? Some of the most innovative clinical trials in the country occur at the NIH itself, at the Warren Magnuson Center in Bethesda, and this institution is now cut off from possibly using cellular products derived from human embryonic cell lines not extant before August 2001. Similarly, the entire Veterans Administration hospital system would be denied access to such future therapies under the Bush policy, because taxpayer money supports the care and the treatment of our soldiers and veterans. Should this most heralded segment of our society, the people responsible for the defense of America, be barred from such medicine?

Kass's distinction between private research and public research also has the unwitting effect of damaging his moral argument, because such a distinction cannot be about morality. If embryonic-stem-cell research is wrong in a federally funded laboratory, then it is wrong also in a privately funded laboratory. If it is the slippery slope to evil in Bethesda, then it is also the slippery slope to evil in Cambridge or Palo Alto or Baltimore.

Kass affirms that we should all "respect the diverse . . . deeply held moral views of the American people." I emphatically agree, but respect does not necessarily translate into law. We respectfully legislate against deeply held moral views all the time. There are pacifists who passionately believe that weapons designed to kill people are immoral. There are many secular and religious leaders who passionately believe that capital punishment for any crime is immoral. Yet there is ample federal legislation that funds numerous types of weapons for killing, and taxpayer money is used in the execution of criminals convicted for federal crimes. The nation routinely confers its "official blessing," through the awarding of federal taxpayer dollars, on practices that many Americans find morally reprehensible. This may be insensitive, but it is the democratic way.

Kass states that taking stem cells from five- to six-day-old human embryos, generally developed during IVF, "is not a morally neutral act. Just as no society can afford to be callous to the needs of suffering humanity, none can afford to be cavalier about how it treats nascent human life." Again, I agree. No one should be cavalier in considering these issues. But why is Kass so sure that the advocates of embryonic-stem-cell research are being morally or philosophically cavalier? Surely there is a significant difference between nascent human life and independent human life. And Kass would not take kindly to the suggestion (which would be unfair, since he is a thoughtful man) that he is being cavalier with independent human life. Anyway, when Kass states that the president's policy of upholding the Dickey amendment "promotes health without violating life or the law of the land," we must note the slight emendation in his language, the disappearance of those rigorous modifying terms "nascent" or "potential." "Violating life" is the phrase that clearly echoes the religious beliefs at the core of the Bush policy and the core of his political base.

There are no guarantees of progress in science. One cannot say with certainty when, or even if, a breakthrough will occur. What is certain is that failure is much more frequent than success. Indeed, failure is often essential to eventual success. In science, we learn most from our misconceptions and our mistakes. And sometimes the most important advances come from the most unexpected places: discoveries made in a worm or in yeast have been key to our understanding of the biology of several human cancers.

The hubris of scientists has no place in arguing for research in human embryonic stem cells. Overselling therapeutic applications is a disservice to desperate patients; and avoiding the ineffable question of what is life is willful ignorance. Scientists who engage in embryonic-stem-cell research have certainly made a moral choice—but it is a supremely defensible moral choice, believing as they do that a greater good will be served by healing the living by means of risking the sacrifice of what may, or may not, be an unborn human soul.

The facts are before us. Human embryonic stem cells provide the potential to ameliorate great human suffering and to save lives. We cannot say when that potential will be realized, only that its realization is much less likely under President Bush's policy. For stem cells are the veritable life of the flesh. Whether or not the prayers of the sick and the dying will be answered through Scripture, they may certainly be addressed by medicine, and legislation, and the judicial process, and the ballot box.

POSTSCRIPT

Is the Ban on Federal Funding of Human Stem Cell Research Justifiable?

Scientists at the University of California, San Diego, reported in *Nature Medicine* (February 2005) that the cell lines currently approved for federally funded research are contaminated with nonhuman molecules from the culture medium used to grow the cells. The presence of sialic acid, which is not found in humans, raises safety problems, which might be addressed by using methods that avoid animal contaminants.

In 2005 President Bush vetoed the Stem Cell Research Enhancement Act, providing federal funds for stem cell research involving embryos created in fertility clinics. There were not enough votes to override the veto, but neither were there enough votes to pass bills opposed to stem cell research.

While the debate about stem cell research continues on the federal level, several states have already passed laws about the practice. According to the National Conference of State Legislatures, "approaches to stem cell research policy range from statutes in California, Connecticut, Maryland, Massachusetts and New Jersey and an executive order in Illinois, which encourage embryonic stem cell research, to South Dakota's law, which strictly forbids research on embryos regardless of the source." States currently funding stem cell research include California, New Jersey, and Ohio, and following the 2006 elections, New York and Wisconsin are likely to move in this direction.

On the international front, in December 2002 Australia's parliament approved stem cell research but limited it to stem cell lines created from embryos left over after infertility treatments. This policy is less restrictive than the U.S. version but not as liberal as the British policy, which allows new stem cell lines to be created. In a November 2004 referendum, Swiss voters approved by a wide margin the government's proposal to permit research on human stem cells. Switzerland is home to many multinational pharmaceutical companies. Research is going on in many other countries as well, each with a different set of rules.

For views opposing stem cell research, see Alo H. Konsen, "Are We Killing the Weak to Heal the Sick? Federally Funded Embryonic Stem Cell Research," in *Health Matrix: Journal of Law-Medicine* (Summer 2002) and Gilbert Meilaender, "The Point of a Ban: Or, How to Think About Stem Cell Research," *Hastings Center Report* (January–February 2001). For views supporting stem cell research, see Michael J. Meyer and Lawrence J. Nelson, "Respecting What We Destroy: Reflections on Human Embryo Research," *Hastings Center Report* (January–February 2001) and Heather Johnson Kukla, "Embryonic Stem Cell

Research: An Ethical Justification," *Georgetown Law Journal* (vol. 90, 2002), pp. 503–543. The Winter 2002 edition of *American Journal of Bioethics* is a special issue on stem cells, as is the March 2004 issue of the *Kennedy Institute of Ethics Journal*. The January–February 2006 issue of the *Hastings Center Report* contains a series of articles on the next set of questions on stem cells.

The President's Council of Bioethics report, "Monitoring Stem Cell Research," issued in January 2004, is available at http://www.bioethics.com. Two members of the President's Council on Bioethics contributed personal viewpoints to the *New England Journal of Medicine* (July 15, 2004). Michael J. Sandel, a professor of government, wrote "Embryo Ethics—The Moral Logic of Stem-Cell Research," and Paul R. McHugh, a psychiatrist, wrote "Zygote and 'Clonote'—The Ethical Use of Embryonic Stem Cells." The Web site of the International Society for Stem Cell Research (http://www.isscr.org) has a section on ethics, which provides links to resources on both sides of the issue.

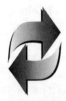

ISSUE 13

Is Genetic Enhancement an Unacceptable Use of Technology?

YES: Michael J. Sandel, from "The Case Against Perfection," *The Atlantic Monthly* (April 2004)

NO: Howard Trachtman, from "A Man Is a Man Is a Man," *The American Journal of Bioethics* (May/June 2005)

ISSUE SUMMARY

YES: Political philosopher Michael J. Sandel believes that using genetic technology to enhance performance, design children, and perfect human nature is a flawed attempt at human mastery, and banishes appreciation of life as a gift.

NO: Physician Howard Trachtman says that the medical community should embrace enhancement as a never-ending quest for health that recognizes that perfection can never be achieved.

Perhaps more than any other people, Americans seem to be obsessed with self-improvement. Each year there is a flood of new books and television commercials promoting ways to be richer, thinner, smarter, happier, healthier, more successful, attractive, or all of the above. Whatever one's presumed character or bodily flaw, there is a remedy. And for parents, there is an additional opportunity (sometimes presented as an obligation) to make one's children richer, thinner, smarter, happier, or all of the above.

Most of these "solutions" are things that individuals do to themselves or with others. Some, such as taking performance-enhancing drugs in sports, involve chemical interventions (see Issue 18). But all at some point encounter the natural limits of an individual's intelligence, physical structure, and inherited or acquired traits, as well as the economic and social context that determines availability and acceptability. A short, slow-moving man is unlikely to become a professional basketball player, no matter how many steroids he takes or how much he trains. Cosmetic surgery can only do so much to alter an aging face or body. Without a natural vocal talent, a woman is unlikely to become an international opera star.

But what if we could change all that? And, if not for ourselves, for our children? The basic idea is not new, and has been practiced for centuries in animal husbandry and agriculture. By breeding for certain characteristics, animals and plants have been created to better meet human purposes. The largest Great Dane and the smallest Pekinese, and all the dog breeds in between, are descended from a handful of wolves tamed by humans in Asia nearly 15,000 years ago. Over the last 500 years humans have practiced breeding techniques that account for the vastly different appearances and characteristics of modern dogs.

Applying these techniques to humans—the theory of eugenics or "better genes"—also has a long but disastrous history. Its advocates, many of them in the United States in the twentieth century, advocated the elimination of "undesirable" people by preventing them from reproducing through involuntary sterilization. In the most malevolent form of eugenics, of course, the Nazi regime in Germany in the 1930s wanted to create a "master race" by encouraging reproduction among blonde, blue-eyed, tall Aryan types and eliminating from the gene pool by murder those from other population groups, such as Jews and gypsies.

While these eugenics methods are not only barbarous and morally corrupt, the idea of enhancing one's capacities and those of future generations has been given new life by scientific advances in genetics. Being able to manipulate genes—the very core of human inheritance—opens up a new world of possibilities. Already animals like sheep and cows have been cloned, that is, reproduced in exact copies. Is it possible to enhance an individual's intelligence or height or beauty—through genetic manipulation? Can a smart person be made smarter? A strong person stronger? Can people be programmed to live two hundred years in good health? Can children be "designed" with particular talents, appearances, and futures? Can "bad" genes—those linked to disease or, more speculatively, criminal tendencies—be eliminated? And if these things are indeed possible, are they a valid use of technology? If these techniques proved to be safe and effective, would they be distributed fairly throughout society?

These questions are at the core of the selections that follow. Political philosopher Michael J. Sandel argues that there is a moral problem with enhancement, whether it is undertaken for one's own benefit or for one's children. These goals express a desire for human mastery over life, which is essentially a gift, and destroys the natural relationship between parents and children. Physician Howard Trachtman, on the other hand, accepts enhancement as a new way of expressing a natural desire to improve health and well-being. He believes that we should not fear progress or try to limit medical manipulations.

YES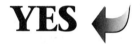

Michael J. Sandel

The Case Against Perfection

Breakthroughs in genetics present us with a promise and a predicament. The promise is that we may soon be able to treat and prevent a host of debilitating diseases. The predicament is that our newfound genetic knowledge may also enable us to manipulate our own nature—to enhance our muscles, memories, and moods; to choose the sex, height, and other genetic traits of our children; to make ourselves "better than well." When science moves faster than moral understanding, as it does today, men and women struggle to articulate their unease. In liberal societies they reach first for the language of autonomy, fairness, and individual rights. But this part of our moral vocabulary is ill equipped to address the hardest questions posed by genetic engineering. The genomic revolution has induced a kind of moral vertigo. . . .

In order to grapple with the ethics of enhancement, we need to confront questions largely lost from view—questions about the moral status of nature, and about the proper stance of human beings toward the given world. Since these questions verge on theology, modern philosophers and political theorists tend to shrink from them. But our new powers of biotechnology make them unavoidable. To see why this is so, consider four examples already on the horizon: muscle enhancement, memory enhancement, growth-hormone treatment, and reproductive technologies that enable parents to choose the sex and some genetic traits of their children. In each case what began as an attempt to treat a disease or prevent a genetic disorder now beckons as an instrument of improvement and consumer choice.

Muscles Everyone would welcome a gene therapy to alleviate muscular dystrophy and to reverse the debilitating muscle loss that comes with old age. But what if the same therapy were used to improve athletic performance? Researchers have developed a synthetic gene that, when injected into the muscle cells of mice, prevents and even reverses natural muscle deterioration. The gene not only repairs wasted or injured muscles but also strengthens healthy ones. This success bodes well for human applications. H. Lee Sweeney, of the University of Pennsylvania, who leads the research, hopes his discovery will cure the immobility that afflicts the elderly. But Sweeney's bulked-up mice have already attracted the attention of athletes seeking a competitive edge. Although the therapy is not yet approved for human use, the prospect of genetically enhanced

From *The Atlantic Monthly*, Volume 293, No. 3, April 2004, excerpts. Copyright © 2004 by Michael J. Sandel. Reprinted by permission.

weight lifters, home-run sluggers, linebackers, and sprinters is easy to imagine. The widespread use of steroids and other performance-improving drugs in professional sports suggests that many athletes will be eager to avail themselves of genetic enhancement. . . .

Memory   Genetic enhancement is possible for brains as well as brawn. In the mid-1990s scientists managed to manipulate a memory-linked gene in fruit flies, creating flies with photographic memories. More recently researchers have produced smart mice by inserting extra copies of a memory-related gene into mouse embryos. The altered mice learn more quickly and remember things longer than normal mice. The extra copies were programmed to remain active even in old age, and the improvement was passed on to offspring.

Human memory is more complicated, but biotech companies, including Memory Pharmaceuticals, are in hot pursuit of memory-enhancing drugs, or "cognition enhancers," for human beings. The obvious market for such drugs consists of those who suffer from Alzheimer's and other serious memory disorders. The companies also have their sights on a bigger market: the 81 million Americans over fifty, who are beginning to encounter the memory loss that comes naturally with age. A drug that reversed age-related memory loss would be a bonanza for the pharmaceutical industry: a Viagra for the brain. Such use would straddle the line between remedy and enhancement. Unlike a treatment for Alzheimer's, it would cure no disease; but insofar as it restored capacities a person once possessed, it would have a remedial aspect. It could also have purely nonmedical uses: for example, by a lawyer cramming to memorize facts for an upcoming trial, or by a business executive eager to learn Mandarin on the eve of his departure for Shanghai.

Some who worry about the ethics of cognitive enhancement point to the danger of creating two classes of human beings: those with access to enhancement technologies, and those who must make do with their natural capacities. And if the enhancements could be passed down the generations, the two classes might eventually become subspecies—the enhanced and the merely natural. But worry about access ignores the moral status of enhancement itself. Is the scenario troubling because the unenhanced poor would be denied the benefits of bioengineering, or because the enhanced affluent would somehow be dehumanized? As with muscles, so with memory: the fundamental question is not how to ensure equal access to enhancement but whether we should aspire to it in the first place.

Height   Pediatricians already struggle with the ethics of enhancement when confronted by parents who want to make their children taller. Since the 1980s human growth hormone has been approved for children with a hormone deficiency that makes them much shorter than average. But the treatment also increases the height of healthy children. Some parents of healthy children who are unhappy with their stature (typically boys) ask why it should make a difference whether a child is short because of a hormone deficiency or because his parents happen to be short. Whatever the cause, the social consequences are the same.

In the face of this argument some doctors began prescribing hormone treatments for children whose short stature was unrelated to any medical problem. By 1996 such "off-label" use accounted for 40 percent of human-growth-hormone prescriptions. Although it is legal to prescribe drugs for purposes not approved by the Food and Drug Administration, pharmaceutical companies cannot promote such use. Seeking to expand its market, Eli Lilly & Co. recently persuaded the FDA to approve its human growth hormone for healthy children whose projected adult height is in the bottom one percentile—under five feet three inches for boys and four feet eleven inches for girls. This concession raises a large question about the ethics of enhancement: If hormone treatments need not be limited to those with hormone deficiencies, why should they be available only to very short children? Why shouldn't all shorter-than-average children be able to seek treatment? And what about a child of average height who wants to be taller so that he can make the basketball team?

Some oppose height enhancement on the grounds that it is collectively self-defeating; as some become taller, others become shorter relative to the norm. Except in Lake Wobegon, not every child can be above average. As the unenhanced began to feel shorter, they, too, might seek treatment, leading to a hormonal arms race that left everyone worse off, especially those who couldn't afford to buy their way up from shortness.

But the arms-race objection is not decisive on its own. Like the fairness objection to bioengineered muscles and memory, it leaves unexamined the attitudes and dispositions that prompt the drive for enhancement. If we were bothered only by the injustice of adding shortness to the problems of the poor, we could remedy that unfairness by publicly subsidizing height enhancements. As for the relative height deprivation suffered by innocent bystanders, we could compensate them by taxing those who buy their way to greater height. The real question is whether we want to live in a society where parents feel compelled to spend a fortune to make perfectly healthy kids a few inches taller.

Sex selection   Perhaps the most inevitable nonmedical use of bioengineering is sex selection. For centuries parents have been trying to choose the sex of their children. Today biotech succeeds where folk remedies failed.

One technique for sex selection arose with prenatal tests using amniocentesis and ultrasound. These medical technologies were developed to detect genetic abnormalities such as spina bifida and Down syndrome. But they can also reveal the sex of the fetus—allowing for the abortion of a fetus of an undesired sex. Even among those who favor abortion rights, few advocate abortion simply because the parents do not want a girl. Nevertheless, in traditional societies with a powerful cultural preference for boys, this practice has become widespread. . . .

It is commonly said that genetic enhancements undermine our humanity by threatening our capacity to act freely, to succeed by our own efforts, and to consider ourselves responsible—worthy of praise or blame—for the things we do and for the way we are. . . .

Though there is much to be said for this argument, I do not think the main problem with enhancement and genetic engineering is that they undermine effort and erode human agency. The deeper danger is that they represent a kind of hyperagency—a Promethean aspiration to remake nature, including human nature, to serve our purposes and satisfy our desires. The problem is not the drift to mechanism but the drive to mastery. And what the drive to mastery misses and may even destroy is an appreciation of the gifted character of human powers and achievements.

To acknowledge the giftedness of life is to recognize that our talents and powers are not wholly our own doing, despite the effort we expend to develop and to exercise them. It is also to recognize that not everything in the world is open to whatever use we may desire or devise. Appreciating the gifted quality of life constrains the Promethean project and conduces to a certain humility. It is in part a religious sensibility. But its resonance reaches beyond religion. . . .

The ethic of giftedness, under siege in sports, persists in the practice of parenting. But here, too, bioengineering and genetic enhancement threaten to dislodge it. To appreciate children as gifts is to accept them as they come, not as objects of our design or products of our will or instruments of our ambition. Parental love is not contingent on the talents and attributes a child happens to have. We choose our friends and spouses at least partly on the basis of qualities we find attractive. But we do not choose our children. Their qualities are unpredictable, and even the most conscientious parents cannot be held wholly responsible for the kind of children they have. That is why parenthood, more than other human relationships, teaches what the theologian William F. May calls an "openness to the unbidden."

May's resonant phrase helps us see that the deepest moral objection to enhancement lies less in the perfection it seeks than in the human disposition it expresses and promotes. The problem is not that parents usurp the autonomy of a child they design. The problem lies in the hubris of the designing parents, in their drive to master the mystery of birth. Even if this disposition did not make parents tyrants to their children, it would disfigure the relation between parent and child, and deprive the parent of the humility and enlarged human sympathies that an openness to the unbidden can cultivate.

To appreciate children as gifts or blessings is not, of course, to be passive in the face of illness or disease. Medical intervention to cure or prevent illness or restore the injured to health does not desecrate nature but honors it. Healing sickness or injury does not override a child's natural capacities but permits them to flourish.

Nor does the sense of life as a gift mean that parents must shrink from shaping and directing the development of their child. Just as athletes and artists have an obligation to cultivate their talents, so parents have an obligation to cultivate their children, to help them discover and develop their talents and gifts. As May points out, parents give their children two kinds of love: accepting love and transforming love. Accepting love affirms the being of the child, whereas transforming love seeks the well-being of the child. Each aspect corrects the excesses of the other, he writes: "Attachment becomes too quietistic if it slackens into mere acceptance of the child as he is." Parents have a duty to promote their children's excellence.

These days, however, overly ambitious parents are prone to get carried away with transforming love—promoting and demanding all manner of accomplishments from their children, seeking perfection. "Parents find it difficult to maintain an equilibrium between the two sides of love," May observes. "Accepting love, without transforming love, slides into indulgence and finally neglect. Transforming love, without accepting love, badgers and finally rejects." May finds in these competing impulses a parallel with modern science: it, too, engages us in beholding the given world, studying and savoring it, and also in molding the world, transforming and perfecting it.

The mandate to mold our children, to cultivate and improve them, complicates the case against enhancement. We usually admire parents who seek the best for their children, who spare no effort to help them achieve happiness and success. Some parents confer advantages on their children by enrolling them in expensive schools, hiring private tutors, sending them to tennis camp, providing them with piano lessons, ballet lessons, swimming lessons, SAT-prep courses, and so on. If it is permissible and even admirable for parents to help their children in these ways, why isn't it equally admirable for parents to use whatever genetic technologies may emerge (provided they are safe) to enhance their children's intelligence, musical ability, or athletic prowess?

The defenders of enhancement are right to this extent: improving children through genetic engineering is similar in spirit to the heavily managed, high-pressure child-rearing that is now common. But this similarity does not vindicate genetic enhancement. On the contrary, it highlights a problem with the trend toward hyperparenting. One conspicuous example of this trend is sports-crazed parents bent on making champions of their children. Another is the frenzied drive of overbearing parents to mold and manage their children's academic careers. . . .

Some see a clear line between genetic enhancement and other ways that people seek improvement in their children and themselves. Genetic manipulation seems somehow worse—more intrusive, more sinister—than other ways of enhancing performance and seeking success. But morally speaking, the difference is less significant than it seems. Bioengineering gives us reason to question the low-tech, high-pressure child-rearing practices we commonly accept. The hyperparenting familiar in our time represents an anxious excess of mastery and dominion that misses the sense of life as a gift. . . .

In a social world that prizes mastery and control, parenthood is a school for humility. That we care deeply about our children and yet cannot choose the kind we want teaches parents to be open to the unbidden. Such openness is a disposition worth affirming, not only within families but in the wider world as well. It invites us to abide the unexpected, to live with dissonance, to rein in the impulse to control. A *Gattaca*-like world in which parents became accustomed to specifying the sex and genetic traits of their children would be a world inhospitable to the unbidden, a gated community writ large. The awareness that our talents and abilities are not wholly our own doing restrains our tendency toward hubris. . . .

There is something appealing, even intoxicating, about a vision of human freedom unfettered by the given. It may even be the case that the allure of that vision played a part in summoning the genomic age into being. It is often assumed that the powers of enhancement we now possess arose as an inadvertent by-product of biomedical progress—the genetic revolution came, so to speak, to cure disease, and stayed to tempt us with the prospect of enhancing our performance, designing our children, and perfecting our nature. That may have the story backwards. It is more plausible to view genetic engineering as the ultimate expression of our resolve to see ourselves astride the world, the masters of our nature. But that promise of mastery is flawed. It threatens to banish our appreciation of life as a gift, and to leave us with nothing to affirm or behold outside our own will.

Howard Trachtman

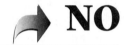 **NO**

A Man Is a Man Is a Man

Every field of human endeavor goes through a period of great anticipation in which the leading lights predict that the end of the discipline is near and that acquisition of new knowledge in the area is almost complete. Thus, at the end of the nineteenth century, physicists were confident that they had natural order of things under control and that mastery of the physical world was just a matter of time. A few decades later, David Hilbert and colleagues asserted that they were closing in on verification of the internal consistency and validity of mathematics and by inference all of philosophy (Goldstein 2005). In the early 1970s, as immunization practice and administration of antibiotics became standard and scourges of earlier eras like smallpox and polio were vanishing, specialists in infectious disease were sure that their field had things well in hand. Finally, after the fall of the Berlin Wall, Francis Fukuyama (1992) wrote confidently that history was at an end and that the global community was entering a phase of prosperity and harmony.

From the privileged vantage point of the early 21st century, we know how grandiose these predictions were. Einstein and his relativistic quanta, Godel and his incompleteness theorem, AIDS and Ebola, and the attack on the World Trade Center demonstrate that nothing ever goes quite exactly according to plan and that human beings still have plenty of work cut out for them.

In light of all of this sobering experience, it is surprising that physicians and bioethicists should have such unrealistic views and apprehensions about prospective therapeutic interventions that may arise from the remarkable advances in genetics or neurobiology. Michael Sandel's (2004) article is representative of this literature and Kamm's (2005) review is an insightful analysis of this position. However, I think it falls short on several practical points that should disarm anxious critics of enhancement.

Enhancement is a new term that is in vogue to describe what doctors have been doing since time immemorial, namely working to improve the lot of the patients they care for. Each medical advance from X-rays to imatinib has always been heralded as the advent of the new millennium only to be replaced by new problems or unexpected complications of old problems (Kantarjian et al. 2002). But, despite rapid approval and grand hopes, no enhancement or treatment has ever turned out to be all it was cracked up to be. Outcomes in real patients hardly ever live up to the exaggerated claims of the advanced sales pitch. With each answer that emerges from a clinical trial, there are even more questions that are raised about optimal efficacy, the best target population, and the appropriate balance of benefits and risks. Longer life spans means more cancer and dementia, more antibiotics mean more virulent organisms, improvements in neonatal care mean more damaged low birth weight survivors. Programs for medical enhancement will never deliver on all great expectations, either good or bad. As such there appears to be no inherent reason to fear enhancement or limit its application.

If enhancement represents the intrinsic nature of man to reach out and control his own fate by manipulating his environment and to reverse any adverse effects of his surroundings, then it is inappropriate to use the term mastery in describing this defining human capacity. Instead of considering enhancement an activity with automatic winners and losers, I suggest that it would clarify the discussion if it was viewed as a hard wired human trait that we all engage in. Some do it better than others but all of us try to enhance our lot in life as best as we can. It is undoubtedly true that knowledge can and will be misdirected and even abused by those interested in self-aggrandizement. However, again this is not a unique feature of the remarkable advances in genomics or imaging technology. The fact that there are Harry Limes in the world does not take away from the benefits of antibiotics. The abuse of erythropoietin by athletes does not detract from the qualitative improvement in the lives of patients with end stage renal disease who are treated with this drug (Schumacher et al. 2001).

Moreover, intent has always been a difficult barometer to gauge the behavior of any professional. Most patients are only interested in getting better or improving their health. They rarely concern themselves with the motivation of the care provider, be it money, fame, fortune, or an altruistic desire to help others. Similarly, physicians rarely question why people want to get better as long as they follow instructions and balance the risks and benefits reasonably in their health care judgments. Even in judging religious behavior, which must comply with extralegal concerns and varying standards of dogma, intent is usually implicitly assumed to be appropriate or ignored provided the outcome is not destructive to the individual or community. One would be hard pressed to see any advantage for the patients if individual doctors or the health profession as a whole got into the business of judging patients' intention when they seek a medical treatment to cure disease or enhance health. If there are any lessons to be drawn from the endless discussions about active and passive euthanasia, it may be that no one is served by making this fine distinction in clinical practice (Kamisar 1969).

Finally, the distinction that is being made between treatment which is justified and permissible *versus* enhancement which smacks of hubris and should be constrained may prove to be irrelevant in real life situations where the boundaries are blurred by rapid advances in medical therapeutics and the definition of disease itself. When is failure to concentrate a sign of disease worthy of treatment and when does it indicate a lazy student who is not willing to work hard enough in school? Is erectile dysfunction an ailment like salmonella enteritis or a failure to perform? If I can confidently help the patient with their problem safely and effectively, I for one would just as soon avoid categorizing their complaint into an acceptable *versus* unacceptable category.

Finally, what is intriguing is that those who frown upon physicians who would dispense treatments that enhance patients rather than treat a disease is the assumption that there will be near unanimous acceptance of the treatment and a groundswell of people requesting the therapy. However, a survey of the history of public health interventions indicates that people, at least in this country, are reluctant to take the words of doctors on faith. Although each advance reported in the press is greeted by the public with great fanfare and anticipation, in reality many treatments are rejected by large segments of the population. Think of the people who refuse immunizations for their child, who place greater credence in alternative medications instead of chemotherapy (Frederickson 2004). There will always be people in search for the quick fix to treat obesity, prevent dementia, or win an Olympic medal. But, I think it is contrary to experience to think that everyone will line up for each new genetic treatment or enhancement. Doctors would do well to remind themselves of how varied their patients really are and that application of any therapeutic advance will still begin with a sensitive dialogue between doctor and patient.

In conclusion, I would encourage the medical community to embrace enhancement as a never ending quest for health that will make us healthier but never perfect. We should not fear progress in diagnostics or try to limit medical manipulations. This is because experience teaches us that they will never meet their goals and always leave us striving for more. I endorse Kamm's proposal to promote education about appropriate utilization of advances in genetics and medical science, insure equitable use of these resources, and maintain surveillance for unanticipated and undesirable consequences. However, as it says in Ethics of the Fathers, "The day is short, the work is hard, the employees are tired, the reward is great, and the boss is pressing" (Babylonian Talmud, Ch. 2, Mishna, 20), But, at the end of the day, we will still be human and knowing that should give us the confidence to proceed.

Acknowledgement

The author wishes to thank Rachel Frank, R.N. for her thoughtful comments about this essay.

References

Frederickson, D. D., T. C. Davis, C. L. Arnould, et al. 2004. Childhood immunization refusal: Provider and parent perceptions. *Family Medicine* 36:431–439.

Fukuyama, F. 1992. *The end of history and the last man.* New York: Free Press.

Goldstein, R. 2005. Incompleteness: The proof and paradox of Kort Godel. New York: W.W. Norton & Co.

Kamisar, Y. 1969. Euthanasia legislation: Some non-religious objections. In *Euthanasia and the right to death,* ed. A. B. Downing, Los Angeles, CA: Nash Publishing Company.

Kamm, F. M. 2005. Is there a problem with enhancement? *Am. J. Bioethics* 5–14.

Kantarjian H., C. Sawyers, A. Hochhaus, et al. 2002. Hematologic and cytogenetic responses to imatinib mesylate in chronic myelogenous leukemia. *New England Journal of Medicine* 346:645–652.

Sandel, M. 2004. The case against perfection. *The Atlantic Monthly* 293(3): 51–62.

Schumacher, Y. O., A. Schmid, and T. Lenz. 2001. Blood testing in sports: Hematological profile of a convicted athlete. *Clinical Journal of Sport Medicine* 11:115–117.

POSTSCRIPT

Is Genetic Enhancement an Unacceptable Use of Technology?

None of the genetic enhancements that arouse either fear or anticipation are possible with current technologies. Some say that they will never be possible since most of the desired or unwelcome characteristics are not controlled by a single gene and are also affected by many other background factors. Still, the future may bring still-undreamed-of possibilities.

The issue of the *American Journal of Bioethics* (vol. 5, no. 3, 2005), from which Howard Trachtman's essay is drawn, also contains several other articles on enhancement. The lead article by Frances M. Kamm, "Is There a Problem with Enhancement?" analyzes Sandel's article from a philosophical perspective.

Julian Savulescu argues that we have a moral obligation to enhance human beings and that "to be human is to strive to be better" ("New Breeds of Humans: The Moral Obligation to Enhance," *Reproductive Medicine Online,* March 2005). In "Enhancements and Justice: Problems in Determining the Requirements of Justice in a Genetically Transformed Society," Ronald A. Lindsay asserts that concern about the "threat of a genetic aristocracy" appears misplaced, given the already existing disparities in society (*Kennedy Institute of Ethics Journal*, vol. 15, no. 1, 2005).

Wondergenes: Genetic Enhancement and the Future of Society by Maxwell J. Mehlman (Indiana University Press, 2003) is an accessible introduction to the social and personal implications of genetic engineering. See also Erik Parens, "Authenticity and Ambivalence: Toward Understanding the Enhancement Debate," *Hastings Center Report* (May–June 2005).

On the Web: "Genetic Enhancement" from the National Human Genome Research Institute http://www.genome.gov/10004767.

Internet References . . .

New Scientist

This site offers pro and con views on the issue of animal experimentation. It also contains letters from readers of *New Scientist* articles on animal experimentation.

http://www.newscientist.com/

Debatabase: Animal Experimentation

This site offers information for those preparing to debate the issue of whether animal experimentation should be allowed. It has arguments, useful Web sites, and books.

http://www.debatabase.org.details.asp?topicID=7

Office for Human Research Protections (OHRP)

OHRP is the government agency charged with protecting the welfare and rights of human research subjects. Its Web site contains regulations and other information on research, including prisoners.

http://www.hhs.gov.ohrp

Human and Animal Experimentation

*T*he goal of scientific research is knowledge that will benefit society. But achieving that goal may subject humans and animals to some risks. Questions arise about not only how research should be conducted but whether or not it should be conducted at all. What, for example, are the justifications for using prisoners in research? This section contends with issues that will shape the future of experimental science.

• Should Animal Experimentation Be Permitted?

• Should Prisoners Be Allowed to Participate in Research?

ISSUE 14

Should Animal Experimentation Be Permitted?

YES: Jerod M. Loeb, et al., from "Human vs. Animal Rights: In Defense of Animal Research," *Journal of the American Medical Association* (November 17, 1989)

NO: Tom Regan, from "Ill-Gotten Gains," in Donald Van DeVeer and Tom Regan, eds., *Health Care Ethics: An Introduction* (Temple University Press, 1987)

ISSUE SUMMARY

YES: Jerod M. Loeb and his colleagues, representing the American Medical Association's Group on Science and Technology, assert that concern for animals, admirable in itself, cannot impede the development of methods to improve the welfare of humans.

NO: Philosopher Tom Regan argues that conducting research on animals exacts the grave moral price of failing to show proper respect for animals' inherent value, whatever the benefits of the research.

In 1865 the great French physiologist Claude Bernard wrote, "Physicians already make too many dangerous experiments on man before carefully studying them in animals." In his insistence on adequate animal research before trying a new therapy on human beings, Bernard established a principle of research ethics that is still considered valid. But in the past few decades this principle has been challenged by another view—one that sees animals not as tools for human use and consumption but as moral agents in their own right. Animal experimentation, according to this theory, cannot be taken for granted but must be justified by ethical criteria at least as stringent as those that apply to research involving humans.

Philosophers traditionally have not ascribed any moral status to animals. Like St. Thomas Aquinas before him, René Descartes, a seventeenth-century French physiologist and philosopher, saw no ethical problem in experimentation on animals. Descartes approved of cutting open a fully conscious animal because it was, he said, a machine more complex than a clock but no more capable of feeling pain. Immanuel Kant argued that animals need not be treated as ends in themselves because they lacked rationality.

Beginning in England in the nineteenth century, antivivisectionists (people who advocate the abolition of animal experimentation) campaigned, with varying success, for laws to control scientific research. But the internal dissensions in the movement and its frequent lapses into sentimentality made it only partially effective. At best the antivivisectionists achieved some legislation that mandated more humane treatment of animals used for research, but they never succeeded in abolishing animal research or even in establishing the need for justification of particular research projects.

The more recent movement to ban animal research, however, is both better organized politically and more rigorously philosophical. The movement, often called animal liberation or animal rights, is similar in principle to the civil rights movement of the 1960s. Just as blacks, women, and other minorities sought recognition of their equal status, animal advocates have built a case for the equal status of animals.

Peter Singer, one of the leaders of this movement, has presented an eloquent case that we practice not only racism and sexism in our society but also "speciesism." That is, we assume that human beings are superior to other animals; we are prejudiced in favor of our own kind. Experimenting on animals and eating their flesh are the two major forms of speciesism in our society. Singer points out that some categories of human beings—infants and mentally retarded people—rate lower on a scale of intelligence, awareness, and self-consciousness than some animals. Yet we would not treat these individuals in the way we do animals. He argues that "all animals are equal" and that the suffering of an animal is morally equal to the suffering of a human being.

Proponents of animal research counter that such views are fundamentally misguided, that human beings, with the capacity for rational thought and action, are indeed a superior species. They contend that, while animals deserve humane treatment, the good consequences of animal research (i.e., knowledge that will benefit human beings) outweigh the suffering of individual animals. No other research techniques can substitute for the reactions of live animals, they declare.

In the selections that follow, Jerod M. Loeb and his colleagues reaffirm the American Medical Association's defense of animal research because it is essential for medical progress and it would be unethical to deprive humans and animals of advances in medicine that result from this research. Tom Regan disputes the view that benefit to humans justifies research on animals. Pointing to their inherent value, he says that "whatever our gains, they are ill-gotten," and he calls for an end to such research.

YES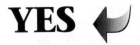

Jerod M. Loeb, et al.

Human vs. Animal Rights: In Defense of Animal Research

Research with animals is a highly controversial topic in our society. Animal rights groups that intend to stop all experimentation with animals are in the vanguard of this controversy. Their methods range from educational efforts directed in large measure to the young and uninformed, to promotion of restrictive legislation, filing lawsuits, and violence that includes raids on laboratories and death threats to investigators. Their rhetoric is emotionally charged and their information is frequently distorted and pejorative. Their tactics vary but have a single objective—to stop scientific research with animals.

The resources of the animal rights groups are extensive, in part because less militant organizations of animal activists, including some humane societies, have been infiltrated or taken over by animal rights groups to gain access to their fiscal and physical holdings. Through bizarre tactics, extravagant claims, and gruesome myths, animal rights groups have captured the attention of the media and a sizable segment of the public. Nevertheless, people invariably support the use of animals in research when they understand both sides of the issue and the contributions of animal research to relief of human suffering. However, all too often they do not understand both sides because information about the need for animal research is not presented. When this need is explained, the presentation often reveals an arrogance of the scientific community and an unwillingness to be accountable to public opinion.

The use of animals in research is fundamentally an ethical question: is it more ethical to ban all research with animals or to use a limited number of animals in research under humane conditions when no alternatives exist to achieve medical advances that reduce substantial human suffering and misery? . . .

Animals in Scientific Research

Animals have been used in research for more than 2000 years. In the third century BC, the natural philosopher Erisistratus of Alexandria used animals to study bodily function. In all likelihood, Aristotle performed vivisection on animals. The Roman physician Galen used apes and pigs to prove his theory that veins carry blood rather than air. In succeeding centuries, animals were

From *Journal of the American Medical Association,* vol. 262, no. 19, November 17, 1989, pp. 2716–2720.

employed to confirm theories about physiology developed through observation. Advances in knowledge from these experiments include demonstration of the circulation of blood by Harvey in 1622, documentation of the effects of anesthesia on the body in 1846, and elucidation of the relationship between bacteria and disease in 1878.[1] In his book *An Introduction to the Study of Experimental Medicine* published in 1865, Bernard[2] described the importance of animal research to advances in knowledge about the human body and justified the continued use of animals for this purpose.

In this century, many medical advances have been achieved through research with animals.[3] Infectious diseases such as pertussis, rubella, measles, and poliomyelitis have been brought under control with vaccines developed in animals. The development of immunization techniques against today's infectious diseases, including human immunodeficiency virus disease, depends entirely on experiments in animals. Antibiotics that control infection are always tested in animals before use in humans. Physiological disorders such as diabetes and epilepsy are treatable today through knowledge and products gained by animal research. Surgical procedures such as coronary artery bypass grafts, cerebrospinal fluid shunts, and retinal reattachments have evolved from experiments with animals. Transplantation procedures for persons with failed liver, heart, lung, and kidney function are products of animal research.

Animals have been essential to the evolution of modern medicine and the conquest of many illnesses. However, many medical challenges remain to be solved. Cancer, heart disease, cerebrovascular disease, dementia, depression, arthritis, and a variety of inherited disorders are yet to be understood and controlled. Until they are, human pain and suffering will endure, and society will continue to expend its emotional and fiscal resources in efforts to alleviate or at least reduce them.

Animal research has not only benefited humans. Procedures and products developed through this process have also helped animals.[4,5] Vaccines against rabies, distemper, and parvovirus in dogs are a spin-off of animal research, as are immunization techniques against cholera in hogs, encephalitis in horses, and brucellosis in cattle. Drugs to combat heartworm, intestinal parasites, and mastitis were developed in animals used for experimental purposes. Surgical procedures developed in animals help animals as well as humans.

Research with animals has yielded immeasurable benefits to both humans and animals. However, this research raises fundamental philosophical issues concerning the rights of humans to use animals to benefit humans and other animals. If these rights are granted (and many people are loath to do so), additional questions arise concerning the way that research should be performed, the accountability of researchers to public sentiment, the nature of an ethical code for animal research, and who should compose and approve the code. Today, some animal activists are asking whether humans have the right to exercise dominion over animals for any purpose, including research. Others suggest that because humans have dominion over other forms of life, they are obligated to protect and preserve animals and ensure that they are not exploited. Still others agree that animals can be used to help people, but only under circumstances that are so structured as to be unattainable by most researchers. These attitudes may all differ, but their consequences are similar. They all threaten to diminish or stop animal research.

Challenge to Animal Research

Challenges to the use of animals to benefit humans are not new—their origins can be traced back several centuries. With respect to animal research, opposition has been vocal in Europe for more than 400 years and in the United States for at least 100 years.[6]

Most of the current arguments against research with animals have historic precedents that must be grasped to understand the current debate. These precedents originated in the controversy between Cartesian and utilitarian philosophers that extended from the 16th to the 18th centuries.

The Cartesian-utilitarian debate was opened by the French philosopher Descartes, who defended the use of animals in experiments by insisting the animals respond to stimuli in only one way—"according to the arrangement of their organs."[7] He stated that animals lack the ability to reason and think and are, therefore, similar to a machine. Humans, on the other hand, can think, talk, and respond to stimuli in various ways. These differences, Descartes argued, make animals inferior to humans and justify their use as a machine, including as experimental subjects. He proposed that animals learn only by experience, whereas humans learn by "teaching-learning." Humans do not always have to experience something to know that it is true.

Descartes' arguments were countered by the utilitarian philosopher Bentham of England. "The question," said Bentham, "is not can they reason? nor can they talk? but can they suffer?"[8] In utilitarian terms, humans and animals are linked by their common ability to suffer and their common right not to suffer and die at the hands of others. This utilitarian thesis has rippled through various groups opposed to research with animals for more than a century.

In the 1970s, the antivivisectionist movement was influenced by three books that clarified the issues and introduced the rationale for increased militancy against animal research. In 1971, the anthology *Animals, Men and Morals*, by Godlovitch et al.,[9] raised the concept of animal rights and analyzed the relationships between humans and animals. Four years later, *Victims of Science*, by Ryder,[10] introduced the concept of "speciesism" as equivalent to fascism. Also in 1975, Singer[11] published *Animal Liberation: A New Ethic for Our Treatment of Animals*. This book is generally considered the progenitor of the modern animal rights movement. Invoking Ryder's concept of speciesism, Singer deplored the historic attitude of humans toward nonhumans as a "form of prejudice no less objectionable than racism or sexism." He urged that the liberation of animals should become the next great cause after civil rights and the women's movement.

Singer's book not only was a philosophical treatise; it also was a call to action. It provided an intellectual foundation and a moral focus for the animal rights movement. These features attracted many who were indifferent to the emotional appeal based on a love of animals that had characterized antivivisectionist efforts for the past century. Singer's book swelled the ranks of the antivivisectionist movement and transformed it into a movement for animal rights. It also has been used to justify illegal activities intended to impede animal research and instill fear and intimidation in those engaged in it. . . .

Defense of Animal Research

The issue of animal research is fundamentally an issue of the dominion of humans over animals. This issue is rooted in the Judeo-Christian religion of western culture, including the ancient tradition of animal sacrifice described in the Old Testament and the practice of using animals as surrogates for suffering humans described in the New Testament. The sacredness of human life is a central theme of biblical morality, and the dominion of humans over other forms of life is a natural consequence of this theme.[12] The issue of dominion is not, however, unique to animal research. It is applicable to every situation where animals are subservient to humans. It applies to the use of animals for food and clothing; the application of animals as beasts of burden and transportation; the holding of animals in captivity such as in zoos and as household pets; the use of animals as entertainment, such as in sea parks and circuses; the exploitation of animals in sports that employ animals, including hunting, racing, and animal shows; and the eradication of pests such as rats and mice from homes and farms. Even provision of food and shelter to animals reflects an attitude of dominion of humans over animals. A person who truly does not believe in human dominance over animals would be forced to oppose all of these practices, including keeping animals as household pets or in any form of physical or psychological captivity. Such a posture would defy tradition evolved over the entire course of human existence.

Some animal advocates do not take issue with the right of humans to exercise dominion over animals. They agree that animals are inferior to humans because they do not possess attributes such as a moral sense and concepts of past and future. However, they also claim that it is precisely because of these differences that humans are obligated to protect animals and not exploit them for the selfish betterment of humans.[13] In their view, animals are like infants and the mentally incompetent, who must be nurtured and protected from exploitation. This view shifts the issues of dominion from one of rights claimed by animals to one of responsibilities exercised by humans.

Neither of these philosophical positions addresses the issue of animal research from the perspective of the immorality of not using animals in research. From this perspective, depriving humans (and animals) of advances in medicine that result from research with animals is inhumane and fundamentally unethical. Spokespersons for this perspective suggest that patients with dementia, stroke, disabling injuries, heart disease, and cancer deserve relief from suffering and that depriving them of hope and relief by eliminating animal research is an immoral and unconscionable act. Defenders of animal research claim that animals sometimes must be sacrificed in the development of methods to relieve pain and suffering of humans (and animals) and to affect treatments and cures of a variety of human maladies.

The immeasurable benefits of animal research to humans are undeniable. One example is the development of a vaccine for poliomyelitis, with the result that the number of cases of poliomyelitis in the United States alone declined from 58,000 in 1952 to 4 in 1984. Benefits of this vaccine worldwide are even more impressive.

Every year, hundreds of thousands of humans are spared the braces, wheelchairs, and iron lungs required for the victims of poliomyelitis who survive this infectious disease. The research that led to a poliomyelitis vaccine required the sacrifice of hundreds of primates. Without this sacrifice, development of the vaccine would have been impossible, and in all likelihood the poliomyelitis epidemic would have continued unabated. Depriving humanity of this medical advance is unthinkable to almost all persons. Other diseases that are curable or treatable today as a result of animal research include diphtheria, scarlet fever, tuberculosis, diabetes, and appendicitis.[3] Human suffering would be much more stark today if these diseases, and many others as well, had not been amendable to treatment and cure through advances obtained by animal research.

Issues in Animal Research

Animal rights groups have several stock arguments against animal research. Some of these issues are described and refuted herein.

The Clinical Value of Basic Research

Persons opposed to research with animals often claim that basic biomedical research has no clinical value and therefore does not justify the use of animals. However, basic research is the foundation for most medical advances and consequently for progress in clinical medicine. Without basic research, including that with animals, chemotherapeutic advances against cancer (including childhood leukemia and breast malignancy), beta-blockers for cardiac patients, and electrolyte infusions for patients with dysfunctional metabolism would never have been achieved.

Duplication of Experiments

Opponents of animal research frequently claim that experiments are needlessly duplicated. However, the duplication of results is an essential part of the confirmation process in science. The generalization of results from one laboratory to another prevents anomalous results in one laboratory from being interpreted as scientific truth. The cost of research animals, the need to publish the results of experiments, and the desire to conduct meaningful research all function to reduce the likelihood of unnecessary experiments. Furthermore, the intense competition of research funds and the peer review process lessen the probability of obtaining funds for unnecessary research. Most scientists are unlikely to waste valuable time and resources conducting unnecessary experiments when opportunities for performing important research are so plentiful. . . .

The Use of Primates in Research

Animal activists often make a special plea on behalf of nonhuman primates, and many of the sit-ins, demonstrations, and break-ins have been directed at primate research centers. Efforts to justify these activities invoke the premise that primates are much like humans because they exhibit suffering and other emotions.

Keeping primates in cages and isolating them from others of their kind is considered by activists as cruel and destructive of their "psychological well-being." However, the opinion that animals that resemble humans most closely and deserve the most protection and care reflects an attitude of speciesism (i.e., a hierarchical scheme of relative importance) that most activists purportedly abhor. This logical fallacy in the drive for special protection of primates apparently escapes most of its adherents.

Some scientific experiments require primates exactly because they simulate human physiology so closely. Primates are susceptible to many of the same diseases as humans and have similar immune systems. They also possess intellectual, cognitive, and social skills above those of other animals. These characteristics make primates invaluable in research related to language, perception, and visual and spatial skills.[14] Although primates constitute only 0.5% of all animals used in research, their contributions have been essential to the continued acquisition of knowledge in the biological and behavioral sciences.[15]

Do Animals Suffer Needless Pain and Abuse?

Animal activists frequently assert that research with animals causes severe pain and that many research animals are abused either deliberately or through indifference. Actually, experiments today involve pain only when relief from pain would interfere with the purpose of the experiments. In any experiment in which an animal might experience pain, federal law requires that a veterinarian must be consulted in planning the experiment, and anesthesia, tranquilizers, and analgesics must be used except when they would compromise the results of the experiment.[16]

In 1984, the Department of Agriculture reported that 61% of research animals were not subjected to painful procedures, and another 31% received anesthesia or pain-relieving drugs. The remaining 8% did experience pain, often because improved understanding and treatment of pain, including chronic pain, were the purpose of the experiment.[14] Chronic pain is a challenging health problem that costs the United States about $50 billion a year in direct medical expenses, lost productivity, and income.[15]

Alternatives to the Use of Animals

One of the most frequent objections to animal research is the claim that alternative research models obviate the need for research with animals. The concept of alternatives was first raised in 1959 by Russell and Burch[17] in their book, *The Principles of Humane Experimental Technique*. These authors exhorted scientists to reduce the pain of experimental animals, decrease the number of animals used in research, and replace animals with nonanimal models whenever possible.

However, more often than not, alternatives to research animals are not available. In certain research investigations, cell, tissue, and organ cultures and computer models can be used as adjuncts to experiments with animals, and occasionally as substitutes for animals, at least in preliminary phases of the investigations. However, in many experimental situations, culture techniques and computer models are wholly inadequate because they do not encompass the physiological complexity of the whole animal. Examples where animals are essential to research include development of a vaccine against human immunodeficiency virus, refinement of organ transplantation techniques, investigation of mechanical devices as replacements for and adjuncts to physiological organs, identification of target-specific pharmaceuticals for cancer diagnosis and treatment, restoration of infarcted myocardium in patients with cardiac disease, evolution of new diagnostic imaging technologies, improvement of methods to relieve mental stress and anxiety, and evaluation of approaches to define and treat chronic pain. These challenges can only be addressed by research with animals as an essential step in the evolution of knowledge that leads to solutions. Humans are the only alternatives to animals for this step. When faced with this alternative, most people prefer the use of animals as the research model.

Comment

Love of animals and concern for their welfare are admirable characteristics that distinguish humans from other species of animals. Most humans, scientists as well as laypersons, share these attributes. However, when the concern for animals impedes the development of methods to improve the welfare of humans through amelioration and elimination of pain and suffering, a fundamental choice must be made. This choice is present today in the conflict between animal rights activism and scientific research. The American Medical Association made this choice more than a century ago and continues to stand squarely in defense of the use of animals for scientific research. In this position, the Association is supported by opinion polls that reveal strong endorsement of the American public for the use of animals in research and testing.[18] . . .

The American Medical Association believes that research involving animals is absolutely essential to maintaining and improving the health of people in America and worldwide.[6] Animal research is required to develop solutions to human tragedies such as human immunodeficiency virus disease, cancer, heart disease, dementia, stroke, and congenital and developmental abnormalities. The American Medical Association recognizes the moral obligation of investigators to use alternatives to animals whenever possible, and to conduct their research with animals as humanely as possible. However, it is convinced that depriving humans of medical advances by preventing research with animals is philosophically and morally a fundamentally indefensible position. Consequently, the American Medical Association is committed to the preservation of animal research and to the conduct of this research under the most humane conditions possible.[19,20]

References

1. Rowan AN, Rollin BE. Animal research-for and against: a philosophical, social, and historical perspective. *Perspect Biol Med.* 1983; 27:1–17.

2. Bernard C, Green HC, trans. *An Introduction to the Study of Experimental Medicine.* New York, NY: Dover Publications Inc; 1957.

3. Council on Scientific Affairs. Animals in research. *JAMA,* 1989; 261:3602–3606.

4. Leader RW, Stark D. The importance of animals in biomedical research. *Perspect Biol Med.* 1987; 30:470–485.

5. Kransney JA. Some thoughts on the value of life. *Buffalo Physician,* 1984; 18:6–13.

6. Smith SJ, Evans RM, Sullivan-Fowler M, Hendee WR. Use of animals in biomedical research: historical role of the American Medical Association and the American physician. *Arch Intern Med.* 1988; 148:1849–1853.

7. Descartes R. *'Principles of Philosophy,' Descartes: Philosophical Writings.* Anscombe E, Geach PT, eds. London, England: Nelson & Sons; 1969.

8. Bentham J. *Introduction to the Principles of Morals and Legislation.* London, England: Athlone Press; 1970.

9. Godlovitch S, Godlovitch, Harris J. *Animals, Men and Morals.* New York, NY: Taplinger Publishing Co Inc; 1971.

10. Ryder R. *Victims of Science.* London, England: Davis-Poynter; 1975.

11. Singer P. *Animal Liberation: A New Ethic for Our Treatment of Animals.* New York, NY: Random House Inc; 1975.

12. Morowitz HJ, Jesus, Moses, Aristotle and laboratory animals. *Hosp Pract.* 1988; 23:23–25.

13. Cohen C. The case for the use of animals in biomedical research. *N Engl J Med.* 1986; 315: 865–870.

14. *Alternatives to Animal Use in Research, Testing, and Education.* Washington, DC: Office of Technology Assessment; 1986. Publication OTA-BA-273.

15. Committee on the Use of Laboratory Animals in Biomedical and Behavioral Research. *Use of Laboratory Animals in Biomedical and Behavioral Research.* Washington, DC: National Academy Press; 1988.

16. *Biomedical Investigator's Handbook.* Washington, DC: Foundation for Biomedical Research; 1987.

17. Russell WMS, Burch RL. *The Principles of Humane Experimental Technique.* Springfield, Ill: Charles C Thomas Publisher; 1959.

18. Harvey LK, Shubat SC. *AMA Survey of Physician and Public Opinion on Health Care Issues.* Chicago, Ill: American Medical Association; 1989.

19. Smith SJ, Hendee WR. Animals in research. *JAMA* 1988; 259:2007–2008.

20. Smith SJ, Loeb JM, Evans RM, Hendee WR. Animals in research and testing; who pays the price for medical progress? *Arch Ophthalmol.* 1988; 106:1184–1187.

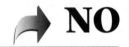

Ill-Gotten Gains

The Story

Late in 1981 a reporter for a large metropolitan newspaper (we'll call her Karen to protect her interest in remaining anonymous) gained access to some previously classified government files. Using the Freedom of Information Act, Karen was investigating the federal government's funding of research into the short- and long-term effects of exposure to radioactive waste. It was with understandable surprise that, included in these files, she discovered the records of a series of experiments involving the induction and treatment of coronary thrombosis (heart attack). Conducted over a period of fifteen years by a renowned heart specialist (we'll call him Dr. Ventricle) and financed with federal funds, the experiments in all likelihood would have remained unknown to anyone outside Dr. Ventricle's sphere of power and influence had not Karen chanced upon them.

Karen's surprise soon gave way to shock and disbelief. In case after case she read of how Ventricle and his associates took otherwise healthy individuals, with no previous record of heart disease, and intentionally caused their heart to fail. The methods used to occasion the "attack" were a veritable shopping list of experimental techniques, from massive doses of stimulants (adrenaline was a favorite) to electrical damage of the coronary artery, which, in its weakened state, yielded the desired thrombosis. Members of Ventricle's team then set to work testing the efficacy of various drugs developed in the hope that they would help the heart withstand a second "attack." Dosages varied, and there were the usual control groups. In some cases, certain drugs administered to "patients" proved more efficacious than cases in which others received no medication or smaller amounts of the same drugs. The research came to an abrupt end in the fall of 1981, but not because the project was judged unpromising or because someone raised a hue and cry about the ethics involved. Like so much else in the world at that time, Ventricle's project was a casualty of austere economic times. There simply wasn't enough federal money available to renew the grant application.

One would have to forsake all the instincts of a reporter to let the story end there. Karen persevered and, under false pretenses, secured an interview with Ventricle. When she revealed that she had gained access to the file, knew in detail the largely fruitless research conducted over fifteen years, and was incensed about his work, Ventricle was dumbfounded. But not because Karen had unearthed the file. And not even because it was filed where it was (a "clerical error," he assured her). What surprised Ventricle was that anyone would think there was a serious ethical question to be raised about what he had done. Karen's notes of their conversation include the following:

Ventricle: But I don't understand what you're getting at. Surely you know that heart disease is the leading cause of death. How can there be any ethical question about developing drugs which *literally* promise to be life-saving?

Karen: Some people might agree that the goal—to save life—is a good, a noble end, and still question the means used to achieve it. Your "patients," after all, had no previous history of heart disease. *They* were healthy before you got your hands on them.

Ventricle: But medical progress simply isn't possible if we wait for people to get sick and then see what works. There are too many variables, too much beyond our control and comprehension, if we try to do our medical research in a clinical setting. The history of medicine shows how hopeless that approach is.

Karen: And I read, too, that upon completion of the experiment, assuming that the "patient" didn't die in the process—it says that those who survived were "sacrificed." You mean killed?

Ventricle: Yes, that's right. But always painlessly, always painlessly. And the body went immediately to the lab, where further tests were done. Nothing was wasted.

Karen: And it didn't bother you—I mean, you didn't ever ask yourself whether what you were doing was wrong? I mean . . .

Ventricle: (interrupting): My dear young lady, you make it seem as if I'm some kind of moral monster. I work for the benefit of humanity, and I have achieved some small success, I hope you will agree. Those who raise cries of wrongdoing about what I've done are well intentioned but misguided. After all, I use animals in my research—chimpanzees, to be more precise—not human beings.

The Point

The story about Karen and Dr. Ventricle is just that—a story, a small piece of fiction. There is no real Dr. Ventricle, no real Karen, and so on. But there *is* widespread use of animals in scientific research, including research like our imaginary Dr. Ventricle's. So the story, while its details are imaginary—while it is, let it be clear, a literary device, not a factual account—is a story with a point. Most people reading it would be morally outraged if there actually were a Dr. Ventricle who did coronary research of the sort described on otherwise healthy human beings. Considerably fewer would raise a morally quizzical eyebrow when informed of such research done on animals, chimpanzees, or whatever. The story has a point, or so I hope, because, catching us off-guard, it brings this difference home to us, gives it life in our experience, and, in doing so, reveals something about ourselves, something about our own constellation of values. If we think what Ventricle did would be wrong if done to human beings but all right if done to chimpanzees, then we must believe that there are different moral standards that apply to how we may treat the two—human beings and chimpanzees. But to acknowledge this difference, if acknowledge it we do, is only the beginning, not the end, of our moral thinking. We can meet the challenge to think well from the moral point of view only if we are able to cite a *morally relevant difference* between humans and chimpanzees, one that illuminates in a clear, coherent, and rationally defensible way why it would be wrong to use humans, but not chimpanzees, in research like Dr. Ventricle's. . . .

The Law

Among the difference between chimps and humans, one concerns their legal standing. It is against the law to do to human beings what Ventricle did to his chimpanzees. It is not against the law to do this to chimps. So, here we have a difference. But a morally relevant one?

The difference in the legal status of chimps and humans would be morally relevant if we had good reason to believe that what is legal and what is moral go hand in glove: where we have the former, there we have the latter (and maybe vice versa too). But a moment's reflection shows how bad the fit between legality and morality sometimes is. A century and a half ago, the legal status of black people in the United States was similar to the legal status of a house, corn, a barn: they were property, other people's property, and could legally be bought and sold without regard to their personal interests. But the legality of the slave trade did not make it moral, any more than the law against drinking, during the era of that "great experiment" of Prohibition, made it immoral to drink. Sometimes, it is true, what the law declares illegal (for example, murder and rape) is immoral, and vice versa. But there is no necessary connection, no pre-established harmony between morality and the law. So, yes, the legal status of chimps and humans differs; but that does not show that their moral status does. Their difference in legal status, in other words, is not a morally relevant difference and will not morally justify using these animals, but not humans, in Ventricle's research.

The Value of the Individual

[An] alternative vision [to utilitarian value] consists in viewing certain individuals as themselves having a distinctive kind of value, what we will call "inherent value." This kind of value is not the same as, is not reducible to, and is not commensurate either with such values as preference satisfaction or frustration (that is, mental states) or with such values as artistic or intellectual talents (that is, mental and other kinds of excellences or virtues). We cannot, that is, equate or reduce the inherent value of an individual to his or her mental states or virtues, and neither can we intelligibly compare the two. In this respect, the three kinds of value (mental states, virtues, and the inherent value of the individual) are like proverbial apples and oranges.

They are also like water and oil: they don't mix. It is not only that [a man's] inherent value is not the same as, not reducible to, and not commensurate with *his* satisfaction, pleasures, intellectual and artistic skills, etc. In addition, *his* inherent value is not the same as, is not reducible to, and is not commensurate with the valuable mental states or talents of *other* individuals, whether taken singly or collectively. Moreover, and as a corollary of the preceding, the individual's inherent value is in all ways independent both of his or her usefulness relative to the interest of others and of how others feel about the individual (for example, whether one is liked or admired, despised or merely tolerated). A prince and a pauper, a streetwalker and a nun, those who are loved and those who are forsaken, the genius and the retarded child, the artist and the philistine, the most generous philanthropist and the most unscrupulous used car salesman—all have inherent value, according to the view recommended here, and all have it equally. . . .

What Difference Does It Make?

To view the value of individuals in this way is not an empty abstraction. To the question, "What difference does it make whether we view individuals as having equal inherent value, or as utilitarians do, as lacking such value, or, as perfectionists do, as having such value but to varying degree?"—our response to this question must be, "It makes all the moral difference in the world!" Morally, we are *always* required to treat those who have inherent value in ways that display proper respect for their distinctive kind of value, and though we cannot on this occasion either articulate or defend the full range of obligations tied to this fundamental duty, we can note that we fail to show proper respect for those who have such value whenever we treat them as if they were mere receptacles of value or as if their value was dependent on, or reducible to, their possible utility relative to the interests of others. In particular, therefore, Ventricle would fail to act as duty requires—would, in other words, do what is morally wrong—if he conducted his coronary research on competent human beings, without their informed consent, on the grounds that this research just might lead to the development of drugs or surgical techniques that would benefit others. That would be to treat these human beings as mere receptacles or as mere medical resources for others, and though Ventricle might be able to do this and get away with it, and though others might benefit as a result, that would not alter the nature of the grievous wrong he would have done. And it would be wrong, not because (or only if) there were utilitarian considerations, or contractarian considerations, or perfectionist considerations against his doing his research on these human beings, but because it would mark a failure on his part to treat them with appropriate respect. To ascribe inherent value to competent human beings, then, provides us with the theoretical wherewithal to ground our moral case against using competent human beings, against their will, in research like Ventricle's.

Who Has Inherent Value?

If inherent value could nonarbitrarily be limited to competent humans, then we would have to look elsewhere to resolve the ethical issues involved in using other individuals (for example, chimpanzees) in medical research. But inherent value can only be limited to competent human beings by having the recourse to one arbitrary maneuver or another. Once we recognize that we have direct duties to competent and incompetent humans as well as to animals such as chimpanzees; once we recognize the challenge to give a sound theoretical basis for these duties in the case of these humans and animals; once we recognize the failure of indirect duty, contractarian, and utilitarian theories of obligation; once we recognize that the inherent value of competent humans precludes using them as mere resources in such research; once we recognize that perfectionist vision of morality, one that assigns degrees of inherent value on the basis of possession of favored virtues, is unacceptable because of its inegalitarian implications, and once we recognize that morality simply will not tolerate double standards, then we cannot, except arbitrarily, withhold ascribing inherent value, to an equal degree, to incompetent humans and animals such as chimpanzees. All have this value, in short, and all have it equally. All considered, this is an essential part of the most adequate total vision of morality. Morally, none of those having inherent value may be used in Ventricle-like research (research that puts them at risk of significant harm in the name of securing benefits for others, whether those benefits are realized or not). And none may be used in such research because to do so is to treat them as if their value is somehow reducible to their possible utility relative to the interests of others, or as if their value is somehow reducible to their value as "receptacles." What contractarianism, utilitarianism, and the other "isms" discussed earlier will allow is not morally tolerable.

Hurting and Harming

The prohibition against research like Ventricle's, when conducted on animals such as chimps, cannot be avoided by the use of anesthetics or other palliatives used to eliminate or reduce suffering. Other things being equal, to cause an animal to suffer is to harm that animal—is, that is, to diminish that individual animal's welfare. But these two notions—harming on the one hand and suffering on the other—differ in important ways. An individual's welfare can be diminished independently of causing her to suffer, as when, for example, a young woman is reduced to a "vegetable" by painlessly administering a debilitating drug to her while she sleeps. We mince words if we deny that harm has been done to her, though she suffers not. More generally, harms, understood as reductions in an individual's welfare, can take the form either of *inflictions* (gross physical suffering is the clearest example of a harm of this type) or *deprivations* (prolonged loss of physical freedom is a clear example of a harm of this kind). Not all harms hurt, in other words, just as not all hurts harm.

Viewed against the background of these ideas, an untimely death is seen to be the ultimate harm for both humans and animals, such as chimpanzees, and it is the ultimate harm for both because it is their ultimate deprivation or loss—their loss of life itself. Let the means used to kill chimpanzees be as "humane" (a cruel word, this) as you like. That will not erase the harm that an untimely death is for these animals. True, the use of anesthetics and other "humane" steps lessens the wrong done to these animals, when they are "sacrificed" in Ventricle-type research. But a lesser wrong is not a right. To do research that culminates in the "sacrifice" of chimpanzees or that puts these and similar animals at risk of losing their life, in the hope that we might learn something that will benefit others, is morally to be condemned, however "humane" that research may be in other respects.

The Criterion of Inherent Value

It remains to be asked, before concluding, what underlies the possession of inherent value. Some are tempted by the idea that life itself is inherently valuable. This view would authorize attributing inherent value to chimpanzees, for example, and so might find favor with some people who oppose using these animals in research. But this view would also authorize attributing inherent value to anything and everything that is alive, including, for example, crabgrass, lice, bacteria, and cancer cells. It is exceedingly unclear, to put the point as mildly as possible, either that we have a duty to treat these things with respect or that any clear sense can be given to the idea that we do.

More plausible by far is the view that those individuals have inherent value who are *the subjects of a life*—who are, that is, the experiencing subjects of a life that fares well or ill for them over time, those who have *an individual experiential welfare*, logically independent of their utility relative to the interests or welfare of others. Competent humans are subjects of a life in this sense. But so, too, are those incompetent humans who have concerned us. And so, too, and not unimportantly, are chimpanzees. Indeed, so too are the members of many species of animals: cats and dogs, monkeys and sheep, cetaceans and wolves, horses and cattle. Where one draws the line between those animals who are, and those who are not, subjects of a life is certain to be controversial. Still there is abundant reason to believe that the members of mammalian species of animals do have a psychophysical identity over time, do have an experiential life, do have an individual welfare. Common sense is on the side of viewing these animals in this way, and ordinary language is not strained in talking of them as individuals who have an experiential welfare. The behavior of these animals, moreover, is consistent with regarding them as subjects of a life, and the implications of evolutionary theory are that there are many species of animals whose members are, like the members of the species *Homo sapiens*, experiencing subjects of a life of their own, with an individual welfare. On these grounds, then, we have very strong reason to believe, even if we lack conclusive proof, that these animals meet the subject-of-a-life criterion.

If, then, those who meet this criterion have inherent value, and have it equally relative to all who meet it, chimpanzees and other animals who are subjects of a life, not just human beings, have this value *and* have neither more nor less of it than we do. (To hold that they have less than we do is to land oneself in the inegalitarian swamp of perfectionism.) Moreover, if, as has been argued, having inherent value morally bars others from treating those who have it as mere receptacles or as mere resources for others, then any and all medical research like Ventricle's, done on these animals in the name of possibly benefitting others, stands morally condemned. And it is not only cases in which the benefits for others do not materialize that are condemnable; also to be condemned are cases, such as the research done on chimps regarding hepatitis, for example, in which the benefits for others are genuine. In these cases, as in others like them in the relevant respects, the ends do not justify the means. The *many millions* of mammalian animals used each year for scientific purposes, including medical research, bear mute, tragic testimony to the narrowness of our moral vision.

Conclusions

This condemnation of such research probably is at odds with the judgment that most people would make about this issue. If we had good reason to assume that the truth always lies with what most people think, then we could look approvingly on Ventricle-like research done on animals like chimps in the name of benefits for others. But we have no good reason to believe that the truth is to be measured plausibly by majority opinion, and what we know of the history of prejudice and bigotry speaks powerfully, if painfully, against this view. Only the cumulative force of informed, fair, rigorous argument can decide where the truth lies, or most likely lies, when we examine a controversial moral question. Although openly acknowledging and, indeed, insisting on the limitations of the arguments . . . , these arguments make the case, in broad outline, against using animals such as chimps in medical research such as Ventricle's. . . .

Those who oppose the use of animals such as chimps in research like Ventricle's and who accept the major themes advanced here, oppose it, then, not because they think that all such research is a waste of time and money, or because they think that it never leads to any benefits for others, or because they view those who do such research as, to use Ventricle's, words, "moral monsters," or even because they love animals. Those of us who condemn such research do so because this research is not possible except at the grave moral price of failing to show proper respect for the value of the animals who are used. Since, whatever our gains, they are ill-gotten, we must bring to an end research like Ventricle's, whatever our losses. A fair measure of our moral integrity will be the extent of our resolve to work against allowing our scientific, economic, health, and other interests to serve as a reason for the wrongful exploitation of members of species of animals other than our own.

POSTSCRIPT

Should Animal Experimentation Be Permitted?

$\mathbf{I}$n 1985 Congress passed the Health Research Extension Act, which directed the National Institutes of Health (NIH) to establish guidelines for the proper care of animals to be used in biomedical and behavioral research. The NIH regulations implementing the law require institutions that receive federal grants to establish Animal Care and Use Committees. The Office of Science and Technology Policies' "Principles for the Utilization and Care of Vertebrate Animals Used in Testing, Research and Training," *Federal Register* (May 20, 1985) serves as the basis for the U.S. government's policy. The NIH's *Guide for the Care and Use of Laboratory Animals,* rev. ed. (1985) offers explicit instructions.

In February 1993 a federal judge ruled that the Department of Agriculture's standards on the treatment of laboratory dogs and primates were not stringent enough and that the agency had failed to put into effect the 1985 law. Charles R. McCarthy, in "Improved Standards for Laboratory Animals?" *Kennedy Institute of Ethics* (vol. 3, no. 3, 1993), asserts that this ruling actually lowers the standard for the care of laboratory animals.

Although they do not recommend a complete ban on animal research, some authors have argued that current practices in animal research must be reevaluated and better regulated. See, for example, *Lives in the Balance: The Ethics of Using Animals in Biomedical Research* edited by Jane A. Smith and Kenneth M. Boyd (Oxford University Press, 1991) and *In the Name of Science: Issues in Responsible Animal Experimentation* by F. Barbara Orlans (Oxford University Press, 1993).

For an opposing view, see the Office of Technology Assessment's *Alternatives to Animal Use in Research, Testing, and Education* (Government Printing Office, 1986). Richard P. Vance analyzes what he believes are erroneous myths held by supporters of animal research in "An Introduction to the Philosophical Presuppositions of the Animal Liberation/Rights Movement," *Journal of the American Medical Association* (October 7, 1992). Also see John P. Gluck, Tony Dipasquale, and F. Barbara Orlans, *Applied Ethics in Animal Research* (Purdue University Press, 2002); and Cass R. Sunstein and Martha C. Nussbaum, eds., *Animal Rights: Current Debates and New Directions* (Oxford University Press, 2004).

ISSUE 15

Should Prisoners Be Allowed to Participate in Research?

YES: Institute of Medicine Committee on Ethical Considerations for Revisions to DHHS Regulations for Protection of Prisoners Involved in Research, from *Ethical Considerations for Research Involving Prisoners* (June 2006)

NO: Silja J.A. Talvi, from "End Medical Experimentation on Prisoners Now," inthesetimes.com (September 26, 2006)

ISSUE SUMMARY

YES: The Institute of Medicine Committee believes that the current protections for prisoners rely too much on their vulnerability as a category and should be revised to consider the potential risks and benefits of each study, thus allowing prisoners to participate in some kinds of research.

NO: Silja J.A. Talvi, an investigative journalist, believes that all prison research should end because prison medical care is so poor and there is such a high potential for abuse.

Prisoners are, by definition, a captive population, which makes them both desirable as a research population and vulnerable as research subjects. The history of the use of prisoners as research subjects in the United States is an example of how changes in societal values and context affect ethical decision making.

Among the first examples of medical experimentation involving prisoners were the 1906 cholera studies in Bilibid Prison in Manila, Philippines. Dr. Richard P. Strong, an American physician, conducted the experiments on inmates scheduled for execution. Because a vial of bubonic plague serum was inadvertently substituted for the cholera virus, 13 inmates died. In a study of pellagra in Rankin Farm prison in Mississippi, Dr. Joseph Goldberger induced the disease by substituting a diet rich in calories but low in protein in a group of healthy prisoners. After these prisoners became seriously ill, they were granted pardons for participating in the experiment.

Although there were occasional and largely nonscientific incidents in the early part of the twentieth century, medical experimentation in prisons became widespread during World War II. Beginning in 1944, for example, hundreds of prisoners in Stateville Prison in Illinois participated in experiments to find treatments for malaria, a disease that threatened Allied forces in the Pacific. Participation in studies like these was acclaimed as a patriotic act, not a forced or abusive one, even though prisoners suffered serious and long-lasting effects.

After the war, the revelations of the atrocities committed by Nazi physicians in the guise of medical experimentation shocked the world. Interestingly, defense lawyers for these doctors cited the American cholera and pellagra studies, as well as others, to show that the use of prisoners as research subjects had American antecedents. This defense did not succeed, however, and the doctors were found guilty. As its first principle, the Nuremberg Code issued in 1947 declared that the only acceptable experimental subjects are those who are "so situated as to be able to exercise free power of choice." Most countries interpreted this as a complete ban on the use of prisoners for research.

In the United States, however, the broad institutional arrangements set up for wartime research were turned to other medical and military aims. With huge investments by the National Institutes of Health, pharmaceutical companies, and the U.S. Army, prison research expanded to include a broad range of clinical studies on disease ranging from athlete's foot to syphilis. By the early 1970s, the Food and Drug Administration estimated that 90 percent of all investigational drugs were first tested on prisoners. Radiation experiments, trials of mind-altering drugs, chemical warfare agents all became part of the prison research agenda, hidden from public scrutiny.

By the 1970s public awareness of abuses in research involving many categories of subjects led to investigations and calls for reform. The National Commission for the Protection of Human Subjects of Biomedical and Behavioral Research issued a report on prisoner research, which did not call for a complete ban on the practice, but recommended stringent rules to protect prisoners. Among the rules is a requirement that a prisoner advocate be part of the reviewing body. By then pharmaceutical companies, wary of the adverse publicity and the costs, had largely abandoned prisons as a research site.

In the 1990s, as HIV/AIDS, hepatitis C, and other diseases related to drug use became more common among prisoners, some advocates who had previously opposed prisoner research sought ways to make experimental treatments available to prisoners. The pendulum began to swing back toward acceptance of some kinds of research. The debate, however, is far from closed.

In the following selections, a committee convened by the Institute of Medicine presents the case for looking beyond protectionism to evaluating risk. While agreeing that protections are essential, they believe that new conditions require a more open view toward access to research. Opposing this view, Silja J.A. Talvi declares that prisoner research should be banned altogether, because the potential for abuse is so high and because prisons fail to provide good medical care.

YES ↵

Ethical Considerations for Research Involving Prisoners

The Ethical Framework for Research Involving Prisoners

In 1976, the National Commission for the Protection of Human Subjects of Biomedical and Behavioral Research (NCPHSBBR) addressed the ethics of research with prisoners in a document entitled *Report and Recommendations: Research Involving Prisoners*. The commission focused on respect for persons and justice as the two key ethical considerations that would guide their recommendations. . . .

An Updated Ethical Framework

The [Committee on Ethical Considerations for Revisions to DHHS Regulations for Protection of Prisoners Involved in Research] developed a new ethical framework that utilizes the ethical principles applied by the national commission in the 1976 [report], with several new, important components. The framework builds on the principles of respect for persons and justice by shifting from a categorical approach to review to a risk-benefit analysis approach, and by adding a derivative of justice, called collaborative responsibility to research proposal development.

Ideas about justice and respect for persons have evolved over the past three decades. To construct a comprehensive ethical framework for thinking about research in prisons, this chapter explores recent research ethics scholarship. Changes in the way these principles have been conceptualized have influenced the shape of our recommendations. However, before beginning to address how this new ethical framework is different than that of the original commission, it is important to stress that it does not deviate from their core ethical principles.

Respect for persons requires that research subjects be treated as autonomous individuals. . . . It is clear that prisoners are still an extremely vulnerable population, with severely restricted autonomy; thus, this issue requires special attention. Prisoners still need to be protected from the risk of coercion, undue inducement, and exploitation. The historical pattern of research abuses in prisons underscores the need to have an ethical framework that, first and foremost, is concerned with the welfare of prisoners. Similarly, justice still requires a careful consideration of the fair distribution of burdens and benefits. Prisoners, as a vulnerable population, are in jeopardy of receiving a disproportionate share of the risk associated with human subjects research. As stated by the National Bioethics Advisory Commission, "In research involving human subjects, risk is a central organizing principle, a filter through which protocols must pass (NBAC, 1998, p. 89). Like the original commission, our recommendations start with a baseline ethical concern for the protection of prisoners.

Respect for Persons

In this section, the committee expresses its support for a broadened view of the principle of respect for persons, to consider more than a narrow focus on informed consent issues, which are still vital but not the whole picture. It also suggests a shift from a categorical approach to research review to a risk-benefit approach.

An expanded view of respect for persons   In accord with its emphasis on the principle of respect for persons, the original commission's report focused on informed consent. Although informed consent is still an ethically important means of ensuring respect for the right of persons to engage in autonomous decision making, recent scholarship has questioned the myopia caused by such a narrow focus.

Kahn, Mastroianni, and Sugarman (1998) are the editors of a volume that captures a major research ethics reform agenda in its title: *Beyond Consent: Seeking Justice in Research*. One question the editors raise is whether research ethics has been too concerned with informed consent to the neglect of other matters. There seems to be agreement from a variety of perspectives that informed consent forms have consumed too much time and energy. Critics of the preoccupation with forms are not necessarily interested in shifting attention away from informed consent. Rather, they may emphasize that documentation should be but a part of an informed consent process that involves opportunities for questions and answers and allows time for reflection before a decision is made, and that more attention should be paid to ameliorating basic power and knowledge differentials, which may undermine information sharing, understanding, and voluntariness. One proposal for reform advises simply raising the consciousness of investigators and ancillary personnel. Another suggests the use of external measures such as third-party monitoring to guard against deficiencies. This could be accomplished by the integration of third-party research subject advocates in the informed consent process, especially for studies that are considered unusually sensitive or risky or that involve subjects with impaired autonomy. . . .

A more fundamental question is whether too much weight has been placed on informed consent in the framework of research ethics and research regulation. As noted previously, the National Research Act charge to the commission focused on informed consent issues, so the centrality of consent issues in the report is neither surprising nor necessarily indicative of a judgment on the part of the commissioners that the most compelling issues in research with prisoners are those of consent.

An alternate perspective, discussed by Emanuel et al. (2000), focuses on directing attention to risks and to risk-benefit analysis. According to this view, only health-related benefits derived from the research can be counted as benefits to individual subjects, meaning that extraneous benefits, such as payments or medical services unrelated to the research, are excluded in this analysis. Further, although the process of weighing risks against benefits is inherently subjective, the analysis should be based on data permitting identification of the types of potential harms and benefits, their probability of occurrence, and their long-term consequences. For example, a placebo-controlled trial of new antiemitic therapy for patients undergoing chemotherapy could be rejected because the investigators failed to give adequate weight to the discomfort associated with nausea and vomiting and failed to take steps to minimize this potential harm by using available antiemitic agents in the control group (Emanuel et al., 2000).

These questions about an undue focus on informed consent influence our recommendations. More attention needs to be paid to risks and risk-benefit analysis rather than the formalities of an informed consent document. The ethical risks associated with research involving prisoners cannot be solved by focusing only on the informed consent document.

The role of protectionism   A risk-benefit paradigm is necessarily more flexible than the current categorical approach. Although some might view this flexibility as opening the door for potential abuses, this new approach should actually increase the protection of prisoners involved in research.

This committee, like the original commission, is focused on the protection of prisoners as our core ethical concern. However, there are many approaches one can take to accomplish this goal, involving different levels of protective oversight mechanisms. One scholar outlines three types of protectionism:

> Weak protectionism is the view that this problem is best resolved through the judgment of virtuous scientists. Moderate protectionism accepts the importance of personal virtue but does not find it sufficient. Strong protectionism is disinclined to rely, to any substantial degree, on the virtue of scientific investigators for purposes of subject protection (Moreno, 2001)

The movement over time has been from weaker to stronger forms of protectionism as a means of addressing a fundamental problem, specifically, the tension between protecting the interests of subjects and promoting scientific progress. Strong protectionism sharply limits investigator discretion and demands external assurances through measures such as third-party monitors of consent, conflict-of-interest committees, and other procedures. These external assurances can be associated with costs, thus leading to an ethical critique of strong protectionism. For example, an emphasis on external assurances may weaken the sense of personal moral responsibility on the part of investigators. Similarly, rigid external assurances, like those seen in the current regulations, can direct attention away from an analysis of risks and benefits, where the key ethical issues can be found.

Simultaneously, there has been a countervailing force in the march toward strong protectionism, exemplified in the push by AIDS activists for greater access to clinical trials and by progressives for the inclusion of women and children in research studies. More recently, there has been a similar movement to ensure that racial/ethnic minority groups are included in research. These tendencies form one basis for a somewhat different reading of the history. This reading indicates a trend away from viewing certain types of research participation (especially clinical trials) as mostly risky or burdensome toward viewing them as mostly beneficial.

This represents a change in thinking about distributive justice. The commission focused on the equitable distribution of risks and worried that prisoners would bear more than their fair share. However, an equally valid case can be made for attention to the distribution of benefits. For example, Mastroianni and Kahn (2001) wrote that, in the 1970s, federal "policies emphasized the protection of human subjects from the risks of harm in research, and justice was seen as part of this protection," but since the early 1990s "justice as applied in research ethics has emphasized the need to ensure access to the potential benefits that research has to offer" (Mastroianni and Kahn, 2001).

Some fundamental changes in the nature of the research conducted with human subjects provide support for this account of the recent history of research practices. For example, although the paradigmatic studies with prisoners in the period leading up to the report were studies in which investigators induced disease to learn more about it, biomedical research is more likely now to be discussed in terms of clinical trials comparing alternative beneficial treatments. The last several years have also seen the publication of studies comparing the outcome between patients who participate in clinical trials and those who receive standard care outside such trials; the results have tended to favor the former (Agrawal and Emanuel, 2003).

The two accounts can be reconciled in several ways. Increased protectionism is quite visible over the past century, whereas movements demanding greater access to clinical trials are far more recent. Further, protectionism as distrust of individual investigators can coexist with a view that participation in research subject to external oversight can often offer benefits to individuals and groups. One can simultaneously believe that the piling on of more rules and oversight bodies at some point becomes counterproductive and that human subjects are presently inadequately protected. Indeed, many modern ethicists seem to hope for a reawakening of scientific conscience rather than additional fortifications to the citadel of regulations.

This committee concurs. The critique of strong protectionism, combined with a new understanding of research as a potential benefit, requires a reexamination of the current regulations. Advances in ethical thinking about protectionism suggest a new regulatory model. In particular, the committee rejects strong protectionism because it discounts the notion that researchers can be trusted to act virtuously in the protection of subjects. Researchers have responsibility for protecting subjects in their studies, especially those who are most vulnerable. However, given the troubling history of research abuses in prisons, weak protectionism is not an option. The recommendations in this chapter, and throughout this report, reflect a moderate protectionist stance, acknowledging that robust protections are needed but that they need not be rigid or absolute.

This position should not be perceived as a call for the relaxation of prison research ethics. Justice and respect for persons are as vital today as they were three decades ago; research still must be constrained by these ethical principles. The prison continues to be a setting in which it may be difficult to avoid contamination through contact with what will often be a culture of, at best, deprivation and dysfunction and, at worst, corruption, brutality, and degradation (Hornblum, 1997, 1998; Murphy, 2005; Rhodes, 2005).

Perhaps some unease is appropriate about removing what prisoners themselves, given full information and understanding, might regard as acceptable or even desirable options in light of their circumstances, circumstances that are unlikely to be changed for the better by research bans. A prisoner's ability to participate in research need not be completely precluded.

The original commissioners talked to actual prisoner-subjects during a fact-finding visit to Jackson State Prison on November 14, 1975. The prison, in southern Michigan, was at the time home to one of the largest nontherapeutic biomedical research programs in the country. The report notes that commission members spoke with a representative sample of research participants and nonparticipants selected by commission staff from a master list of all prisoners and found that, overall, participants valued the opportunity to participate in research and felt they were sufficiently informed and free to enroll or withdraw at will, and nonparticipants did not object to this opportunity being available to others (NCPHSBBR, 1976).

This message continues to be articulated today. This committee visited one prison and one prison medical facility to discuss experimentation with current prisoners and peer educators. . . . The prisoners actively expressed the desire to have access to research. They stated they would feel they had a choice as to whether to participate and that they know their rights when it comes to study participation. The prisoners and peer educators at those site visits also echoed the sentiment that prisoners possess sufficient autonomy to make informed decisions about whether to participate in a given study.[1]

This, combined with the myopic emphasis on informed consent, is why the current categorical regulatory approach should be abandoned in favor of a risk-benefit paradigm. The following recommendations strive to acknowledge that, in limited circumstances, the potential benefit of a research protocol can justify research involving prisoners. These limited circumstances cannot be captured by a rigid categorical approach but need to be rooted in a risk-benefit analysis that grapples with the balance between a need for protection and access to potentially beneficial research protocols.

Note

1. Of course, this survey only represents the views of a limited sample of prisoners. Although many inmates might share these opinions, others might feel that their circumstances do not permit the exercise of autonomy. This emphasizes the need for setting specific collaboration, discussed in detail later.

References

Agrawal M, Emanuel E. 2003. Ethics of phase 1 oncology studies: reexamining the arguments and data. *Journal of the American Medical Association* 290:1075–1082.

Emanuel EJ, Wendler D, Grady C. 2000. What makes clinical research ethical? *Journal of the American Medical Association* 283:2701–2711.

Hornblum AM. 1997. They were cheap and available: prisoners as research subjects in twentieth century America. *British Medical Journal* 315:1437–1441.

Homblum AM. 1998. *Acres of Skin: Human Experiments at Holmesburg Prison.* New York: Routledge.

Kahn JP, Mastroianni AC, Sugarman J, eds. 1998. *Beyond Consent: Seeking Justice in Research.* New York: Oxford University Press.

Mastroianni A, Kahn J. 2001. Swinging on the pendulum. *Hastings Center Report* 31(3):21–28.

Moreno JD. 1998. Convenient and captive populations. In: Kahn JP, Mastroianni AC, Sugarman J, eds. *Beyond Consent: Seeking Justice in Research.* New York: Oxford University Press. Pp. 111–130.

Moreno JD. 2001. Goodbye to all that: the end of moderate protectionism in human subjects research. *Hastings Center Report* 31(3):9–17.

Murphy D. 2005. Health care in the federal bureau of prisons: fact or fiction. *California Journal of Health Promotion* 3(2):23–37.

NBAC (National Bioethics Commission). 1998. *Research Involving Persons with Mental Disorders That May Affect Decisionmaking Capacity, Volume I: Report and Recommendations of the National Bioethics Advisory Commission.* P. 89.

NCPHSBBR (National Commission for the Protection of Human Subjects of Biomedical and Behavioral Research). 1976. *Report and Recommendations: Research Involving Prisoners.* Washington, DC: NCPHSBBR.

Rhodes, LA. 2005. Pathological effects of the supermaximum prison. *American Journal of Public Health.* 95(10):1692–1695.

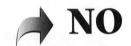

End Medical Experimentation on Prisoners Now

One of the most powerful movies ever to be made about the Holocaust was the 2003 made-for-TV movie, *Out of the Ashes,* which highlighted the sickening crucible faced by medical professionals held captive in the Third Reich's torture-and-killing camps.

Medical experimentation on Jewish and Roma (Gypsy) women was one of Dr. Josef Mengele's favorite forms of entertainment. In the movie, Dr. Gisella Perl (Christine Lahti) faces an ethical crisis when she is forced to comfort a young pregnant Roma woman and then stand by and watch as Mengele, the Angel of Death, marks up and slices open her stomach without the benefit of anesthesia. Mengele's sadistic detachment as he walks away from the remains of the dead woman and her fetus is agonizingly contrasted with Perl's helplessness and trauma.

Perl's story is real. Millions died, and thousands were experimented on (and then usually murdered) in the name of the Nazi "science" of eugenics. And it is because of such treatment that in 1947, the Nuremberg Code spelled out an unequivocal position on the experimentation of people in captivity: The human subject of medical experimentation "should have legal capacity to give consent . . . [and] should be so situated as to be able to exercise free power of choice, without the intervention of any element of force, fraud, deceit, duress, over-reaching or other ulterior form of constraint or coercion."

Strange thing about this country of ours—we always seem to be able to justify the "legitimate" exceptions to international law and agreements.

From the '40s through the early '70s, the United States officially sanctioned the use of prisoners in medical experiments, including the injection of typhoid fever, herpes, malaria, TB and a host of sexually transmitted diseases. In the name of science, doctors have dosed prisoners with LSD, placed them in extreme isolation to develop "mind control" techniques, and, in Washington State between 1963 and 1973, radiated their testicles and then sliced them open. (This last case brought about one of the few successful lawsuits by prisoners against medical experimentation.)

In 1976, things seemed to change for the better. The National Commission for the Protection of Human Subjects of Biomedical and Behavioral Research released a scathing report that led to new protections of human research subjects. The specific protections for prisoners, in a section known as Subpart C, accompanied similar protections for the disabled, children and other vulnerable populations.

Now, things may be changing again to allow for more medical experimentation on prisoners. In August, the influential Institute of Medicine (IOM), presented a report, "Ethical Considerations for Research Involving Prisoners," to federal officials that recommended increasing research on prison populations. Such research, the report said, provided a way of "improving the health of prisoners and the conditions in which they live." In an August 21 editorial, *USA Today* heartily agreed.

The report also raised valid concerns about consent, safeguards, prisoner privacy and access to adequate health care while in prison. It also called for the expansion of the definition of "prisoners" to include all of the nearly 7 million persons under some form of adult correctional supervision.

The IOM said that "respect for persons and justice should still be the basis for the conduct and regulation of prisoners today." In reaction, a *New York Times* editorial two days later observed that: "The country should move slowly on this issue. The savage and dishonorable legacy of drug testing in prison makes it imperative that any change be carried out carefully, with maximum transparency and concern for inmate safety."

But the United States has already been moving far too slowly on this issue. A 1978 federal regulation stated that prisoners can participate in federally-funded research only if the "experiment poses no more than 'minimal' risk," which it defined as a "risk of physical or psychological harm that is no greater in probability and severity than that ordinarily encountered in the daily lives, or in the routine medical, dental or psychological examinations of healthy persons." While that would seem to make a certain amount of sense, federal oversight and monitoring of medical experimentation has been incredibly sloppy and disorganized, even according to those who have been responsible for that oversight. "What we've got from the regulatory standpoint is a mess," said Dr. Thomas Puglisi, the former director of compliance for the Office of Protection from Research Risks—now the Office of Human Research Protections (OHRP)—at a medical research summit in March 2001. "I couldn't say that when I worked for the federal government, but I can say that now."

And it's worth noting that the only national oversight is of clinical trials in prisons that receive federal funds. Pharmaceutical companies that want to fund their own studies have no oversight body outside of what a prison or state might deem minimally necessary. A national database of medical experimentation on prisoners does not exist. Research studies don't even always end up being published—particularly when they fail, sometimes causing serious injury or death to their human subjects.

These are among the most severe obstacles facing journalists who try to find out more about what's going on, as I discovered while pursuing a January 2002 cover story for *In These Times,* "The Prison as Laboratory."

In investigating that story, I found that the number of experimental studies on youth and adults in correctional facilities was increasing. Many of the studies clearly and egregiously violated the existing regulations on "minimal" risk to their subjects, according to FOIA documents I received from the OHRP.

Simply put, medical experimentation on prisoners in the United States never went away. Researchers just got savvier about keeping their prison studies out of the public eye, often turning to pharmaceutical funding, which allows them to experiment with as little notice, oversight or intervention as possible.

Last year, the OHRP Secretary's Advisory Committee on Human Research Protections (SACHRP) asked its Subpart C subcommittee (addressing prisoner safeguards) to determine whether existing regulations were still "adequate," as well as to investigate the prevalence of medical testing on prisoners.

In the internal document submitted by that subcommittee to SACHRP, more than 1,000 studies related to prisoners or incarceration came up as "hits" on a PUBMED database search. Of the 79 studies that appeared to be conducted entirely in prison settings, 63 percent had to do with socio-behavioral research revolving around substance abuse, mental illness and disease risk behaviors.

The report noted the lack of real, centralized information on medical testing on prisoners, and added "much of the research in correctional settings is graduate student research of uncertain quality."

Medical testing in prisons should be brought to a halt—at the very least until quality prison health care for every single inmate is a reality. Genuine preventative and interventionist care for people outside of prison who cannot afford medical insurance should also be a priority.

"Before prisoners can freely make decisions about their medical care and treatment they first must have access to medical care and treatment that meets with community standards," says Paul Wright, editor of *Prison Legal News*. "Every day prisoners around the country are dying of medical neglect because they are not provided with simple, known and available medical care. It is laughable to think that somehow cutting-edge medical treatment is suddenly going to be made available to prisoners. The people carrying out the drug testing have a fiduciary duty to enrich their shareholders and employers, not provide the best medical care for prisoners."

In the current system, prisoners' lives are already endangered. In light of this country's legacy of medically abusing captive populations—and to honor the memory, intent and purpose of the creation of the Nuremberg Code—prison experimentation simply needs to come to an end.

POSTSCRIPT

Should Prisoners Be Allowed to Participate in Research?

The most vivid denunciation of prisoner research is Allen M. Holmblum's book *Acres of Skin: Human Experiments at Holmesberg Prison* (Taylor & Francis, 1998). Holmblum describes the experiments that took place at Holmesberg Prison in Philadelphia from the mid-1940s to 1974 and attacks the pharmaceutical industries that used inmates as cheap sources of research material.

Jonathan D. Moreno, a philosopher and former member of the Clinton administration's Advisory Committee on Human Radiation Experiments, describes the twentieth-century history of chemical and biological experimentation in *Undue Risk: Secret State Experiments on Humans* (W. H. Freeman, 2001).

One study of mentally ill prisoners and a control group of healthy prisoners concluded that "a very high percentage of particularly vulnerable, mentally ill prisoners demonstrated adequate capacity to consent to research" (D. J. Moser, et al., "Coercion and Informed Consent in Research Involving Prisoners," *Comprehensive Psychiatry,* January–February 2004) found that "all controls and all but one of the prisoners demonstrated adequate capacity to consent to research."

The U.S. Office of Human Research Protections guidelines on prisoner research can be found at http://www.hhs.gov/ohrp/humansubjects/guidance/prisoner. htm. Also see Chapter 9: History of Prison Research Regulation, issued by the Advisory Committee on Human Radiation Experiments, at http://www.eh.doe. gov/ohre/roadmap/achre/chap9_4.html.

Internet References . . .

Organ Donation

This site provides current statistics and background information on the allocation of transplantable organs in the United States.

http://www.organdonor.gov

Kaiser Family Foundation

This research organization's Web site has reports and data about health care coverage in the United States, including state data on medicaid.

http://www.kff.org/

World Anti-Drug Doping Agency

This international organization has information for athletes, coaches, fans, and others about the use of drugs in sports.

http://www.wada-ama.org

Bioethics and Public Policy

*I*n its modern infancy, biomedical ethics was almost exclusively concerned with issues relating to individual doctor-patient relationships. Questions of resource allocation and public policy did occur, but mostly within the context of whether or not a patient could pay for certain kinds of care. In the past several decades, as medical care costs have skyrocketed, the issues concerning equitable distribution of scarce resources have become paramount. As medical care became more costly, it became less accessible to the uninsured and to the underinsured (people who have some employment-based health insurance but not enough to cover their own illnesses or those of their families). In this new world of market-driven health care, some old problems of resource allocation and public policy take on new urgency. How far should commercialism extend? The threat of war and bioterrorism have created new dilemmas for military doctors and policy makers as they struggle to define a balance between protecting the public's health in case of an attack and preserving the basic liberties that Americans prize so highly. This section takes up these issues.

- Should Federally Funded Health Care Be Tied to Following Doctors' Orders?

- Does Military Necessity Override Medical Ethics?

- Should Performance-Enhancing Drugs Be Banned From Sports?

- Should There Be a Free Market in Body Parts?

- Should Pharmacists Be Allowed to Deny Prescriptions on Grounds of Conscience?

- Should Public Health Override Powers Over Individual Liberty in Combating Bioterrorism?

ISSUE 16

Should Federally Funded Health Care Be Tied to Following Doctors' Orders?

YES: **State of West Virginia,** from *Medicaid Redesign Proposal* (November 7, 2005)

NO: **Gene Bishop and Amy C. Brodkey,** from "Personal Responsibility and Physician Responsibility—West Virginia's Medicaid Plan," *New England Journal of Medicine* (August 24, 2006)

ISSUE SUMMARY

YES: The State of West Virginia believes that penalizing Medicaid recipients who do not follow doctors' orders or maintain healthy lifestyles will lead to improved health outcomes and in the long term reduce the state's costs.

NO: Physicians Gene Bishop and Amy C. Brodkey believe that the plan is unfair because it places responsibility on patients for factors that may be out of their control and holds them to a higher standard than other patients.

Two of the most urgent problems facing American health care today are its high costs and poor outcomes. The United States spends more than any other country on health care—nearly $2 trillion a year—and yet it is consistently lower than other developed countries on public health indicators like infant mortality. Even though American health care is justly celebrated for its remarkable technological advances in genetics and organ transplantation, for example, it has done less well and at far greater cost in delivering primary and chronic care.

The current system of delivering health care is based on an acute care model, which was designed to treat serious and usually sudden episodes of illness or trauma, keep the patient in the hospital until he or she had recovered (or died), and then move on to the next urgent case. Chronic care—treatment of slow, degenerative, disabling but not usually life-threatening diseases—requires a different model, one that involves the patient in a more active role. For example, diabetes, one of the most common conditions, can be treated but the patient must also follow a strict diet, test blood sugar several times a day, administer drugs accurately, and be monitored frequently by a doctor or nurse. Many people find it hard to adhere to all these requirements because it means a change in the lifestyle to which they and their families have grown accustomed over years. Other habits harmful to one's health, like smoking, are difficult to stop without continuous support.

For many years there has been a debate about the appropriate ethical balance between "personal responsibility"—the idea that people must take control of their own health by following sensible diets, exercising, not smoking, and seeing their doctor regularly—and the obligation of the medical system to take care of all people who are ill, regardless of the cause. For the most part this debate has focused on money—whether smokers, for example, should pay higher health insurance premiums, or whether people whose diseased livers stemmed from alcohol abuse should be able to receive the scarce resource of a transplantable liver.

In 2005 the debate took a new turn, driven both by economics and a renewed emphasis on personal responsibility by federal and state government officials. The federal Deficit Reduction Act of 2005 gave states new options to control their portion of the costs of Medicaid—the federal-state program for poor people. About 46 million people, including 18.4 million children, were enrolled in Medicaid in 2003, and the combined federal-state costs were $278.3 billion.

Although the state portion of Medicaid costs varies by the population and the condition of the economy, as people move in and out of jobs with health insurance coverage, Medicaid costs continue to be a major drain on state budgets. West Virginia, a poor state ranked near the bottom of all states in terms of its population's health status, took advantage of the DFA to propose to the Centers for Medicare and Medicaid Services (CMS) a new plan that in their view would do two important things: improve health outcomes by giving Medicaid recipients incentives to follow healthy lifestyles and penalizing them if they failed to do so; and in the long term control costs by better management of chronic diseases like heart disease, diabetes, and hypertension. CMS quickly approved the proposal, and it went into effect in a pilot phase in three rural West Virginia counties late in 2006.

In 2002 about 183,000 children and 60,000 parents were enrolled in the state's Medicaid program. About two-thirds of the adults were women. To be eligible for Medicaid in West Virginia, a parent must have an income below 37 percent of the poverty line ($6,142 per year for a family of three in 2006). Children can be covered at somewhat higher income levels. Under the plan, about 160,000 of these children and adults without disabilities will be offered an "enhanced" benefit package including mental health counseling, long-term diabetes management, and cardiac rehabilitation, prescription drugs and home health visits if needed, as well as antismoking and nutrition classes. If they choose not to sign up, they will get only the basic package of services required by federal law but will be limited to four prescriptions a month and will not receive the other enhanced benefits. If they sign up but don't comply with the agreement, they will lose the enhanced benefits.

The first of the following two selections presents the agreements that West Virginia's Medicaid patients are asked to sign. In response, physicians Gene Bishop and Amy C. Brodkey criticize the plan because it fails to appreciate the many reasons individuals are unable to adhere to doctor's orders and may actually result in denial of needed health care. In their view, poor people on Medicaid are being held to a higher standard than people with other forms of health insurance.

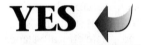

YES

Medicaid Redesign Proposal

Introduction

The goals of the West Virginia comprehensive Medicaid Redesign proposal are to:

- streamline administration;
- tailor services to meet the needs of enrolled populations;
- coordinate care, especially for members with chronic conditions; and
- provide members with opportunity and incentives to be responsible for maintaining and improving their health and their family's health.

Prevention, personal responsibility and disease management are hallmarks of the redesign. In the prevention arena, non-traditional services such as nutrition counseling and weight loss programs will be added to the benefits package. West Virginia will introduce Healthy Rewards Accounts, which provide the incentive for members to make healthy decisions and use health care services appropriately. The Redesign will also focus upon establishing a medical home for all members. . . .

Healthy Rewards Accounts

Two of the expected outcomes of the West Virginia Medicaid Redesign includes improving the health of Medicaid members and more efficient use of state and federal resources. A tool to assist in that effort is a new West Virginia-designed concept known as *Healthy Rewards Accounts*. The premise of these accounts is based on Consumer Directed Health (CDH) now used in the private sector.

In the private sector, employers establish high deductible employee benefit plans. Along with these plans are health reimbursement accounts funded by the employer. These accounts are used to finance a portion of out-of-pocket medical expenses incurred by employees. If a person spends wisely or has no claims, the ending balance may be carried year-to-year.

While a high deductible account would not be applicable for the Medicaid program, the idea of incentives or disincentives for member behavior is appropriate. Unlike private insurance, Medicaid does not allow large meaningful or enforceable co-payments. Under this concept, if a certain class of pharmaceuticals has two equal choices, and 'A' will cost the state $1.00 and 'B' will cost the state $50.00; it would be in the best interest of the state and the member to share the savings if the member chooses 'A'; the least expensive option.

From Medicaid State Plan Amendment, May 3, 2006. Copyright © 2006 by West Virginia Bureau of Medical Services, Center for Medicaid and Medicare Services. Reprinted by permission.

Currently, if the member and his or her health care provider want 'B', the person will get 'B', with no consequence for the member or the provider. This is a situation that must be changed. . . .

West Virginia intends to establish a Healthy Rewards Account for all Medicaid members who have the ability and capability to partner in their personal health decisions and this will be the first target population. . . .

Disincentives

Some examples of member behavior West Virginia Medicaid intends to target with disincentives are:

- non-emergent use of emergency services;
- missed medical appointments;
- non-compliance with the preferred drug list; and
- smoking . . .

There is a perception in the provider community that West Virginia Medicaid members have a high no-show rate. This leads to two concerns. First, providers become frustrated and refuse to treat Medicaid members. Secondly and more importantly, many medical conditions require compliance checks and follow-up visits. If a patient does not follow up, the result can be negative health outcomes or hospitalization leading to higher costs. After missing a predetermined number of visits, a certain amount of credit will be deducted from the Healthy Rewards Account.

The final disincentive in the first phase would be for failure to choose from the preferred drug list. Medicaid will move to a multi-tiered co-payment structure with non-preferred drugs having higher co-payments deducted from the Healthy Rewards Accounts.

Incentives

The first phase incentive programs would be limited to the following care management or wellness initiatives: prenatal care, well-child checkups and vaccinations, cardiovascular, asthma and diabetes care as well as tobacco cessation. As the program develops, additional disease states may be included. . . .

By bringing members into partnership with their health care providers, West Virginia Medicaid hopes to foster more active member participation in their health care. Not only will they become better informed, they will become involved in programs that will improve quality of life for themselves and their families.

West Virginia Medicaid Member Agreement

Member Rights

1. **I understand** that the information I provide is confidential and the Medicaid Program and my health plan only will release the information for purposes related to the administration of the Medicaid Program.

2. **I understand** that I have a right to be in charge of my health care. I understand that I have a right to see my medical records. I will be a part of all decisions about my health care. I can talk freely and honestly with my health care provider and ask him or her any questions I have about my or my children's illness and treatment.
3. **I understand** that I will be treated fairly and with respect. I will get the care and treatment I need as soon as possible. I understand that I cannot be treated differently because I am in the Medicaid Program or because of my age, sex, race, national origin, illness or health condition.
4. **I understand** that I have a right to know about all laws, regulations, rules and requirements about the Medicaid Program and my health plan.
5. **I understand** that I can call or write to my health plan about any questions or tell them about problems I am having by calling (304) 558-XXXX or writing to XXXX.
6. **I understand** that as a Medicaid member that I have a Right to appeal any decision and to receive a prompt Fair Hearing before the Department of Health and Human Resources, Board of Review. I can request a fair hearing by calling (304) 558-XXXX or writing to XXX.

Member Responsibilities

1. **I understand** that it is my responsibility to follow the rules and requirements of the West Virginia Medicaid program and my health plan. I understand that it is my responsibility to take the best care of myself and my children.
2. **I will cooperate** with the Medicaid Program and my health plan and provide them with accurate and timely information about myself and my family members. I will notify the Medicaid Program of any changes in my life situation. Changes may include, but are not limited to:

   a. change in address or phone number;
   b. someone moving in or out of my home;
   c. getting or losing a job;
   d. any changes in earnings, income or assets; and
   e. any changes in health status such as becoming pregnant, being diagnosed with a disease or achieving my health improvement goals.

3. **I understand** that it is my responsibility to do what is necessary to stay healthy. I understand that smoking, using drugs illegally, drinking too much alcohol, and being overweight are bad for my health. I promise to try not to do these things. I will go to the special programs as my health care provider advises in order to improve and maintain my health including exercise and nutrition programs.
4. **I promise** to examine the booklets and materials my health care provider gives me about how to be a healthy person or have them explained to me by my health care provider. I will ask my health care provider questions if I do not understand his or her instructions or if I do not understand the material I have read.

5. **I understand** that it is my responsibility to select a medical home. If I do not select a medical home in 45 days, one will be selected for me. I understand it is my responsibility to go to that medical home when I or any of my family members get sick. I understand that I should go to my health care provider at least once a year for a check up, and to take my children more often when the health care provider advises me to. I will listen to the health care provider when I or my children are sick, and do what the health care provider tells me to do; including taking the medications he/she gives me. I will show up on time when I or my children have an appointment to see the health care provider. If I must cancel when I have an appointment, I will call to tell my health care provider I cannot come. I will only do this when there is a very good reason. If I miss three consecutive appointments, I understand I will be assessed a penalty.

6. If I hold up my part of this agreement and I meet the health improvement goals set by my doctor, I understand that I may receive an award or have to pay less for my medical appointments and my medicines.

7. If I do not hold up my part of this agreement, I understand that I may be excluded from the special benefit programs and may be excluded from incentive programs.

8. **I will** go to the hospital emergency room only when I feel it is a medical emergency. Whenever, I am sick I will call my doctor first and go see him or her. If I cannot talk to my doctor or someone in the doctor's office and it is an emergency, then I will go to the hospital.

West Virginia Medicaid Responsibilities and Acknowledgment

1. **DHHR will** work with you and your health care provider to develop a health improvement plan and make any changes that may be needed.

2. **DHHR will** support your health improvement plan by providing information, guidance and services.

3. **DHHR will** encourage you to take the lead in determining the plan to achieve your health improvement goals.

4. **DHHR will** give you timely notice before anything negative happens to your benefits and will provide the opportunity for a Fair Hearing on any issue related to your benefits or to your health improvement plan.

5. **As a representative of DHHR,** I have carefully explained the above information and acknowledge the responsibilities of the Department

_____   _____
Income Maintenance Worker Signature   Date

Member Acknowledgment

I understand the information contained in this document and agree to follow this, my West Virginia Medicaid Member Agreement.

_____   _____
West Virginia Medicaid Member Signature   Date

Member Agreement

In order to be a **responsible parent** I agree to . . .

1. NOT smoke
2. take my children to all of their check-ups
3. make sure my children get all of their shots
4. take my children to the dentist
5. follow all of the safety guidelines recommended by my health care provider

In order to be a **healthy woman** I must . . .

1. see my health care provider every year for a check-up
2. see the dentist every 6 months
3. have advanced directives on my medical records so that it is clear what my wishes are if I get hurt and cannot state my wishes
4. get all of my shots
5. have a female pap test and breast exam every year starting at age 18 (or when I first become sexually active)
6. have a mammogram regularly, as instructed by my health care provider, starting at age 40
7. have colorectal cancer screening starting at age 50 (age 40 if colon cancer runs in my family)
8. have my cholesterol checked starting at age 25
9. make sure I have a complete skin exam by my health care provider at my check-up
10. NOT smoke or use alcohol in excess
11. maintain a healthy weight (body mass index less than 25)
12. take control of my health and know my health status
13. know my family health history because it can affect my health

In order to be a **healthy man** I must . . .

1. see my health care provider every year for a check-up
2. see the dentist every 6 months
3. have advanced directives on my medical records so that it is clear what my wishes are in case I get hurt and cannot state my wishes
4. have colorectal cancer screening completed every year starting at age 50 (age 40 if colon cancer runs in my family)
5. talk to my provider about screening for prostate cancer starting at age 50 (age 40 if prostate cancer runs in my family)
6. have my cholesterol checked starting at age 25
7. make sure I have a complete skin exam by my health care provider at my check-ups
8. NOT smoke or use alcohol in excess
9. maintain a healthy weight (body mass index less than 25)
10. take control of my health and know my health status
11. know my family health history because it could affect my health

If I have **diabetes** ("sugar") I must . . .

1. know what a Hemoglobin A1C is (average sugar over 3 months)

2. know my Hemoglobin A1C (a number from 4-15)
3. know my goal for my Hemoglobin A1C (less than 7)
4. get my blood checked regularly (about every three months)
5. know my blood pressure and my blood pressure goals (less than 130/80)
6. know my cholesterol and what my goals are (total less than 200, LDL less than 70, HDL more than 40)
7. follow a diabetic (low sugar) diet
8. take all of my medicines
9. exercise at least three times a week for about an hour
10. see my provider every three months (unless they instruct me otherwise)
11. see a diabetic instructor twice a year
12. get a complete foot check every year
13. make sure I understand the effects diabetes has on my heart, kidneys, eyes, legs
14. see the eye doctor every year
15. get all of my shots

To Be a Healthy Person—Know Your Numbers!

Body Mass Index (BMI)—an accurate way to know if I am a healthy weight

Cholesterol (total, LDL, HDL, triglycerides)

Blood Pressure

Hemoglobin A1C (HgA1C) if you are a diabetic

Gene Bishop and
Amy C. Brodkey

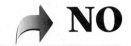 **NO**

Personal Responsibility and Physician Responsibility—West Virginia's Medicaid Plan

Mary Jones is your 53-year-old patient with diabetes and obesity. These conditions developed after she began to take an atypical antipsychotic drug for schizophrenia. Jones signed a treatment contract stating that she will keep all her medical appointments, attend diabetes education classes, and lose weight. She attended one class but became paranoid and left halfway through it, and she has gained 5 lb. You gave her educational materials to read, but you have discovered that she doesn't understand them. She has just missed her second consecutive appointment with you; last time, she didn't have bus fare. Neither her glycated hemoglobin nor her blood lipids are at target levels. You are now legally obligated to report this information to your state Medicaid agency, and Jones may lose her mental health benefits and some of her prescription coverage as a result.

This scenario is no Orwellian fantasy: West Virginia is planning to ask residents who are eligible for Medicaid because of low income to sign documents outlining "member responsibilities and rights." By signing these documents, they agree, among other things, to take their medications, keep their appointments, and avoid unnecessary emergency room visits. Patients who don't uphold their end of the bargain will have some benefits reduced or eliminated. In the first year, the state will track four indicators: whether patients participate in health care screenings and adhere to health improvement programs as directed by their health care providers, whether they keep their medical appointments, and whether they take their medications.[1] The plan does not specify standards for determining successful adherence to these criteria.

As part of a trend emphasizing "personal responsibility" for health status, the plan has implications far beyond its effects on needy West Virginians. This strategy will have important consequences for practicing physicians. Its speedy approval by the Centers for Medicare and Medicaid Services (CMS) demonstrates the agency's enthusiasm for such an approach. Under the Deficit Reduction Act of 2005, Idaho and Kentucky have submitted plans with similar philosophies. When the West Virginia plan was approved, CMS administrator Mark McClellan stated, "Medicaid enrollees in West Virginia will now become

From *New England Journal of Medicine*, August 24, 2006, pp. 756–758. Copyright © 2006 by Massachusetts Medical Society. All rights reserved. Reprinted by permission.

part of an emerging trend in health care that empowers patients to make educated, consumer-driven decisions related to their own treatment."[2]

Personal responsibility is a laudable goal with intuitive appeal and an established place in the lexicon of American culture and values, but used in this context, it is at odds with current models of the doctor–patient relationship. Physicians and patients negotiate treatment, taking into account the dynamic tension between desirable behaviors and achievable ones. Failure leads to renegotiation. Reasons for missed appointments are many—sick children, depression, business meetings that run late, and just plain forgetfulness. An exploration of the reason may improve future behavior, whereas humiliation and punishment may result in decreased adherence to treatment. Treatment negotiations are both individual and ever changing. The West Virginia plan is a blunt instrument that takes the therapeutic contract outside of the medical encounter, and there is a paucity of evidence to support this approach to improving health-related behaviors.

The plan also raises fundamental issues of fairness. First, it places responsibility on patients for factors that may be out of their control. Persons who depend on public transportation or transportation provided by Medicaid can attest to the unreliability of these systems. Primary care offices have limited evening and weekend hours, forcing patients to visit emergency rooms. And at least 75 percent of the beneficiaries who may be affected are children, who will have to depend on their parents or guardians for adherence to the rules.

Second, the plan holds Medicaid patients to a standard of behavior that is not required of other patients. An editorial in a West Virginia newspaper said, "All the state is asking is that patients take their medications, follow their doctors' orders, and show up on time for their appointments."[3] As physicians, we know how rare such behavior is. Even under the ideal circumstances of a clinical trial, the rate of compliance with medication ranges from 43 percent to 78 percent, and there is no consensual standard for what constitutes adequate adherence.[4] Privately insured patients may reject their physicians' advice without losing their health benefits—and they may have the confidence to express that disagreement overtly, leading to renegotiation—whereas poorer and often less well-educated Medicaid patients may simply choose silently not to comply.

There are well-understood reasons why Medicaid beneficiaries have poorer health indicators and higher rates of noncompliance than many other patients. Poverty results in reduced access to child care, transportation, healthful foods, and exercise facilities, as well as lower literacy, more life crises, and higher rates of untreated psychiatric illnesses. People with fewer experiences of success are less likely than others to believe that they can change their health status. This plan asks the most vulnerable population to do more with less ability to accomplish what we ask of them.

The plan makes explicit the belief that persons must behave according to set norms in order to deserve health care and health insurance. What physician has not sighed in frustration over the patient who continues to smoke after angioplasty? Yet while promoting healthful behaviors, we continue to offer care. The West Virginia plan risks the application of an actuarial value to every behavior. Is riding a bicycle to work good for your health because of exercise or bad for your health because of the risk of accidents? Is it irresponsible to refuse to take a medication if it makes you ill and you cannot reach your physician to ask for advice?

The plan asks physicians to violate all three fundamental principles enumerated in the Physician Charter on Medical Professionalism: the primacy of patient welfare, the principle of patient autonomy, and the principle of social justice.[5] It raises potential conflicts by placing physicians in a reporting situation in which the public health is not at issue, possibly asking them to harm their patients or their relationships with patients. As physicians become agents of the state, poor patients' distrust of the medical system can only increase. Although the plan's member agreement mentions the patient's right "to decide things about my health care and the health care of my children," it does not recognize that noncompliance can be an expression of disagreement with the physician. The plan promotes discrimination not only on the basis of socioeconomic status, but also on the basis of diagnosis: surely, people with mental illnesses who have trouble managing activities of daily living such as keeping appointments will be discriminated against under a plan that rescinds their mental health benefits because of such lapses.

It is unclear what steps will be taken if physicians do not comply with reporting requirements. The four indicators require data collection from physicians' offices. This requirement for additional documentation is an unfunded administrative mandate that could actually decrease physician participation in the Medicaid program.

In the face of both increasing health care costs and numbers of uninsured persons, states will continue to seek ways to control Medicaid costs. Clinicians often abstain from policy discussions until it is too late for them to have an impact. But who is better able to provide evidence of the misguided nature of such plans? What physician would recommend that a person with diabetes who misses appointments lose the ability to attend diabetes education classes? What physician wants to be faced with a child with asthma whose benefits have been reduced to four prescriptions per month when she gets pneumonia and an antibiotic makes five? In an era of "personal responsibility," physicians must assume the responsibility of speaking out about how such policies affect their practices and their patients' health.

Notes

1. West Virginia Medicaid State Plan Amendment as approved by the Center for Medicaid and Medicare Services. (Accessed August 2, 2006. . . .)

2. Daly R. Mental health experts wary about law on Medicaid changes. Psychiatric News. Vol. 41. No. 11. June 2, 2006:10. (Arlington, Va.: American Psychiatric Publishing.)

3. Medicaid changes are common sense. Charleston Daily Mail. June 2, 2006:P4A.

4. Osterberg L, Blaschke T. Adherence to medication. N Engl J Med 2005;353: 487–497.

5. Medical professionalism in the new millenium: a physician charter. Ann Intern Med 2002;136:243–6.

POSTSCRIPT

Should Federally Funded Health Care Be Tied to Following Doctors' Orders?

A 2006 public opinion poll found that a large majority (87 percent) of Americans believed that health insurance premiums should not vary by health status. However, a majority (60 percent) believed that smokers should pay more, and almost a third (29 percent) felt that people who are obese should pay more. Interestingly, only a small number (12 percent) felt that people with family histories of heart disease should pay more, even though heart disease is also linked to lifestyle (Marc L. Berk, Daniel S. Gaylin, and Claudia L. Schur, "Exploring the Public's View on the Health Care System: A National Survey on the Issues and Options," *Health Affairs,* November 14, 2006).

In Great Britain, the Norfolk and Newcastle-under-Lyme primary care trusts (the basic source of health care under the National Health Service), both under severe financial stress, have decided to refuse to provide some kinds of nonemergency surgery like hip and knee replacements to smokers. Earlier the East Suffolk primary care trust refused to perform these operations on obese patients until they lose weight.

As part of a health reform package, the German government proposed in October 2006 to penalize cancer patients who failed to undergo regular screening by making them pay more toward their treatments (*British Medical Journal*, October 28, 2006). These patients would have to pay 2 percent of their gross income, rather than the 1 percent others with a chronic disease are required to pay. Germans who do not have regular dental checkups are already required to contribute to the cost of their treatment. The cancer screening requirement is controversial partly because there are questions about the usefulness of some recommended screening tests.

Judith Solomon of the Washington-based Center on Budget and Policy Priorities released a report that claims the West Virginia's Medicaid changes are unlikely to reduce state costs or improve beneficiaries' health (www.cbpp.org/5-31-06health.htm).

See also Erik Eckholm, "Medicaid Plan Prods Patients Toward Health" (*New York Times*, December 1, 2006). For individual state statistics on health status and spending, see http://www.kaiserstatehealthfacts.org.

ISSUE 17

Does Military Necessity Override Medical Ethics?

YES: Michael L. Gross, from "Bioethics and Armed Conflict: Mapping the Moral Dimensions of Medicine and War," *Hastings Center Report* (November/December 2004)

NO: M. Gregg Bloche and Jonathan H. Marks, from "When Doctors Go to War," *New England Journal of Medicine* (January 6, 2005)

ISSUE SUMMARY

YES: Political scientist Michael L. Gross argues that war brings military and medical values into conflict, and that military necessity often overwhelms a physician's other moral obligations, such as relieving suffering.

NO: M. Gregg Bloche, a physician and lawyer, and Jonathan H. Marks, a British barrister, stress that physicians remain physicians even in the military and that there is an urgent moral challenge in managing the conflict, not denying it.

As long as human beings have engaged in war, medical personnel have tended the wounded and dying. However, for centuries, the available techniques, skills, and medications were not very effective against grave battlefield wounds.

Although from the earliest times there were attempts to set limits for the proper conduct of combatants in war, serious attempts to set ethical parameters for the conduct and protection of medical personnel began in the nineteenth century. Two events are particularly important for consideration of ethical issues. First, in the United States in 1865, Captain Henry Wirz, a Confederate physician who commanded the infamous Andersonville prison in Georgia, was tried for a series of offenses alleging inhumane conduct against Union prisoners of war. He claimed in his defense that "superior orders" mitigated his behavior. Nevertheless, he was convicted and hanged.

In Europe, around the same time, Henri Dunant, a Swiss banker, was shocked by the carnage of the Battle of Solferino, which took place on June 24, 1859. A conference Dunant helped organize in 1864 in Geneva, Switzerland, led to the creation of the International Red Cross. It also established the principle that the sick and wounded, as well as medical personnel, facilities, and transport, were to be considered neutral. This international agreement was the first Geneva Convention, and for his efforts Dunant was awarded the first Nobel Peace Prize.

In 1949, after World War II, this agreement was updated by three other international agreements collectively called the Geneva Conventions. They concern the casualties of naval warfare, the treatment of prisoners, and the protection of civilians from deportation, hostage taking, torture, and discrimination in treatment. Sixty nations, including the United States, signed. The Geneva Conventions states that medical personnel are to be regarded as "noncombatants," and are forbidden to engage in or be parties to acts of war. Furthermore, the wounded and sick of all parties must be respected, protected, treated humanely, and cared for by the belligerents. No physical or moral coercion is allowed against protected persons, in particular to obtain information from them or from third parties.

The Nuremberg Code of 1949, another influential document, followed World War II. The revelations at the Nuremberg, Germany, trial of Nazis who carried out brutal and lethal experiments on prisoners were particularly shocking because these men were physicians, sworn to heal and prevent suffering. Their experiments, such as exposing individuals to freezing water until they died, were conducted to gain knowledge that might assist the German military.

Just as medicine has changed dramatically in the past century, so has warfare. Guerrilla warfare, terrorism, unclear objectives, vastly superior weapons, the blurring of lines between civilian and military participants and targets, attacks on hospitals and ambulances—all have altered the way in which political and ideological struggles are waged. The question is, has this new type of warfare also changed the ethics of military medicine?

In 2004, this question was brought to the forefront of public and professional opinion because of revelations and allegations about mistreatment of prisoners in the U.S.-led war in Afghanistan and Iraq and in the treatment of detainees at Guantanamo Bay, Cuba, an American naval base. Widely circulated photographs of abuses at Abu Ghraib prison in Iraq showed degrading and abusive behavior by American troops. According to Steven H. Miles, a physician and human rights advocate, "Government documents show that the U.S. military medical system failed to protect detainees' human rights, sometimes collaborated with interrogators or abusive guards, and failed to properly report injuries or deaths caused by beatings."

In October 2004, the World Medical Association, a physician organization, reaffirmed its 1982 declaration that medical ethics are the same whether a nation is at war or at peace. But does this statement reflect reality? Michael L. Gross believes that it does not because war brings military and medical values into conflict and that sometimes states sacrifice the lives of many to save some intangible national asset that embodies its common vision of the good. M. Gregg Bloche and Jonathan H. Marks do not deny that a conflict exists, but stress that physicians remain physicians even in the military and that their expertise should not be used to do harm.

YES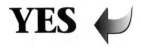

Michael L. Gross

Bioethics and Armed Conflict: Mapping the Moral Dimensions of Medicine and War

Medical ethics in time of armed conflict are identical to medical ethics in time of peace," declares the World Medical Association.[1] Were this the case, wartime and peacetime medicine would turn on the same principles and present similar dilemmas. But war fundamentally transforms the major principles and central issues that engage bioethics. A patient's rights to life and self-determination contract; human dignity strains under the barrage of military necessity; and the interests of the state and political community may outweigh considerations of patients' welfare. Also, actors and interests multiply. Combatants and noncombatants, enemies and allies, states and individuals, citizens and soldiers, prisoners of war, the wounded and the dying, those who can return to combat duty and those who cannot—all of these litter the battlefield.

Armed conflict augments the general principles of bioethics with those peculiar to the conduct of war. For instance, states are obliged to recognize noncombatant immunity, minimize collateral damage, and adhere to a principle of proportionality when fighting threatens to take the lives of civilians and destroy their property. If difficult bioethical dilemmas arise when fundamental moral principles conflict, war adds novel dimensions of its own, as competing bioethical principles must contend not only with one another, but also with the overriding "reason of state" and military necessity that animate any issue of military ethics and may overwhelm other fundamental moral obligations.

Medical ethics in war are not identical to medical ethics in times of peace. Moreover, the nature of war is itself changing as conflicts between nation-states and sub-state actors—guerillas, insurgent ethnic groups, and international terrorist organizations—replace conventional war between sovereign nations. The changing modes of warfare create difficulties for the established conventions of war. They also create new dilemmas for medical personnel, who may be called upon to lend their expertise to the prosecution of war rather than simply to relieve the suffering it causes.

Medical and Military Ethics

In contrast to medical ethics, a wide range of agents, interests, and principles characterize military ethics. Whereas bioethics turns its attention to the patient, either as an individual or class of individuals, military ethics focuses on the rights and interests of three distinct actors: combatants, noncombatants, and the state. The 1949 Geneva Conventions define noncombatants as "persons taking no active part in the hostilities." These include civilians— "people who do not bear arms"—as well as prisoners of war and wounded soldiers. Combatants, on the other hand, bear arms and belong to military organizations that oversee compliance with international law; they include uniformed soldiers, irregulars, members of militia, and guerillas. This definition excludes terrorists who defy international law by intentionally targeting civilian populations.

Alongside individual actors stands the nation-state or political community with interests of its own. Nationstates are internationally recognized sovereign bodies, while political communities reflect the underlying linguistic, historical, ethnic, or religious groups that state or sub-state actors may represent. Representing a "collective way of life" or national ethos, states and political communities are "super-personalities" with a range of interests not necessarily identical to, and possibly in conflict with, the interests of their members.

In spite of divergent actors and interests, the ethics of medicine and armed conflict share norms anchored in the right to life, autonomy, dignity, and utility. The right to life, a central feature of contemporary political theory, grounds a state's obligation to safeguard the lives of its citizens, while liberty interests secure political self-determination and its close cousin, medical autonomy. Dignity is of more recent political interest than either the right to life or self-determination, although it is certainly an integral part of Kant's discussion of autonomy and an enduring aspect of medical ethics. Enshrined in post-war humanitarian law, dignity turns on the inherent worth of any person by virtue of being human. First among Rawls's primary goods, dignity is a correlate of self-esteem, a function of the value and confidence one places in one's own life plans, and the respect others accord their fellow men and women as they pursue their vision of the good.[2] Degradation, humiliation, illtreatment, and debasement invariably cripple self-esteem and make it impossible for individuals to formulate, much less realize, the goals that will make them better people.

Despite the supreme value we attach to life, liberty, and dignity, they sometimes conflict. One way of avoiding these conflicts is to invoke a "utility maximizing" principle, according to which one should act so as to bring about the outcome that best promotes human welfare. Bioethics, which has largely resigned itself to the difficulties of using multiple first principles, places utility maximization alongside other principles. Military ethics, on the other hand, elevates utility in a way that may run roughshod over other fundamental principles, as utility allows military necessity to trump other moral constraints on military action.

The Right to Life in Medicine and War

Most countries hold that the right to life obligates the state to protect its citizens' life and well-being, and that this entails, among other things, the provision of medical care, particularly acute care. Liberty interests and the right to self-determination also secure the right to medical care, since access to adequate and basic medical care is necessary if a person is to exercise liberty. The sick, after all, make poor citizens. The state's duty to protect life is not absolute, however, and contemporary medical practice generally allows individuals to withdraw or withhold life-sustaining care when the quality of life deteriorates badly.

War fundamentally abridges an individual's right to life together with the state's concomitant duty to protect life. Combatants lose their right to life as they gain the right to kill. Whether they pose an immediate threat or man a desk, fight for a just cause or engage in open aggression, soldiers are perpetually at risk. Noncombatants, too, find their lives subject to the constraints of permissible harm, as the principle of noncombatant immunity provides only limited protection from the destruction and devastation of armed conflict.

Just as war impinges on one's right to life, it undermines each actor's right to medical care. Enemy soldiers' right to medical care is a function of the threat they pose. Deprived of their right to life, enemy combatants have no intrinsic right to medical care. Once wounded and no longer a threat, however, they regain their right to life and to medical care. This is the moral significance of *hors de combat* (literally "out of combat"), the special status accorded combatants who are no longer a threat. Yet once wounded enemy soldiers recover sufficiently to pose a threat, their status reverts again to that of enemy combatant.

If the enemy's right to medical treatment is contingent upon the threat they pose, the right of one's own wounded soldiers to receive medical care is contingent upon their "salvage value"—that is, the likelihood that they will return to duty. "Salvage," a criterion of medical care unique to war, largely replaces "quality of life."[3] During war, medical personnel do not treat individual soldiers as discrete patients, but as components of a fighting force, a living collective entity. To maintain this force, medical personnel bear an obligation to salvage soldiers and return as many to duty as quickly as possible. Salvage speaks to a specific and *objective* measure of quality of life distinct from the patient's own, subjective evaluation. Salvageable soldiers may not invoke quality of life to refuse treatment, however painful or onerous, if it will return them to military duty. Those beyond salvage, on the other hand, may not appeal to any right to life to secure medical care when resources are scarce. Combatants who are critically wounded and unlikely to return to duty revert to a noncombatant status and lose their privileged claim to scarce medical resources.

War significantly restricts noncombatants' rights as well. Although civilians are generally immune from the ravages of combat, they remain vulnerable to "collateral harm," that is, to unintended but proportionate harm that noncombatants suffer as the unavoidable outcome of a legitimate military operation.

This is the original context of the much-vaunted doctrine of double effect, which prohibits adversaries from intentionally harming noncombatants.[4] Though it is subject to considerable controversy and conflicting interpretation, the doctrine subordinates a noncombatant's right to life, and access to medical care, to the imperatives peculiar to war, most notably those concerning military necessity and scarcity of resources.

In the final analysis, each set of actors—enemy wounded, unsalvageable friendly soldiers, and civilians—has a fundamentally different claim to medical treatment contingent on the threat they pose, their salvage value, and military necessity, respectively. Further, the status of each actor is not stable, and constant shifting from one status to another plays havoc with medical ethics.

During war, neither combatants nor noncombatants enjoy the same right to life as ordinary patients. Moreover, the state has a life of its own and will wage war to preserve its right to life and common good. Sometimes the common good reflects the welfare of many citizens, but during war the state rarely sacrifices a few lives to save many. Instead, it sacrifices the lives of many to save some intangible national asset that embodies its common vision of the good life and the collective goods that it believes are worth saving.

Autonomy and Self-Determination in Medicine and War

As ordinary citizens, patients command the right of political and medical self-determination. The former embraces such commonly accepted political rights as representation, movement, and free speech, while the latter encompasses the well-known principles of autonomy and patient self-determination: informed consent, privacy, and confidentiality. War complicates and attenuates these principles. Regardless of a nation's state of war, military service limits, if not alters, the nature of autonomy. Autonomy no longer denotes "self-rule"— that is, rule of one's self for the good of oneself—for the good of the self is not a concern of anyone in the military. Rather, autonomy gives way to benign paternalism as others (officers, for example) rule one's self for the good of the state and its armed forces.

As a consequence, civil liberties—be they freedom of speech, movement, or assembly—face distinct limits, and autonomy in medical decisionmaking largely disappears. Informed consent, confidentiality, and privacy are all curtailed, and as a result, bioethical questions largely settled during peacetime emerge with renewed vigor during war.

Noncombatants find that war tears their liberties apart in a similar manner. During war, nations will often abridge civil liberties, including the rights of free speech, assembly, and representation, to safeguard national security and protect the state's sovereignty and territorial integrity. The patient rights of noncombatants, on the other hand, should remain secure and intact. An occupying power, for example, must provide medical care to civilian populations under its control. Exigencies may occasionally prevent this, but there is nothing to indicate that military medical personnel are relieved of their duty to guarantee informed consent, privacy, and confidentiality. On the contrary, developments since World War Two render it imperative to take particular care with the medical rights of occupied peoples to prevent the kind of abuses that characterized Nazi medical experimentation. This, of course, was the intent of the Geneva Conventions and the post-war Nuremberg Code.[5] These prohibit medical experiments contrary to a person's medical interests. Interestingly enough, wartime medicine brings the principles of autonomy and self-determination to the fore far more urgently than peacetime medicine. The same is true for human dignity and self-esteem.

Dignity and Self-Esteem During War

While war curtails the right to life and autonomy of all but the state itself, human dignity should remain unaffected by the vagaries of armed conflict. Dignity entails respect for personhood and a commitment to non-humiliation. For most medical practitioners, neither principle is particularly controversial. However, dignity and self-esteem are among the first casualties of armed conflict. Humanitarian law embraces absolute rights untouched by war, the threat of war, or any other public emergency, and prohibits humiliation, torture, slavery, cruel and inhuman treatment, crushing poverty, ignorance, and political impotence.[6] During armed conflict there is a great temptation to inflict all this and more upon one's enemy, and humanitarian law exists to insure that human rights do not go the way of civil liberties in time of war.

Human rights are inviolable, however, only insofar as they do not conflict, and during war it is not difficult to imagine conflicts between holders of competing rights. Freedom from ill-treatment may conflict with the right to life, leading a state to consider sacrificing the dignity of some to protect the lives of others. This is the hard problem of interrogational torture, and it often draws medical personnel into its web.[7] While torture is an extreme example, tension between life and dignity and the costs of maintaining each are at the heart of many bioethical dilemmas in war.

War exacerbates these tensions because individual and collective interests are often incommensurable and difficult to reconcile. There is, then, during times of war a tendency to turn to the principle of utility and maximize the interests of state above all else. . . .

Bioethics *or* Armed Conflict?

As citizens evaluate the arguments surrounding patient rights, neutrality, and unconventional warfare, and more generally assess the moral implications of going to war, they may quickly confront conflicting duties. Familial duties, small group loyalties, and professional obligations are all thrown off track when states go to war, impose military service, and partake in armed violence. Individuals often identify with a nation's reasons for going to war and subordinate their other moral obligations to their civic duties. Often, indeed, they seem willing to risk their own lives and take those of others. They will desist, if at all, only when higher moral principles compel them to pursue conscientious objection or civil disobedience when they perceive wars to be unjust.

In times of war every citizen, regardless of profession, has the same obligation to weigh reason of state and evaluate humanitarian principles. Nevertheless, one is sometimes tempted to ask whether medical personnel have a unique obligation to resolve dilemmas during war in a way that is consistent with their professional obligations. While one might not expect an individual's professional obligations to assume overriding importance as one contemplates the intractable ethical and moral questions of war, a medical practitioner's duties seem, to many, to be different. In each case above, it appears at first glance that physicians have a special duty to avoid some non-caregiving uses of medical expertise, even if these are militarily justified. Although international law permits certain types of nonlethal weapons, and assuming one could provide reasonable grounds to justify the policy of the Egyptian government, medical personnel must nonetheless refuse to develop these weapons systems because their professional obligation to "do no harm" requires them to use their expertise solely to promote human good. Similarly, health care professionals may be expected to uphold patient rights and medical neutrality regardless of military necessity.

But this conclusion, if correct, seems to push medicine into a moral class of its own. It allows medical personnel to invoke professional duties in order to avoid causing harm while ordinary citizens must subordinate their professional duties to reason of state when conditions merit. Those who believe medicine answers a "higher calling" may find this conclusion attractive. Yet it confuses professional duties with humanitarian obligations. When the WMA prohibited medical participation in chemical and biological warfare, it declared: "It is the privilege of the medical doctor to practice medicine in the service of humanity, to preserve and restore bodily and mental health without distinction as to persons, to comfort and ease the suffering of his or her patients. The utmost respect for human life is to be maintained even under threat, and no use made of any medical knowledge contrary to the laws of humanity."[8]

The WMA, however, uses the word "humanity" in two distinct senses, and this, perhaps, sums up the difficulty facing the medical profession during war. "Service of humanity" refers to beneficence and the imperative to preserve and restore human health. This is a professional obligation and, in principle, no different from those duties that obligate other professions that serve different human needs and that may fall before reason of state during war. The "laws of humanity," in contrast, invoke humanitarian law and respect for human rights. They are inviolable insofar as they do not conflict with one another, and, in spite of the tendency sometimes to conflate the laws of humanity and medicine's professional duty of beneficence, the two are not synonymous. Preserving this distinction is important. While one would not expect a physician or anyone else to use his or her knowledge contrary to the laws of humanity, there is sometimes room to ask whether any individual, physicians included, may violate another person's "bodily and mental health." This is the question we all face in the shadow of armed conflict.

References

1. *World Medical Association Regulations in Time of Armed Conflict*, amended by the 35th World Medical Assembly, Venice Italy, October 1983.

2. J. Rawls, *A Theory of Justice* (Cambridge, Mass.: Harvard University Press, 1971): 440.

3. *Emergency War Surgery NATO Handbook*, part 3, chapter 12. . . . Ordinary triage classifies the wounded so all will receive optimum care, while mass casualty triage treats the injured according to salvage value when the injured overwhelm available medical facilities and not all can be treated.

4. A. McIntyre, "Doing Away with Double Effect," *Ethics* 111 (2001): 219–55; W.S. Quinn, "Actions, Intentions and Consequences: The Doctrine of the Double Effect," *Philosophy and Public Affairs* 18 (1989): 334–51; J. McMahan, "Revising the Doctrine of Double Effect," *Journal of Applied Philosophy* 11, 2 (1994): 201–212.

5. First and Second Geneva Convention, common article 12, Third Geneva Convention, article 13, Fourth Geneva Convention, article 32; Geneva, 1949. These prohibit medical experiments contrary to a person's medical interests. Requirements stipulating informed consent did not enter international law until 1966. United Nations, "International Covenant on Civil and Political Rights," article 7. Adopted and opened for signature, ratification, and accession by General Assembly resolution 2200A (XXI) of December 16, 1966, entry into force March 23, 1976. . . . Also, L.C. Green, *The Contemporary Law of Armed Conflict*, Second Edition (Manchester, England: University of Manchester Press, 2000): 234–39.

6. United Nations, "International Covenant on Civil and Political Rights." The only non-derogable rights during war or public emergency are the right to life; freedom from torture, slavery, servitude, and retroactive legislation; freedom of conscience; the right to recognition before the law; and the right not to be imprisoned for breach of contract.

7. M.L. Gross, "Doctors in the Decent Society: Medical Care, Torture and Ill-Treatment," *Bioethics* 18, 2 (2004): 181–203.

8. World Medical Association, *Declaration on Chemical and Biological Weapons*.

M. Gregg Bloche and
Jonathan H. Marks

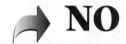 **NO**

When Doctors Go to War

When military forces go into combat, they are typically accompanied by medical personnel (physicians, physician assistants, nurses, and medics) who serve in noncombat roles. These professionals are bound by international law to treat wounded combatants from all sides and to care for injured civilians. They are also required to care for enemy prisoners and to report any evidence of abuse of detainees. In exchange, the Geneva Conventions protect them from direct attack, so long as they themselves do not become combatants.

Recently, there have been accounts of failure by U.S. medical personnel to report evidence of detainee abuse, even murder, in Iraq and Afghanistan.[1] There have also been claims, less well supported, that medics and others neglected the clinical needs of some detainees. The Department of Defense says it is investigating these allegations, though no charges have been brought against caregivers.

But Pentagon officials deny another set of allegations: that physicians and other medical professionals breached their professional ethics and the laws of war by participating in abusive interrogation practices. The International Committee of the Red Cross (ICRC) has concluded that medical personnel at Guantanamo Bay shared health information, including patient records, with army units that planned interrogations.[2] The ICRC called this "a flagrant violation of medical ethics" and said some of the interrogation methods used were "tantamount to torture."[2] The Pentagon answered that its detention operations are "safe, humane, and professional" and that "the allegation that detainee medical files were used to harm detainees is false."[2]

Our own inquiry into medical involvement in military intelligence gathering in Iraq and Guantanamo Bay has revealed a more troublesome picture. Recently released documents and interviews with military sources point to a pattern of such involvement, including participation in interrogation procedures that violate the laws of war. Not only did caregivers pass health information to military intelligence personnel; physicians assisted in the design of interrogation strategies, including sleep deprivation and other coercive methods tailored to detainees' medical conditions. Medical personnel also coached interrogators on questioning technique.

Physicians who did such work tend not to see these practices as unethical. On the contrary, a common understanding among those who helped to plan interrogations is that physicians serving in these roles do not act as physicians and are therefore not bound by patient-oriented ethics. In an interview, Dr. David Tornberg, Deputy Assistant Secretary of Defense for Health Affairs, endorsed this view. Physicians assigned to military intelligence, he contended, have no doctor–patient relationship with detainees and, in the absence of life-threatening emergency, have no obligation to offer medical aid.

Most people we interviewed who had served or spent time in detention facilities in Iraq or Guantanamo Bay reported being told not to talk about their experiences and impressions. Dr. David Auch, commander of the medical unit that staffed Abu Ghraib during the time of the abuses made notorious by soldiers' photographs, said military intelligence personnel told his medics and physician assistants not to discuss deaths that occurred in detention. Physicians who cared for so-called high-value detainees were especially hesitant to share their observations.

Yet available documents, the consistency of multiple confidential accounts, and confirmation of key facts by persons who spoke on the record make possible an understanding of the medical role in military intelligence in Iraq and Guantanamo. They also shed light on how those involved tried to justify this role in ethical terms.

In testimony taken in February 2004, as part of an inquiry into abuses at Abu Ghraib (and recently made public under the freedom of Information Act and posted on the Web site of the American Civil Liberties Union [ACLU] . . . , Colonel Thomas M. Pappas, chief of military intelligence at the prison, described physicians' systematic role in developing and executing interrogation strategies. Military intelligence teams, Pappas said, prepared individualized "interrogation plans" for detainees that included a "sleep plan" and medical standards. "A physician and a psychiatrist," he added, "are on hand to monitor what we are doing."

What was in these interrogation plans? None have become public, though Pappas's testimony indicates that he showed army investigators a sample, including a sleep deprivation schedule. However, a January 2004 "Memorandum for Record" (also available on the ACLU Web site) lays out an "Interrogation and Counter-Resistance Policy" calling for aggressive measures. Among these approaches are "dietary manipulation—minimum bread and water, monitored by medics"; "environmental manipulation—i.e., reducing A.C. [air conditioning] in summer, lower[ing] heat in winter"; "sleep management—for 72-hour time period maximum, monitored by medics"; "sensory deprivation—for 72-hour time period maximum, monitored by medics"; "isolation—for longer than 30 days"; "stress positions"; and "presence of working dogs."

Physicians collaborated with prison guards and military interrogators to put such approaches into practice. "Typically," said Pappas, military intelligence personnel give guards "a copy of the interrogation plan and a written note as to how to execute [it]. . . . The doctor and psychiatrist also look at the files to see what the interrogation plan recommends; they have the final say as to what is implemented." The psychiatrist would accompany interrogators to the prison and "review all those people under a management plan and provide feedback as to whether they were being medically and physically taken care of," said Pappas. These practices, he conceded, were without precedent. "The execution of this type of operation . . . is not codified in doctrine," he said. "Except for Guantanamo Bay, this sort of thing was a first."

At both Abu Ghraib[3] and Guantanamo,[2] "behavioral science consultation teams" advised military intelligence personnel on interrogation tactics. These teams, each of which included psychologists and a psychiatrist, functioned more formally at Guantanamo; staff shortages and other administrative difficulties reduced their role at Abu Ghraib.

A slide presentation prepared by medical ethics advisors to the military as a starting point for internal discussion poses a hypothetical case that, we were told, is a "thinly veiled" account of actual events. A physician newly deployed to "Irakistan" must decide whether to post physician assistants and medics behind a one-way mirror during interrogations. A military police commander tells the doctor that "the way this worked with the unit here before you was: We'd capture a guy; the medic would screen him and ensure he was fit for interrogation. If he had questions he'd check with the supervising doctor. The medic would get his screening signed by the doc. After that, the medic would watch over the interrogation from behind the glass."[4]

Interrogation facilities at Abu Ghraib included a one-way mirror, according to internal FBI documents obtained and made public by the ACLU in December. Draft rules of conduct, now under review, would permit army medical personnel to attend interrogations but would give them a right to refuse on ethical grounds.

Military intelligence interrogation units also had access to detainees' medical records and to clinical caregivers in both Iraq and Guantanamo Bay. "They couldn't conduct their job without that info," Tornberg told us. Caregivers, he said, have only a limited doctor–patient relationship with detainees and "make it very clear to the individuals that their medical information will not be protected . . . To the extent it is military-relevant . . ., that information can be used."

In helping to plan and execute interrogation strategies, did doctors breach medical ethics? Military physicians and Pentagon officials make a case to the contrary. Doctors, they argue, act as combatants, not physicians, when they put their knowledge to use for military ends. A medical degree, Tornberg said, is not a "sacramental vow"—it is a certification of skill. When a doctor participates in interrogation, "he's not functioning as a physician," and the Hippocratic ethic of commitment to patient welfare does not apply. According to this view, as long as the military maintains a separation of roles between clinical caregivers and physicians with intelligence-gathering responsibilities, assisting interrogators is legitimate.

Military physicians point to civilian parallels, including forensic psychiatry and occupational health, in arguing that the medical profession sometimes serves purposes at odds with patient welfare. They argue, persuasively in our view, that the Hippocratic ideal of undivided loyalty to patients fails to capture the breadth of the profession's social role. This role encompasses the legitimate needs of the criminal and civil justice systems, employers' concerns about workers' fitness for duty, allocation of limited medical resources, and protection of the public's health.

But the proposition that doctors who serve these social purposes don't act as physicians is self-contradictory. Their "physicianhood"—encompassing technical skill, scientific understanding, a caring ethos, and cultural authority—is the reason they are called on to assume these roles. The forensic psychiatrist's judgments about personal responsibility and competence rest on his or her moral sensibility and grasp of mental illness. And the military physician's contributions to interrogation—to its effectiveness, lawfulness, and social acceptance in a rights-respecting society—arise from his or her psychological insight, clinical knowledge, and perceived humanistic commitment.

In denying their status as physicians, military doctors divert attention from an urgent moral challenge—the need to manage conflict between the medical profession's therapeutic and social purposes. The Hippocratic ethical tradition offers no road map for resolving this conflict, but it provides a starting point. The therapeutic mission is the profession's primary role and the core of physicians' professional identity. If this mission and identity are to be preserved, there are some things doctors must not do. Consensus holds, for example, that physicians should not administer the death penalty, even in countries where capital punishment is lawful. Similarly, when physicians are involved in war, some simple rules should apply.

Physicians should not use drugs or other biologic means to subdue enemy combatants or extract information from detainees, nor should they aid others in doing so. They should not be party to interrogation practices contrary to human rights law or the laws of war, and their role in legitimate interrogation should not extend beyond limit setting, as guardians of detainees' health.[5] This role does not carry patient care responsibilities, but it requires physicians to tell detainees about health problems they find and to make treatment available. It also demands that physicians document abuses and report them to chains of command. By these standards, military medicine has fallen short.

The conclusion that doctors participated in torture is premature, but there is probable cause for suspecting it. Follow-up investigation is essential to determine whether they helped to craft and carry out the counter-resistance strategies—e.g., prolonged isolation and exposure to temperature extremes—that rise to the level of torture.

But, clearly, the medical personnel who helped to develop and execute aggressive counter-resistance plans thereby breached the laws of war. The Third Geneva Convention states that "[n]o physical or mental torture, nor any other form of coercion, may be inflicted on prisoners of war to secure from them information of any kind whatever." It adds that "prisoners of war who refuse to answer [questions] may not be threatened, insulted, or exposed to any unpleasant or disadvantageous treatment of any kind." The tactics used at Abu Ghraib and Guantanamo were transparently coercive, threatening, unpleasant, and disadvantageous. Although the Bush administration took the position (rejected by the ICRC) that none of the Guantanamo detainees were "prisoners of war," entitled to the full protections of the Third Geneva

Convention, it has acknowledged that combatants detained in Iraq are indeed prisoners of war, fully protected under this Convention.

The Surgeon General of the U.S. Army has begun a confidential effort to develop rules for health care professionals who work with detainees. Such an initiative is much needed, but it ought not to happen behind a veil of secrecy. Ethicists, legal scholars, and civilian professional leaders should participate, and the process should address role conflict in medicine more generally. An Institute of Medicine study committee, broadly representative of competing concerns (including the military's), would be a more suitable venue. To their credit, some military physicians in leadership roles have tried to involve outside ethicists in discussion of duties toward detainees. The Pentagon's civilian leadership has blocked these efforts.

Military physicians, nurses, and other health care professionals have served with courage in Iraq and other theatres of war since September 11, 2001. Some have received serious wounds, and some have died in the line of duty. By most accounts, they have delivered superb care to U.S. soldiers, enemy combatants, and wounded civilians alike. We owe them our gratitude and respect. We would affirm their honor, not besmirch it, by acknowledging the tensions between their Hippocratic and national service commitments and by working with them to map a course between the two.

References

1. Miles SH. Abu Ghraib: its legacy for military medicine. Lancet 2004;364:725–9.
2. Lewis NA. Red Cross finds detainee abuse in Guantanamo. New York Times. November 30, 2004:A1.
3. Joint Interrogation & Debriefing Center. Abu Ghraib, Iraq. 2004. (Accessed December 16, 2004. . . .)
4. Medics, detainee: muddy waters. Presented at the USU Faculty Workshop on Military Healthcare Ethics, 14 October 2004.
5. Principles of medical ethics relevant to the role of health personnel, particularly physicians, in the protection of prisoners and detainees against torture and other cruel, inhuman, or degrading treatment or punishment. Adopted by U.N. General Assembly resolution 37/194 of 18 December 1982. (Accessed December 16, 2004. . . .)

POSTSCRIPT

Does Military Necessity Override Medical Ethics?

Several investigations into abuses of prisoners were launched after Abu Ghraib incidents came to light. In August 2004, the U.S. Army released a report, known as the Fay Report, after one of its chief investigators Maj. Gen. George Fay. The report implicated 27 members of a military intelligence unit in the abuses, in addition to the seven reservist military police previously charged. Among the failures detailed were those of medics who failed to report abuses. Gen. Paul Kern, who supervised the inquiry, said that the report laid out "serious misconduct and a loss of moral values," but stressed that the abusers were a tiny minority of the military personnel.

The debate was joined in 2006 by three authors. Michael Gross expanded this issue into a book, *Bioethics and Armed Conflict: Moral Dilemmas of Medicine and War* (MIT Press). John Yoo, a former assistant attorney general in the U.S. Justice Department, goes even further in his assertion that the Geneva Conventions are outmoded and that presidential authority to counter terrorism is essentially unlimited, in *War by Other Means: An Insider's Account of the War on Terror* (Atlantic Monthly Press). On the other hand, in *Oath Betrayed: Torture, Medical Complicity, and the War on Terror* (Random House, 2006), Steven Miles, a physician, argues that the medical profession's participation in torture and abuses are grossly unethical.

Articles on the conflict between military and medical ethics include Jerome Amir Singh, "American Physicians and Dual Loyalty Obligations in the 'War on Terror,'" *BMC Medical Ethics* (August 1, 2003, http://www.biomedcentral.com); Giovanni Maio, "History of Medical Involvement in Torture—Then and Now," *The Lancet* (May 19, 2001); Leonard S. Rubenstein, "The Medical Community's Response to Torture," *The Lancet* (May 3, 2003); and Edmund G. Howe, "Dilemmas in Military Medical Ethics Since 9/11," *Kennedy Institute of Ethics Journal* (June 2003).

The American Medical Association's policy on torture is available at: http://www.ama-assn.org/ama/pub/category/8421.html. The Geneva Conventions are available at www.genevaconventions.org. The World Medical Association policy on torture is available at www.wma.net/e/policy/t1.htm.

ISSUE 18

Should Performance-Enhancing Drugs Be Banned from Sports?

YES: Thomas H. Murray, from "Drugs, Sports, and Ethics," *Project Syndicate* (July 2004)

NO: Julian Savulescu, Bennett Foddy, and Megan Clayton, from "Why We Should Allow Performance Enhancing Drugs in Sport," *British Journal of Sports Medicine* (December 2004)

ISSUE SUMMARY

YES: Social psychologist Thomas H. Murray contends that performance-enhancing drugs affect the individual athlete's integrity because using banned substances is a dishonest behavior and corrupts a victory.

NO: Philosopher Julian Savulescu and research colleagues Bennett Foddy and Megan Clayton argue that legalizing drugs in sport may be fairer and safer than banning them.

In sports, there are winners and losers. But for many athletes, winning is not enough. Elite athletes want to set records or exceed their prior performances. Athletes of less than elite status aspire to reach that higher level. And even ordinary competitors who know they will never jump as high as Michael Jordan or hit a hockey puck as precisely as Wayne Gretsky want to go farther than their natural talent and motivation might take them. The potential rewards are enormous, not just in personal gratification but also in prestige, career opportunities, and financial success.

For all these different types of sports figures, there is a strong temptation to enhance their performance through the use of drugs. And increasingly they can find some drug that may help them do it. Drug use in sports is not a new phenomenon. Athletes in the original Greek Olympics are believed to have used mushrooms and herbs to make them stronger and faster. In the nineteenth century, French cyclists drank Vin Mariani, a combination of wine and coca leaf extract called "the wine of athletes." Coca leaf, the source of cocaine, made it easier for them to endure the prolonged exertion of cycling.

These potions, however, were mild compared to the modern pharmacopeia available to athletes. In addition to natural substances, prescription drugs used in megadoses, and illegal substances like cocaine and marijuana, there are synthesized forms of human hormones and "designer drugs" for particular purposes.

Concern about drug use in sports in modern times is relatively recent. Steroid use first emerged in the 1964 Olympics. Anabolic androgenic steroids are compounds synthesized from the hormone testosterone, which is present in normal amounts in males. ("Anabolic" means "to build," and "androgenic" means "masculinizing.") Physicians prescribe such steroids to repair damaged tissue, but the doses that athletes use are many times greater than therapeutic ones. Because anabolic steroids build muscle mass, weight lifters, hammer throwers, and other athletes whose performance depends on muscle power are most likely to use them. In females, the results may be not just muscle mass but masculinizing features. In the Montreal Olympics in 1976, East German women swimmers were able to swim faster than other competitors, but they also had deep voices and body hair.

Stimulants such as amphetamines serve a different purpose; they give athletes unusually high levels of alertness, energy, and aggressiveness, characteristics particularly appealing to football players. Other kinds of medical intervention to enhance performance include "blood doping"—storing some of a cyclist's own blood and injecting it before a race to give the maximum number of oxygen-carrying red blood cells. A synthetic substance—erythropoetin (EPO), prescribed to treat anemia in cancer patients—can also be used in this way.

What has been the response of official sports organizations to this growing use of drugs? The World Anti-Doping Agency, an offshoot of the International Olympic Committee, has a 10-page list of banned substances (available at http://www.wada-ama.org). The major categories are anabolic agents, hormones and related substances (such as EPO and human growth hormone), beta-2 agonists (substances that relieve breathing stress, except for athletes who have asthma), agents with anti-estrogenic activity (substances that enhance feminine characteristics), and diuretics and other agents that might mask the presence of drugs by depleting the body of urine. In addition, blood doping, chemical and physical manipulation, and gene doping—a new addition to the armamentarium—are prohibited. Some substances are prohibited in competitions, including stimulants, narcotics, cannabinoids (marijuana and hashish), and other steroids. Certain sports prohibit alcohol or beta-blockers (drugs that lower blood pressure).

Is all this anti-drug activity warranted, or is it an unacceptable invasion of privacy and a losing battle? Why should adults for whom sports is a primary value not be allowed to do whatever they choose to enhance their performance? Can drugs and sport coexist? The two following selections take opposite views. Thomas H. Murray contends that drug use violates the integrity of sport and deprives it of its essential value and meaning. Julian Savulescu, Bennett Foddy, and Megan Clayton, on the other hand, argue that there is nothing inherently wrong in athletes' using drugs to perform at higher levels, and it would be better for all if drug use were legalized and controlled for athletes' safety.

YES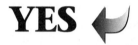

Drugs, Sports, and Ethics

When the Olympic Games return to Greece this summer, the results at the drug testing laboratory may get as much attention as what happens at the Olympic stadium. The history of drugs, and drug control, at the Olympics is discouraging—a farrago of ill-informed rules, outright state-sponsored cheating, and half-hearted and erratic attempts at enforcement.

A new model has recently revived hope for effective drug control by moving testing and enforcement from the direct control of the International Olympic Committee and the national governing bodies to the World Anti-Doping Agency and similar organizations at the national level. The US Anti-Doping Agency, for example, played a central role in uncovering a new synthetic steroid known as THG linked to a California firm catering to Olympic and professional athletes.

But the renewed hope will be frustrated unless we can respond effectively to the ethical challenge. No amount of interdiction will suffice if we do not explain clearly what, precisely, is wrong with using performance enhancing drugs in sport.

There are three compelling reasons to ban such drugs: assuring all athletes that the competition is fair; preserving the integrity of the athlete; and safeguarding what gives sport its meaning and value.

Young Olympians devote their lives to their sport for the opportunity to match themselves against the world's most gifted and dedicated athletes. The difference between gold medalist and also-ran may be measured in fractions of seconds or inches. A tiny advantage can make all the difference. What if that advantage comes from using a performance enhancing drug?

For athletes who want to compete clean, the threat that they may be beaten by a competitor who is not faster, stronger, or more dedicated, but who takes a drug to gain the edge, is profoundly personal. When drugs are prohibited but some athletes use them anyway the playing field tilts in favor of the cheater. If we prohibit drugs in the Olympic Games, we owe it to the athletes to deter, detect, and punish those who cheat.

Integrity seems like an old-fashioned idea, but it is at the heart of who we are and how we live. Performance enhancing drugs affect the individual athlete's integrity in two ways. First, if drugs are banned, then choosing not to use them is a test of one's character. A person of integrity does not behave

From *Project Syndicate*, July 2004. Copyright © 2004 by Project Syndicate. Reprinted by permission.

dishonestly. A person of integrity does not seek to prevail over his competitors by methods that give him an illegitimate advantage.

Second, the concept of integrity implies wholeness, being unbroken, moral soundness and freedom from corruption. When an athlete wins by using a performance enhancing drug, what does that mean for the athlete's own understanding of what happened? Am I the world's best? Or was my supposed victory hopelessly tainted by the drug's effects? The meaning of a drug-aided victory is ambiguous and elusive even for the athlete. It is the result of corruption and brokenness, the very opposite of authentic victory.

What makes a victory authentic? What gives sport its meaning and value? We expect the winning athlete to combine extraordinary natural talents with exemplary effort, training and technique. These are all forms of human excellence. Some we are born with—or not. As much as I loved playing basketball, I was destined never quite to reach six feet in height. An accurate jump shot and the willingness to take punishment never made up for my size and mediocre leaping ability.

Whatever natural abilities we have must be perfected. We achieve this—or not—through a combination of virtues such as fortitude in the face of relentless training, physical courage as we persevere through pain, and cleverness when we outsmart our opponents, along with other factors such as helpful coaching, optimized equipment, and sound nutrition.

Natural talents should be respected for what they are: the occasionally awesome luck of the biological draw. Courage, fortitude, competitive savvy, and other virtues rightfully command our moral admiration. The other factors—equipment, coaching, and nutrition—contribute to an athlete's success but don't evoke the same awe or esteem. When we watch a sprinter set a new Olympic record in the hundred meter dash, it's not the shoes he or she wears that command our admiration. Nor is it the coaching received or the energy bar consumed just before the event.

All of these contribute to the record, just like a good camera was necessary for Ansel Adam's unforgettable photos of the American West, or good marble and sharp chisels for Michelangelo's sculpture of David. But what we care about most, what gives that achievement its meaning and value, is the ineffable combination of remarkable natural talents and extraordinary dedication.

Performance enhancing drugs disguise natural abilities and substitute for the dedication and focus that we admire. Performance enhancing drugs cheapen sport, making winners out of also-rans, and depriving virtuous and superior athletes of the victories that should be theirs.

Getting performance enhancing drugs out of sport will not be easy, and success is not assured. But the effort is worthwhile as long as we care enough about fairness, integrity, and the meaning and value of sport.

Julian Savulescu, Bennett Foddy,
and Megan Clayton

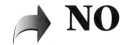

NO

Why We Should Allow Performance Enhancing Drugs in Sport

In 490 BC, the Persian Army landed on the plain of Marathon, 25 miles from Athens. The Athenians sent a messenger named Feidipides to Sparta to ask for help. He ran the 150 miles in two days. The Spartans were late. The Athenians attacked and, although out-numbered five to one, were victorious. Feidipides was sent to run back to Athens to report victory. On arrival, he screamed "We won" and dropped dead from exhaustion.

The marathon was run in the first modern Olympics in 1896, and in many ways the athletic ideal of modern athletes is inspired by the myth of the marathon. Their ideal is superhuman performance, at any cost.

Drugs in Sport

The use of performance enhancing drugs in the modern Olympics is on record as early as the games of the third Olympiad, when Thomas Hicks won the marathon after receiving an injection of strychnine in the middle of the race.[1] The first official ban on "stimulating substances" by a sporting organisation was introduced by the International Amateur Athletic Federation in 1928.[2]

Using drugs to cheat in sport is not new, but it is becoming more effective. In 1976, the East German swimming team won 11 out of 13 Olympic events, and later sued the government for giving them anabolic steroids.[3] Yet despite the health risks, and despite the regulating bodies' attempts to eliminate drugs from sport, the use of illegal substances is widely known to be rife. It hardly raises an eyebrow now when some famous athlete fails a dope test.

In 1992, Vicky Rabinowicz interviewed small groups of athletes. She found that Olympic athletes, in general, believed that most successful athletes were using banned substances.[4]

Much of the writing on the use of drugs in sport is focused on this kind of anecdotal evidence. There is very little rigorous, objective evidence because the athletes are doing something that is taboo, illegal, and sometimes highly dangerous. The anecdotal picture tells us that our attempts to eliminate drugs from sport have failed. In the absence of good evidence, we need an analytical argument to determine what we should do.

From *British Journal of Sports Medicine*, December 2004, pp. 666–667, 670. Copyright © 2004 by BMJ Publishing Group. Reprinted by permission.

Condemned to Cheating?

We are far from the days of amateur sporting competition. Elite athletes can earn tens of millions of dollars every year in prize money alone, and millions more in sponsorships and endorsements. The lure of success is great. But the penalties for cheating are small. A six month or one year ban from competition is a small penalty to pay for further years of multimillion dollar success.

Drugs are much more effective today than they were in the days of strychnine and sheep's testicles. Studies involving the anabolic steroid androgen showed that, even in doses much lower than those used by athletes, muscular strength could be improved by 5–20%.[5] Most athletes are also relatively unlikely to ever undergo testing. The International Amateur Athletic Federation estimates that only 10–15% of participating athletes are tested in each major competition.[6]

The enormous rewards for the winner, the effectiveness of the drugs, and the low rate of testing all combine to create a cheating "game" that is irresistible to athletes. Kjetil Haugen[7] investigated the suggestion that athletes face a kind of prisoner's dilemma regarding drugs. His game theoretic model shows that, unless the likelihood of athletes being caught doping was raised to unrealistically high levels, or the payoffs for winning were reduced to unrealistically low levels, athletes could all be predicted to cheat. The current situation for athletes ensures that this is likely, even though they are worse off as a whole if everyone takes drugs, than if nobody takes drugs.

Drugs such as erythropoietin (EPO) and growth hormone are natural chemicals in the body. As technology advances, drugs have become harder to detect because they mimic natural processes. In a few years, there will be many undetectable drugs. Haugen's analysis predicts the obvious: that when the risk of being caught is zero, athletes will all choose to cheat.

The recent Olympic games in Athens were the first to follow the introduction of a global anti-doping code. From the lead up to the games to the end of competition, 3000 drug tests were carried out: 2600 urine tests and 400 blood tests for the endurance enhancing drug EPO.[8] From these, 23 athletes were found to have taken a banned substance—the most ever in an Olympic games.[9] Ten of the men's weightlifting competitors were excluded.

The goal of "cleaning" up the sport is unattainable. Further down the track the spectre of genetic enhancement looms dark and large.

The Spirit of Sport

So is cheating here to stay? Drugs are against the rules. But we define the rules of sport. If we made drugs legal and freely available, there would be no cheating.

The World Anti-Doping Agency code declares a drug illegal if it is performance enhancing, if it is a health risk, or if it violates the "spirit of sport."[10] They define this spirit as follows.[11] The spirit of sport is the celebration of the human spirit, body, and mind, and is characterised by the following values:

- ethics, fair play and honesty
- health
- excellence in performance
- character and education
- fun and joy
- teamwork
- dedication and commitment
- respect for rules and laws
- respect for self and other participants
- courage
- community and solidarity[11]

Would legal and freely available drugs violate this "spirit"? Would such a permissive rule be good for sport?

Human sport is different from sports involving other animals, such as horse or dog racing. The goal of a horse race is to find the fastest horse. Horses are lined up and flogged. The winner is the one with the best combination of biology, training, and rider. Basically, this is a test of biological potential. This was the old naturalistic Athenian vision of sport: find the strongest, fastest, or most skilled man.

Training aims to bring out this potential. Drugs that improve our natural potential are against the spirit of this model of sport. But this is not the only view of sport. Humans are not horses or dogs. We make choices and exercise our own judgment. We choose what kind of training to use and how to run our race. We can display courage, determination, and wisdom. We are not flogged by a jockey on our back but drive ourselves. It is this judgment that competitors exercise when they choose diet, training, and whether to take drugs. We can choose what kind of competitor to be, not just through training, but through biological manipulation. Human sport is different from animal sport because it is creative. Far from being against the spirit of sport, biological manipulation embodies the human spirit—the capacity to improve ourselves on the basis of reason and judgment. When we exercise our reason, we do what only humans do.

The result will be that the winner is not the person who was born with the best genetic potential to be strongest. Sport would be less of a genetic lottery. The winner will be the person with a combination of the genetic potential, training, psychology, and judgment. Olympic performance would be the result of human creativity and choice, not a very expensive horse race.

Classical musicians commonly use β blockers to control their stage fright. These drugs lower heart rate and blood pressure, reducing the physical effects of stress, and it has been shown that the quality of a musical performance is improved if the musician takes these drugs.[12] Although elite classical music is arguably as competitive as elite sport, and the rewards are similar, there is no stigma attached to the use of these drugs. We do not think less of the violinist or pianist who uses them. If the audience judges the performance to be improved with drugs, then the drugs are enabling the musician to express him or herself more effectively. The competition between elite musicians has rules—you cannot mime the violin to a backing CD. But there is no rule against the use of chemical enhancements.

Is classical music a good metaphor for elite sport? Sachin Tendulkar is known as the "Maestro from Mumbai." The Associated Press called Maria Sharapova's 2004 Wimbledon final a "virtuoso performance."[13] Jim Murrary[14] wrote the following about Michael Jordan in 1996:

> "You go to see Michael Jordan play for the same reason you went to see Astaire dance, Olivier act or the sun set over Canada. It's art. It should be painted, not photographed.
>
>   It's not a game, it's a recital. He's not just a player, he's a virtuoso. Heifetz with a violin. Horowitz at the piano."

Indeed, it seems reasonable to suggest that the reasons we appreciate sport at its elite level have something to do with competition, but also a great deal to do with the appreciation of an extraordinary performance.

Clearly the application of this kind of creativity is limited by the rules of the sport. Riding a motorbike would not be a "creative" solution to winning the Tour de France, and there are good reasons for proscribing this in the rules. If motorbikes were allowed, it would still be a good sport, but it would no longer be a bicycle race.

We should not think that allowing cyclists to take EPO would turn the Tour de France into some kind of "drug race," any more than the various training methods available turn it into a "training race" or a "money race." Athletes train in different, creative ways, but ultimately they still ride similar bikes, on the same course. The skill of negotiating the steep winding descent will always be there. . . .

Test for Health, Not Drugs

The welfare of the athlete must be our primary concern. If a drug does not expose an athlete to excessive risk, we should allow it even if it enhances performance. We have two choices: to vainly try to turn the clock back, or to rethink who we are and what sport is, and to make a new 21st century Olympics. Not a super-Olympics but a more human Olympics. Our crusade against drugs in sport has failed. Rather than fearing drugs in sport, we should embrace them.

In 1998, the president of the International Olympic Committee, Juan-Antonio Samaranch, suggested that athletes be allowed to use non-harmful performance enhancing drugs. This view makes sense only if, by not using drugs, we are assured that athletes are not being harmed.

Performance enhancement is not against the spirit of sport; it is the spirit of sport. To choose to be better is to be human. Athletes should be given this choice. Their welfare should be paramount. But taking drugs is not necessarily cheating. The legalisation of drugs in sport may be fairer and safer.

References

1. House of Commons, Select Committee on Culture, Media and Sport. 2004. Seventh Report of Session 2003–2004, UK Parliament, HC 499–1.

2. House of Commons, Select Committee on Culture, Media and Sport. 2004. Seventh Report of Session 2003–2004, UK Parliament, HC 499–1.

3. Longman, J. 2004. East German Steroids' toll: 'they killed Heidi', *New York Times* 2004 Jan 20, sect D:1.

4. Rabinawicz V. Athletes and drugs: a separate pace? *Psychol Today* 1992;**25**:52–3.

5. Hartgens F, Kuipers H. Effects of androgenic-anabolic steroids in athletes. *Sport Med* 2004;**34**:513–54.

6. IAAF, 2004. . . .

7. Haugen KK. The performance-enhancing drug game. *Journal of Sports Economics* 2004;**5**:67–87.

8. Wilson S. *Boxer Munyasia fails drug test in Athens.* Athens: Associated Press, 2004 Aug 10.

9. Zinser L. With drug-tainted past, few track records fall. *New York Times* 2004 Aug 29, Late Edition, p. 1.

10. WADA. World Anti-Doping Code, Montreal. World Anti-Doping Agency, 2003:16.

11. WADA. World Anti-Doping Code, Montreal. World Anti-Doping Agency, 2003:3.

12. Brantigan CO, Brantigan TA, Joseph N. Effect of beta blockade and beta stimulation on stage fright. *Am J Med* 1982;**72**:88–94.

13. Wilson S. Sharapova beats Williams for title. *Associated Press,* 2004 Jul 3, 09:10am.

14. Murray J. It's basketball played on a higher plane. *Los Angeles Times* 1996 Feb 4 1996, sect C:1.

POSTSCRIPT

Should Performance-Enhancing Drugs Be Banned from Sports?

The controversy surrounding drug use in sports hit American baseball in 2004. In December, San Francisco Giants star hitter Barry Bonds, New York Yankee Jason Giambi, and several other elite athletes were implicated in an investigation of the Bay Area Laboratory Co-operative (BALCO). BALCO was alleged to have created a new and previously undetected illegal steroid tetrahydrogestrinone, known as THG or "the clear," as opposed to another illegal steroid known as "the cream." Baseball officials had generally taken a low-key response to drug use, adopting steroid testing in 2002 but not instituting strict penalties and procedures, which the player's union had opposed.

In January 2005, however, Major League Baseball Commissioner Bud Selig announced a tougher policy. Stating that the league had "zero tolerance" for drug use, Commissioner Selig said that a positive test for a steroid would result in a suspension up to 10 days, a second positive test would bring a 30-day suspension, a third a 60-day penalty, and the fourth a one-year ban. In addition to the previous one mandatory test per season, players will be randomly selected for additional testing both during and after the season. Even so, these penalties are less rigorous than those of the World Anti-Doping Association.

The first global treaty against doping in sports became effective February 2007, after 30 nations ratified an international agreement. (The United States has not ratified the agreement.) The treaty allows governments to take action against the illegal manufacture and supply of doping substances, among other provisions. More information is available at: www.unesco.org/en/antidoping.

Many articles on drugs and sports can be found in newspapers and magazines. For a fuller exposition of Thomas H. Murray's views, see his chapter, "The Ethics of Drugs in Sport," in *Drugs & Performance in Sports*, edited by Richard H. Strauss, M.D. (W. B. Saunders, 1987). Norman Fost, a pediatrician, says appeals to ban drugs are paternalistic and caused more by a displeasure at the loss of innocence in sports than by actual harm ("Banning Drugs in Sports: A Skeptical View," *Hastings Center Report*, August 1986). An unsigned "Opinion" essay in *The Economist* (August 5, 2004) argues that an inflexible anti-doping attitude is unsustainable in a society that uses performance-enhancing drugs so freely for other reasons. See also Gary Wadler and Brian Hainline, *Drugs and the Athlete* (F.A. Davis, 1989) and David R. Mottram, ed., *Drugs in Sport*, 3rd ed. (Routledge, 2002).

ISSUE 19

Should There Be a Free Market in Body Parts?

YES: J. Radcliffe-Richards et al., from "The Case for Allowing Kidney Sales," *The Lancet* (June 27, 1998)

NO: The Institute of Medicine Committee on Increasing Rates of Organ Donation, from *Organ Donation: Opportunities for Action* (2006)

ISSUE SUMMARY

YES: Philosopher J. Radcliffe-Richards and colleagues of the International Forum for Transplant Ethics contend that bans on selling organs remove the only hope of the destitute and dying. Arguments against selling organs are weak attempts to justify the repugnance felt by people who are rich or healthy.

NO: The Institute of Medicine Committee argues that a free market in organs is problematic because in live organ donation both buyers and sellers may not have complete or accurate information, and selling organs of dead people raises concerns about commodification of human bodies.

Human organ transplantation, unachievable at mid-twentieth century and still experimental a few decades ago, has now become routine. Dr. Joseph E. Murray of Brigham and Women's Hospital in Boston performed the first successful kidney transplant in 1954. By the 1980s livers, hearts, pancreases, lungs, and heart-lungs had also been successfully transplanted. Surgical techniques, as well as methods for preserving and transporting organs, had improved over the years. But the most significant advance came from a single drug, cyclosporine, discovered by Jean Borel in the mid-1970s and approved by the Food and Drug Administration in 1983. Cyclosporine suppresses the immune system so that the organ recipient's body does not reject the transplanted organ. However, the drug does not suppress the body's ability to fight infection from other sources.

This achievement has its darker side in that there is a shortage of transplantable organs and many seriously ill people wait for months to receive one. Some die before one becomes available. In 1996 almost 4,000 people on waiting lists died while waiting to receive an organ. According to the United

Network of Organ Sharing (UNOS), the national agency responsible for allocating organs, on December 8, 2006, there were 94,379 patients waiting for transplants. Over 69,000 of these patients were waiting for kidney transplants, and over 17,000 for liver transplants. Heart transplants and lung transplants were the next highest categories, with 2,800 patients each.

By contrast, the UNOS data show that in 2004 only 26,500 transplants were performed, with kidney alone transplants leading the list at 12,575. Of the total transplants, 19,500 came from deceased donors, and almost 7,000 from living donors. Living donors are almost always relatives of the recipient, although there have been several highly publicized cases in which the donor was not related. Like any surgery, transplantation presents risks to the donor but these are usually not grave. A person can live with one kidney, although should that kidney fail, the donor would require regular dialysis (cleansing the blood of toxic substances through a machine) or a transplant.

The shortage of transplantable organs in the U.S. is attributed to many factors: the reluctance of families to approve donation after death, even if the donor has indicated the desire to do so; the reluctance of medical personnel to approach families at a time of crisis; religious objections; and mistrust of the medical system. Despite many educational programs and publicity about donation, Americans seem unwilling either to move to a system of required request (mandated in a few states) or to presume that potential donors would agree to having their organs used for transplantation, unless they had explicitly consented in advance.

The shortage of organs is even more acute in other parts of the world, where cultural or religious objections to removing organs from the deceased remain strong. Organ transplantation is one area in which "technology transfer"—the export of the science and training for the procedure—has been particularly strong. Organ transplant centers have grown rapidly in areas of the world that lack even basic public health measures. However, although some countries have the technology for transplantation, they do not have enough organs to meet the demand.

In the United States, the National Organ Transplant Act (Public Law 98-507), passed in 1984, made it illegal to buy and sell organs. Violators are subject to fines and imprisonment. Congress passed this law because it was concerned that traffic in organs might lead to inequitable access to donor organs with the wealthy having an unfair advantage. (Even with the ban, the wealthy have an advantage in being able to pay for the transplant and the necessary post-transplant supportive services, and thus are more likely to be accepted for a waiting list.)

Although many countries and international medical organizations officially ban the sale of organs as well, the practice goes on. The following selections present opposing views on whether the ban should be reexamined or more aggressively implemented. J. Radcliff-Richards and other members of the International Forum for Transplant Ethics maintain that the ban unfairly punishes both the destitute (whose only hope is selling an organ) and the dying (whose only hope is obtaining one). The Institute of Medicine's committee on transplantable organs argues that selling organs of either living or dead people raises serious questions about the quality of information and the commodification of human bodies.

YES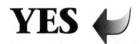

J. Radcliffe-Richards, et al.

The Case for Allowing
Kidney Sales

When the practice of buying kidneys from live vendors first came to light some years ago, it aroused such horror that all professional associations denounced it[1,2] and nearly all countries have now made it illegal.[3] Such political and professional unanimity may seem to leave no room for further debate, but we nevertheless think it important to reopen the discussion.

The well-known shortage of kidneys for transplantation causes much suffering and death.[4] Dialysis is a wretched experience for most patients, and is anyway rationed in most places and simply unavailable to the majority of patients in most developing countries.[5] Since most potential kidney vendors will never become unpaid donors, either during life or posthumously, the prohibition of sales must be presumed to exclude kidneys that would otherwise be available. It is therefore essential to make sure that there is adequate justification for the resulting harm.

Most people will recognise in themselves the feelings of outrage and disgust that led to an outright ban on kidney sales, and such feelings typically have a force that seems to their possessors to need no further justification. Nevertheless, if we are to deny treatment to suffering and dying we need better reasons than our own feelings of disgust.

In this [selection] we outline our reasons for thinking that the arguments commonly offered for prohibiting organ sales do not work, and therefore that the debate should be reopened.[6,7] Here we consider only the selling of kidneys by living vendors, but our arguments have wider implications.

The commonest objection to kidney selling is expressed on behalf of the vendors: the exploited poor, who need to be protected against the greedy rich. However, the vendors are themselves anxious to sell,[8] and see this practice as the best option open to them. The worse we think the selling of a kidney, therefore, the worse should seem the position of the vendors when that option is removed. Unless this appearance is illusory, the prohibition of sales does even more harm than first seemed, in harming vendors as well as recipients. To this argument it is replied that the vendors' apparent choice is not genuine. It is said that they are likely to be too uneducated to understand the risks, and that this precludes informed consent. It is also claimed that, since they are coerced by their economic circumstances, their consent cannot count as genuine.[9]

From *The Lancet*, vol. 351, June 27, 1998, pp. 1950–1952. Copyright © 1998 by The Lancet. Reprinted by permission.

Although both these arguments appeal to the importance of auto-nomous choice, they are quite different. The first claim is that the vendors are not competent to make a genuine choice within a given range of options. The second, by contrast, is that poverty has so restricted the range of options that organ selling has become the best, and therefore, in effect, that the range is too small. Once this distinction is drawn, it can be seen that neither argument works as a justification of prohibition.[7]

If our ground for concern is that the range of choices is too small, we cannot improve matters by removing the best option that poverty has left, and making the range smaller still. To do so is to make subsequent choices, by this criterion, even less autonomous. The only way to improve matters is to lessen the poverty until organ selling no longer seems the best option; and if that could be achieved, prohibition would be irrelevant because nobody would want to sell.

The other line of argument may seem more promising, since ignorance does preclude informed consent. However, the likely ignorance of the subjects is not a reason for banning altogether a procedure for which consent is required. In other contexts, the value we place on autonomy leads us to insist on information and counselling, and that is what it should suggest in the case of organ selling as well. It may be said that this approach is impracticable, because the educational level of potential vendors is too limited to make explanation feasible, or because no system could reliably counteract the mis-information of nefarious middlemen and profiteering clinics. But even if we accepted that no possible vendor could be competent to consent, that would justify only putting the decision in the hands of competent guardians. To justify total prohibition it would also be necessary to show that organ selling must always be against the interests of potential vendors, and it is most unlikely that this would be done.

The risk involved in nephrectomy is not in itself high, and most people regard it as acceptable for living related donors.[10] Since the procedure is, in principle, the same for vendors as for unpaid donors, any systematic difference between the worthwhileness of the risk for vendors and donors presumably lies on the other side of the calculation, in the expected benefit. Nevertheless the exchange of money cannot in itself turn an acceptable risk into an unacceptable one from the vendor's point of view. It depends entirely on what the money is wanted for.

In general, furthermore, the poorer a potential vendor, the more likely it is that the sale of a kidney will be worth whatever risk there is. If the rich are free to engage in dangerous sports for pleasure, or dangerous jobs for high pay, it is difficult to see why the poor who take the lesser risk of kidney selling for greater rewards—perhaps saving relatives' lives,[11] or extricating themselves from poverty and debt—should be thought so misguided as to need saving from themselves.

It will be said that this does not take account of the reality of the ven-dors' circumstances: that risks are likely to be greater than for unpaid donors because poverty is detrimental to health, and vendors are often not given proper care. They may also be underpaid or cheated, or may waste their money through inexperience. However, once again, these arguments apply far more strongly to many other activities by which the poor try to earn money, and which we do not forbid. The best way to address such problems would be by regulation and perhaps a central purchasing system, to provide screening, counselling, reliable payment, insurance, and financial advice.[12]

To this it will be replied that no system of screening and control could be complete, and that both vendors and recipients would always be at risk of exploitation and poor treatment. But all the evidence we have shows that there is much more scope for exploitation and abuse when a supply of desperately wanted goods is made illegal. It is, furthermore, not clear why it should be thought harder to police a legal trade than the present complete ban.

Furthermore, even if vendors and recipients would always be at risk of exploitation, that does not alter the fact that if they choose this option, all alternatives must seem worse to them. Trying to end exploitation by prohibition is rather like ending slum dwelling by bulldozing slums: it ends the evil in that form, but only by making things worse for the victims. If we want to protect the exploited, we can do it only by removing the poverty that makes them vulnerable, or, failing that, by controlling the trade.

Another familiar objection is that it is unfair for the rich to have privileges not available to the poor. This argument, however, is irrelevant to the issue of organ selling as such. If organ selling is wrong for this reason, so are all benefits available to the rich, including all private medicine, and, for that matter, all public provision of medicine in rich countries (including transplantation of donated organs) that is unavailable in poor ones. Furthermore, all purchasing could be done by a central organisation responsible for fair distribution.[12]

It is frequently asserted that organ donation must be altruistic to be acceptable,[13] and that this rules out payment. However, there are two problems with this claim. First, altruism does not distinguish donors from vendors. If a father who saves his daughter's life by giving her a kidney is altruistic, it is difficult to see why his selling a kidney to pay for some other operation to save her life should be thought less so. Second, nobody believes in general that unless some useful action is altruistic it is better to forbid it altogether.

It is said that the practice would undermine confidence in the medical profession, because of the association of doctors with money-making practices. That, however, would be a reason for objecting to all private practice; and in this case the objection could easily be met by the separation of purchasing and treatment. There could, for instance, be independent trusts[12] to fix charges and handle accounts, as well as to ensure fair play and high standards. It is alleged that allowing the trade would lessen the supply of donated cadaveric kidneys.[14] But although some possible donors might decide to sell instead, their organs would be available, so there would be no loss in the total. And in the meantime, many people will agree to sell who would not otherwise donate.

It is said that in parts of the world where women and children are essentially chattels there would be a danger of their being coerced into becoming vendors. This argument, however, would work as strongly against unpaid living kidney donation, and even more strongly against many far more harmful practices which do not attract calls for their prohibition. Again, regulation would provide the most reliable means of protection.

It is said that selling kidneys would set us on a slippery slope to selling vital organs such as hearts. But that argument would apply equally to the case of the unpaid kidney donation, and nobody is afraid that that will result in the donation of hearts. It is entirely feasible to have laws and professional practices that allow the giving or selling only of non-vital organs. Another objection is that allowing organ sales is impossible because it would outrage public opinion. But this claim is about western public opinion: in many potential vendor communities, organ selling is more acceptable than cadaveric donation, and this argument amounts to a claim that other people should follow western cultural preferences rather than their own. There is, anyway, evidence that the western public is far less opposed to the idea, than are medical and political professionals.[15]

It must be stressed that we are not arguing for the positive conclusion that organ sales must always be acceptable, let alone that there should be an unfettered market. Our claim is only that none of the familiar arguments against organ selling works, and this allows for the possibility that better arguments may yet be found.

Nevertheless, we claim that the burden of proof remains against the defenders of prohibition, and that until good arguments appear, the presumption must be that the trade should be regulated rather than banned altogether. Furthermore, even when there are good objections at particular times or in particular places, that should be regarded as a reason for trying to remove the objections, rather than as an excuse for permanent prohibition.

The weakness of the familiar arguments suggests that they are attempts to justify the deep feelings of repugnance which are the real driving force of prohibition, and feelings of repugnance among the rich and healthy, no matter how strongly felt, cannot justify removing the only hope of the destitute and dying. This is why we conclude that the issue should be considered again, and with scrupulous impartiality.

References

1. British Transplantation Society Working Party. Guidelines on living organ donation. *BMJ* 1986; 293: 257–58.

2. The Council of the Transplantation Society. Organ sales. *Lancet* 1985; 2: 715–16.

3. World Health Organization. A report on developments under the auspices of WHO (1987–1991). WHO 1992 Geneva. 12–28.

4. Hauptman PJ, O'Connor KJ. Procurement and allocation of solid organs for transplantation. *N Engl J Med* 1997; 336: 422–31.

5. Barsoum RS. Ethical problems in dialysis and transplantation: Africa. In: Kjellstrand CM, Dossetor JB, eds. Ethical problems in dialysis and transplantation. Kluwer Academic Publishers, Netherlands. 1992: 169–82.

6. Radcliffe-Richards J. Nephrarious goings on: kidney sales and moral arguments. *J Med Philosph*. Netherlands: Kluwer Academic Publishers, 1996; 21: 375–416.

7. Radcliffe-Richards J. From him that hath not. In: Kjellstrand CM, Dossetor JB, eds. Ethical problems in dialysis and transplantation. Netherlands: Kluwer Academic Publishers, 1992: 53–60.

8. Mani MK. The argument against the unrelated live donor, ibid. 164.

9. Sells RA. The case against buying organs and a futures market in transplants. *Trans Proc* 1992; **24:** 2198–202.

10. Daar AD, Land W, Yahya TM, Schneewind K, Gutmann T, Jakobsen A. Living-donor renal transplantation: evidence-based justification for an ethical option. *Trans Reviews* (in press) 1997.

11. Dossetor JB, Manickavel V. Commercialisation: the buying and selling of kidneys. In: Kjellstrand CM, Dossetor JB, eds. Ethical problems in dialysis and transplantation. Netherlands: Kluwer Academic Publishers, 1992: 61–71.

12. Sells RA. Some ethical issues in organ retrieval 1982–1992. *Trans Proc* 1992; **24:** 2401–03.

13. Sheil R. Policy statement from the ethics committee of the Transplantation Society. *Trans Soc Bull* 1995; **3:** 3.

14. Altshuler JS, Evanisko MJ. *JAMA* 1992; **267:** 2037.

15. Guttmann RD, Guttmann A. Organ transplantation: duty reconsidered. *Trans Proc* 1992; **24:** 2179–80.

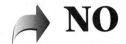 **NO**

Organ Donation:
Opportunities for Action

Why a Free Market in Organs is Problematic

Many economists begin from the position that a market is almost always the best way to allocate a scarce resource. In the standard model of a competitive market economy, markets use prices to allocate scarce resources in an automatic, decentralized fashion. In each market, the price of the good adjusts until the amount that suppliers are willing to sell at the prevailing price equals the amount that consumers are willing to pay. A higher price coaxes out more supply by making it worthwhile for producers to produce more of the good or, if the total amount of the good is fixed, by encouraging the current owners to put more of the good up for sale. On the demand side, a higher price chokes off demand, as some buyers decide that the good is not worth the new price to them.

In this model, the market outcome can be considered both efficient and equitable, provided the distribution of income and assets meets a community standard of fairness. On the demand side, price rations the good to the people who value it the most, that is, those who need it the most, where need is assessed by the people concerned rather than a regulatory body. On the supply side, the supplier is compensated for the cost of production, including a reasonable profit; and in general, resources are directed to the most productive uses. If all markets are perfectly competitive, the resulting distribution of goods is efficient; and because it is the result of voluntary trades from a fair initial distribution of income and assets, it can be argued that it is also equitable.

On the basis of this model, permitting a market in organs could be an equitable and efficient way to achieve an increase in supply that would reduce the number of people on organ transplant waiting lists. However, this conclusion is dependent on the accuracy of the strong assumptions that underlie the theoretical model. When the assumptions do not hold, the normative arguments for the desirability of markets do not hold either. A market process might still be preferable to the available alternatives as an instrument for increasing the organ supply, but the case for it must be built, brick by brick, in light of the actual circumstances. Because the application of the market model

From *Organ Donation: Opportunities for Action,* by The Institute of Medicine Committee on Increasing Rates of Organ Donation (2006), pp. 231–239. Copyright © 2006 by National Academies Press. Reprinted by permission of National Academies Press via Rightslink.

raises different issues on the supply side and the demand side, the chapter will address them separately.

The Supply Side of an Organ Market

The market model's assumptions about supply seem most plausible for living donors. In living donation, a mentally competent adult has an organ (or organ part) that can be supplied to the market at some risk and financial cost. When the person donates the organ or organ part, that is, supplies it at a zero market price, he or she suffers a loss as a result of the discomfort of the operation, the opportunity cost of the time involved, and the long-term health risks. The donor's expectation of a benefit to the recipient is some compensation for this loss, which is why some organs are supplied at a zero price. Reducing the donor's loss by making a financial payment for the organ seems fair, however, and it seems likely that more people would be willing to provide organs as a result. In an efficient market, the additional organs would come from those who require the least financial compensation for the organ and for enduring the donation process.

In evaluating a policy of allowing payment for organs from living donors, two issues that are not assumed in the standard market model become important: distributional inequity and imperfect information. Many people would agree that large, unjust disparities in income and assets exist among Americans. Poor people value extra money more highly because they need it for basic necessities, so the additional organs are likely to come from the poor, a result many find morally troubling. A common economist's response to this concern is, "True, the distribution of income and assets is not fair. But if society cannot (or will not) do anything about it, is it fair to deprive people of an opportunity that they believe would improve their situations? Competent adults should be free to make their own decisions about the medical procedures that they will undergo and the risks that they will take."

This argument is compelling superficially, but it assumes that the organ suppliers have the information and the capacity that they need to make the decision. Information about the long-term risks of donation may not be complete, and the buyers of organs have an incentive to understate the risks. In an unregulated market, organs are likely to come from people who do not fully appreciate the risks that they are taking. Avoiding this result would require the development of complete information for potential living donors and other efforts to ensure that the decisions made by living donors are fully informed, which would require planning and substantial resources. Concerns about inadequate information arise, however, even under the gift model now in place. . . .

The living-donor case is mentioned here mainly to contrast it with the far less straightforward case of obtaining organs from deceased donors. In the latter case, the organs become available only when the person dies. There is no risk to the donor at that point, but a financial payment would not provide any direct benefit to the donor either—the benefit to the donor arises from the interest that the donor had while alive in providing for the well-being of his or her family after death. In practice, the family of the donor often makes the donation decision, and market advocates usually assume that the payment would be made to the family. Essentially, this means that the family is selling a relative's body parts, which raises the issue of cultural norms surrounding the treatment of dead bodies.

Commodification of Dead Bodies

Most societies hold that it is degrading to human dignity to view dead bodies as property that can be bought and sold. . . . [B]odies are supposed to be treated with respect—with funeral rites and burial or cremation—and not simply discarded like worn out household furniture and certainly not sold by the relatives (or anyone else) to the highest bidder. These norms are very powerful. Illicit markets for bodies have existed throughout history; for example, in the 19th century, England had an illicit market in which bodies were dug up in the night by body snatchers and sold for dissection, arguably a socially useful purpose (Richardson, 2000). Buying and selling bodies for dissection was considered a despicable business, however, and even desperately poor people did not willingly sell their relatives' bodies for whatever they could get.

Organ transplantation has provided a compelling justification for using the body parts of deceased individuals, namely, the opportunity to restore life and health to someone on the brink of death. Many people see donating a person's organs for this purpose as a highly meritorious act that honors the sacredness of the body rather than degrades it. At the same time, however, many people regard the act of donating the organs for this purpose as being conceptually and morally distinct from the act of selling the organs (even when the organs are to be used for the same purpose). Currently, the sale of solid organs is prohibited, but the prohibition reflects preexisting and widely accepted cultural norms. In the context of these norms, and the attitudes underlying them, it is not at all clear that the supply of organs from deceased donors would actually increase if sales were made legal. It is possible that the reasons people have for not donating cannot be overcome by money, or that offering money induces some to provide organs while leading an equal or greater number of people who would have provided organs to decide not to. For example, family members may wish to avoid appearing to be profiting from a deceased relative's body, especially if there is any chance of appearing to have participated in a treatment decision that might have hastened death. . . .

Barriers to a Futures Market

Traditionally, the relatives of deceased individuals had the final word about whether organs would be donated, but this has been changing. Because society supports the right of individuals to control what happens to their bodies when they are alive, it is a natural extension to assume that they should also decide what happens to their bodies after death. This adds more intricacy to the application of the market model. Because money is of no use to a corpse, for financial payments to influence the donor's decision, one must introduce a futures market or a bequest motive into the picture.

A futures market is a market in which the commodity bought and sold is the right to sell organs at a future time in the event that a person dies in circumstances that permit organs to be recovered and transplanted. The person receives payment for these contingent organ sale rights while he or she is still alive. Futures markets are inherently complex. In this case, the chances of dying in the appropriate circumstances are low, death may occur far into the future, and it may not be easy to execute the right to the organ at the appropriate moment; therefore, the right to a potential organ is not worth nearly as much as an actual organ at the time of death. What if sellers want to change their minds? Can they rescind their contracts and, if so, on what terms? Also, once the rights to an individual's organs have been sold, the buyer (who would probably be an organ broker) has a financial interest in the seller's death. Some people already worry about receiving suboptimal treatment at the end of life if they are registered organ donors and adding financial interests resulting from the selling of organ rights might add to those concerns. Further, it seems unlikely that there would be enough interested investors to allow a private futures market in organ rights to develop, given the long time horizon required and the uncertainty about the size of the profits.

Alternatively, one can assume that people get satisfaction in life from the knowledge that their heirs will receive inheritances when they die. If this is so, a person could be allowed to spell out his or her wishes for the disposition of his or her body in advance (in a will or in a special organ donor registry) stating whether his or her body should be buried or cremated intact, donated all or in part to a specific organization for a specific purpose, or sold whole or in part with the proceeds forming part of the estate. To the extent that more people would agree to organ removal if they had this option, the supply of organs would increase. This is an empirical question, and as before, there is no certainty of a positive effect. Again, implementation would be complex. For example, a registry would be better than a will, because one cannot wait until the will is probated to determine whether the organs can be sold. . . .

Other Complexities

It has been assumed thus far in the discussion that paying people or their families for organs would increase the supply of organs for transplantation. However, some other complexities of the organ procurement process suggest that the creation of financial incentives for organ donation may be less important for donors and their families than it is for healthcare organizations and the participating healthcare professionals. A family does not simply make the decision to donate (or to honor the decedent's wish to donate) and then it happens automatically. First, the potential donor must be in the process of dying under the right circumstances to be eligible to donate his or her organs. Second, the medical staff must make the family aware of the possibility of organ donation. Only then does the opportunity to say yes or no to donation arise. Many people have not thought much about organ donation before the issue arises, and in any case, they are in an extremely stressful situation. How and when they are told about the opportunity for organ donation and the way in which the request is made can make a significant difference to the relatives' response. Finally, the organs must be removed, the recipients must be identified, and the organs must be transported to their final destinations. These are complex tasks that must be carried out under extreme time pressure.

Many factors—including the structure of financial incentives to the healthcare workers and organizations that carry out these organ transplant-related activities—influence the way in which the process of notification, request, removal, and conveyance to a recipient occurs. If this process is the problem, the introduction of financial payments for organs may simply raise the cost of the transplantation process without having any effect on the number of organs recovered. The efforts and successes of the Organ Donation Breakthrough Collaboratives of the Health Resources and Services Administration suggest that the process is part of the problem and, indeed, is perhaps most of it. . . . The collaboratives have demonstrated that the application of quality improvement methods to the steps in this process can significantly increase the percentage of potential organ donations that are converted into actual donations. There is also potential to increase the organ supply through medical practice changes that make more decedents medically eligible to be organ donors (see the discussion in Chapter 5 on donation after circulatory determination of death), that is, to give more people the opportunity to consent.

The Demand Side of an Organ Market

The demand side of an organ market is also complicated. The simple market model assumes that those who benefit from the use of the good pay for the good, and this is an important element in the normative theory in favor of markets. In the case of organs, advocates for payments for organs from deceased donors generally do not expect the recipients to make the payments. Most people believe that health care is a special kind of commodity that should not be allocated strictly according to an ability to pay because of the unusual importance of health care to the well-being of all people and the uneven distribution of illness among the population. The distribution of health care, especially life-saving health care, should be determined separately from the distribution of other goods and in accord with special ethical principles. This is a major departure from the standard market model and means that even if a fair distribution of income and assets could be arranged, letting health care be determined by voluntary market trades would not yield equitable outcomes, even under the highly unrealistic assumption of the existence of a perfectly competitive market.

In the United States, the result of this societal value judgment is a complex array of private and public policies that are implicitly or explicitly intended to provide people with care that they would not receive if all health care were distributed through unregulated private markets. Unfortunately, there is no general, transparent consensus on the nature and extent of health-care services that people should be able to receive without regard to the ability to pay and how the cost of that care should be distributed across the population. The unfortunate result is a financing system that distributes both care and cost arbitrarily in a manner that meets no rational standard of efficiency or equity.

The U.S. healthcare system does not guarantee access to life-saving treatments such as organ transplantations, and the ability to pay does play a role in the distribution of this important good. Few people pay directly for organ transplantation, which is expensive even without payment for the organs. People in need of organs rely on public or private insurance to pay the cost of acquiring the organs and transplanting them, and a transplant is not received unless insurance coverage or access to charity care is available (the so-called green screen).

Given this system of healthcare financing (or any system that might replace it), what would the demand side of a market for organs look like? Presumably, most of the actual buyers would be the healthcare organizations that perform transplantations. They would compete with one another for the available organs, the price would settle down at the market-clearing price, and the cost of organs would become part of the total charge to a third-party payer for an organ transplant. This market would inevitably be very complex.

So far the chapter has referred to "the price" of an organ, but an actual market would have multiple prices for organs because organs are highly differentiated products. For example, hearts differ from kidneys and kidneys differ from one another along many medically significant dimensions. Organ recipients also differ from one another, and matching an organ with the right recipient is important in achieving the benefits of transplantation. This means that the kidney market or the heart market would actually be a whole set of interconnected markets for goods that are close substitutes for each other (e.g., kidneys or hearts from people of different ages, with different blood types, or different human leukocyte antigen factors). The price of a kidney would therefore actually be a price structure for all the different kinds of kidneys. This price structure would result from the interaction of the array of kidneys available with the variety of patients in need of a kidney at any point in time and the trade-offs among kidney characteristics that are medically possible for transplantation into various patients.

Of course, the original suppliers and the end users of the organs do not have the medical knowledge to make sophisticated sales and purchase decisions, and even if they did, they are hardly in the best physical condition to apply their knowledge at the time of donation or transplantation. Like the rest of the healthcare market, this market would be characterized by complicated agency relationships (situations in which decisions are made by an expert on someone else's behalf). The various potential agents here would include the transplant recipient's physician, the organ donor's physician, the healthcare organizations in which the organ recovery and the transplantation occur, a specialized organ "broker" such as the United Network for Organ Sharing (UNOS), the private and public third-party payers that pay for the transplantation-related care, and so on.

Real-world markets in which differentiated products are sold under circumstances of imperfect information and intricate agency relationships do exist, and such markets can be superior to other methods of allocation. In the case of organs, however, it is interesting to note that a nonmarket process for allocating organs to recipients and managing waiting lists has been in place since the beginning of the transplantation era. The Organ Procurement and Transplantation Network system grew up in response to a perceived need to manage the organ allocation process within the transplantation community, although it has come to have substantial government involvement. There is ongoing pressure to adjust the process to make it more efficient and equitable, with the usual difficulties in defining exactly what efficiency and equity mean in such a complicated context. There is also recognition that financial and other incentives should be aligned with ultimate goals, but little enthusiasm for relying completely on an unregulated market process exists.

In summary, in a hypothesized market for organs, the good to be sold is highly differentiated and must be matched to the final user in many ways. The process of making an organ available requires skilled labor and technology. The good is highly perishable, and recovery and transfer to the final user must be accomplished under extreme time pressure. The good has unique cultural significance that would powerfully influence the response of suppliers to market incentives, even in the absence of the existing legal constraints on their behavior. Imperfect information issues are significant, and the end user is not in a position to act as an informed buyer. The need for information, skilled labor and technology, and third-party payment means that the market transactions involve complex agency relationships. With all of these departures from the standard assumptions of the market model, organ transplantation occurs in a world of imperfect markets when it comes to evaluating efficiency. A perfectly functioning market and a fair distribution of income and assets would not likely produce equity in the current healthcare system. As a society, it is not clear what an equitable distribution of health care and its cost would look like, but it is generally agreed that the distribution of organ transplants should not be totally determined by the ability to pay.

Given all of these factors, the committee doubts that it would even be possible to have a well-functioning free market in organs from deceased donors. If such a market existed, there is no certainty that it would produce a greater supply of organs. Moreover, a free market in organs would deviate substantially from prevailing norms in the United States regarding the nature of health care and the fair distribution of organs for transplantation, norms that have been developed within various communities of stakeholders and that are now well entrenched.

POSTSCRIPT

Should There Be a Free Market in Body Parts?

UNOS policies prohibit designating donated organs for a group—that is, limiting a donation to patients who are white, black, Catholic, male, or any other category. In "Members First: The Ethics of Donating Organs and Tissues to Groups," Timothy F. Murphy and Robert M. Veatch raise questions about the implications of the activities of LifeSharers, a voluntary organization whose members agree that their organs will be donated first to other members (*Cambridge Quarterly of Healthcare Ethics*, vol. 15, 2006). In the same issue, Barbro Bjorkman argues against selling of organs and calls instead for a "virtue ethics" approach in his article, "Why We Are Not Allowed to Sell That Which We Are Encouraged to Donate."

An intermediate approach is described in "Compensated Kidney Donation: An Ethical Review of the Iranian Model" by Alireza Bagheri (*Kennedy Institute of Ethics Journal*, vol. 16, no. 3, 2006). In this program donors receive compensation for their time taken from work, travel, and other expenses. While supporting this concept, the author warns that it does not have secure enough measures to prevent a direct monetary relationship between donors and recipients.

In the fall 2004 issue of the *American Journal of Bioethics*, David Steinberg proposes a new method for allocating organs for transplantation ("An 'Opting In' Paradigm for Kidney Transplantation"). His proposal would reward people who agree to donate their kidneys after they die by giving them preferences for a kidney should they need one while alive. Twenty-one commentaries follow the article.

As alternatives to paid organ donations, Francis Delmonico and colleagues proposed donor medals of honor, reimbursement for funeral expenses, organ exchanges, medical leaves for organ donation, and other mechanisms, in "Ethical Incentives—Not Payment—for Organ Donation," *The New England Journal of Medicine* (June 20, 2002).

From a United Kingdom perspective Charles Erin and John Harris, however, have proposed an "ethical market" in organs. In their proposal, the market would be confined to a specific area, and only citizens from that area could buy and sell organs. One purchaser, probably a government agency, would buy all organs and distribute them according to some order of medical priority. Individuals would not be allowed to enter the market directly. See "An Ethical Market in Human Organs," *British Medical Journal* (July 20, 2002).

The most controversial consideration in the allocation of transplantable organs in the United States is whether the organs should be allocated nationally or locally. The Department of Health and Human Services (DHHS) proposed in March 1998 that current geographic disparities in the allocation of scarce organs should be addressed by creating national uniform criteria for determining a patient's medical status and eligibility for placement on a waiting list. Under the current system, local centers have first chance at organs in their region, even though patients in other areas may have greater medical need or have been on the waiting list longer.

This proposal was received enthusiastically by the large transplant centers, which attract the most ill and most affluent recipients, who can travel to the center and remain for months. However, it was criticized by smaller transplant centers, which rely on local recipients and the value of being able to tell potential donors or their families that the organs will be given to a local resident. Congress asked the Institute of Medicine (IOM), an independent agency, to study the impact of the rule. The IOM's report, issued in July 1999, agreed that organs should be allocated on the basis of medical need across wider geographical areas. A Special Section of *The Cambridge Quarterly of Healthcare Ethics* (vol. 10, 2001) contains several articles discussing this and other aspects of organ allocation in the United States.

For more information on organ transplantation, see Courtney S. Campell, "The Selling of Organs, the Sharing of Self," *Second Opinion* (vol. 19, no. 2, 1993); Stuart J. Youngner, Renee C. Fox, and Laurence J. O'Connell, eds., *Organ Transplantation: Meanings and Realities* (University of Wisconsin Press, 1996); and the title essay in Arthur Caplan, *If I Were a Rich Man, Could I Buy a Pancreas?* (Indiana University Press, 1992). In the same issue of the *Kennedy Institute of Ethics Journal* in which Gill and Sade's article appeared, Cynthia Cohen presents a critique of their arguments in "Public Policy and the Sale of Human Organs" (pp. 47 64). She believes that "public resistance to the sale of human body parts, no matter how voluntary or well informed, is ground in the conviction that such a practice would diminish human dignity."

The various reports on transplantation issued by the Institute of Medicine are available at http://www.nap.edu.

ISSUE 20

Should Pharmacists Be Allowed to Deny Prescriptions on Grounds of Conscience?

YES: Donald W. Herbe, from "The Right to Refuse: A Call for Adequate Protection of a Pharmacist's Right to Refuse Facilitation of Abortion and Emergency Contraception," *Journal of Law and Health* (2002/2003)

NO: Julie Cantor and Ken Baum, from "The Limits of Conscientious Objection—May Pharmacists Refuse to Fill Prescriptions for Emergency Contraception?" *New England Journal of Medicine* (November 4, 2004)

ISSUE SUMMARY

YES: Law student Donald W. Herbe asserts that pharmacists' moral beliefs concerning abortion and emergency contraception are genuinely fundamental and deserve respect. He proposes that professional pharmaceutical organizations lead the way to recognizing a true right of conscience, which would eventually result in universal legislation protecting against all potential ramifications of choosing conscience.

NO: Julie Cantor, a lawyer, and Ken Baum, a physician and lawyer, reject an absolute right to object, as well as no right to object, to these prescriptions but assert that pharmacists who cannot or will not dispense a drug have a professional obligation to meet the needs of their customers by referring them elsewhere.

Under U.S. law and practice, a person who objects on grounds of conscience or religious belief to performing certain acts has considerable protections. To force someone to perform an act totally forbidden by his or her religion would be a profound violation of ethical and human rights. But there are limits to exercising this right. Right now there is no military draft in the United States; however, all young men must register with the Selective Service Agency on their eighteenth birthday. If there were to be a military draft, a conscientious objector would have to demonstrate that he has a strongly held religious or moral belief, not just a political one, against participation in the military. Conscientious objectors could request alternative community service, such as caring for the elderly, or serving in the military as a noncombatant, for example, as a medic. In the Vietnam War, some conscientious objectors were jailed for their refusal to serve.

Conscientious objection has ethical implications for medical personnel as well. Physicians, for example, may refrain from performing procedures that are legal but repugnant to them on moral grounds. Just as in the military example, there are limits. Physicians cannot ethically refuse to provide life-saving or emergency treatment to a person on the grounds that the individual is a murderer or has committed an act that violates the physician's religion. They can refuse to perform abortions on grounds of conscience, but ethical codes require them to refer patients to another provider. Nurses have less discretion than physicians because they are employees of hospitals and are subject to disciplinary action. Nevertheless, they too can establish grounds for refusing to assist in an abortion procedure, sterilization, or the withdrawal of life-sustaining treatment.

The issue is murkier, however, when it comes to pharmacists, who are generally self-employed, or pharmacy employees. They do not directly participate in the acts they find objectionable, but they make those acts possible by dispensing medications. What are their options and obligations?

Birth control pills and emergency contraception medications, which are basically high doses of regular birth control pills taken to prevent pregnancy after unprotected sexual intercourse, have been on the market for years. Some pharmacists object to dispensing these medications. The issue became much more controversial when in September 2000 the Food and Drug Administration (FDA) approved the drug mifepristone as safe and effective. This drug, formerly known as RU-486 after Russel Uclaf, its initial French manufacturer, had been marketed in Europe for several years. Mifepristone is a synthetic steroid that blocks progesterone, preventing an implanted fertilized egg from developing. It must be taken within 49 days of conception and followed within 48 hours by a second drug, misoprostol, related to the hormone prostaglandin. Taken together, the two drugs act as a chemical form of early abortion. Emergency contraception, on the other hand, is not a form of abortion, since no conception has taken place.

And it is here that some pharmacists have drawn the line. Believing strongly that abortion is immoral, they want the legal right to exercise their religious beliefs and ethical right by refusing to dispense the drugs for this purpose and to be protected from losing their jobs, or other repercussions. Should they be allowed to do so and without referring women to another, more willing pharmacist?

The following selections present different points of view. Donald Herbe sees the exercise of conscientious objection as fundamental to pharmacists' human rights and calls for legislation to protect them from any kind of repercussions or discrimination. While recognizing that pharmacists have a legitimate interest in avoiding conflicts of conscience, Julie Cantor and Ken Baum believe that because pharmacists are licensed and have a professional obligation to serve the public, they must make alternative options available to customers who seek legal prescription drugs they find objectionable.

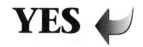

YES

Donald W. Herbe

The Right to Refuse: A Call for Adequate Protection of a Pharmacist's Right to Refuse Facilitation of Abortion and Emergency Contraception

Introduction

The ability to convince an individual, through the art of honest persuasion, of the righteousness of a belief is celebrated; however, in failure of such persuasion, compelling that person to act contradictory to their retained ideal is detestable. The free will to reject a movement or disagree with a practice is the sort of liberty this Nation was founded upon, yet today the potential exists that many in the pharmaceutical profession will be forced into behaviors repugnant to their basic standards of goodness and morality. The proliferation of abortive and contraceptive drug therapies has thrust many pharmacists into roles as facilitators of practices they oppose on fundamental levels without a corresponding ability to opt out of such action.

When a patient desires drug therapies that, in the eyes of the pharmacist, are likely to destroy an unborn human life, the pro-life pharmacist is left in an unsettling position: accommodate the patient and breach basic moral principles *or* adhere to conscience and risk liability and disciplinary action.

Section I: Anti-Reproduction Pills and the Pharmacist's Role

The Pills

On September 28, 2000, the Food and Drug Administration (FDA) approved the drug mifepristone, formerly known as RU-486, for use in the United States as an abortifacient. Mifepristone had previously been approved and is currently used in some European countries, including France, England, and Sweden. Although mifepristone has other potential uses, such as postcoital

From *Journal of Law and Health*, vol. 17, issue 1, 2002/2003, pp. excerpts from 77–103. Copyright © 2002 by Donald W. Herbe. Reprinted by permission.

contraception and daily-use birth control, its FDA approved use is as an early pregnancy abortifacient.

Mifepristone acts as an anti-hormone and precludes a woman's uterus from retaining an *implanted* fertilized egg. The drug blocks progesterone, an essential hormone in the acceptance and retention of an implanted egg within a woman's uterus; and, when taken in concurrence with misoprostol, induces a spontaneous abortion. The fact that the mifepristone abortion regimen acts to destroy an implanted egg as opposed to a fertilized yet not implanted egg, is what distinguishes it from emergency contraception.

Drugs used post-coitally with the intent to prevent the development of a pregnancy are referred to as emergency contraception. This labeling as emergency contraception is a bit conclusory, as the definition of whether use of such drugs is contraception or abortion lies at the heart of the controversy over them. However, for purposes of convenience and clarity, this Note will refer to drug regimens consumed post-intercourse for the purpose of preventing the onset or continuance of pregnancy as emergency contraception (EC), as that is the term that has been attached to them in modern medical, social, and political arenas.

Notwithstanding this controversy, the physical and biological effects of orally administered EC, often referred to as the morning-after pill, are not in dispute. EC may prevent the development of a pregnancy by inhibiting any of four successive biological events, either pre or post fertilization, necessary to establish and maintain a pregnancy. EC works before fertilization by either suppressing ovulation, like regular birth-control pills, or preventing fertilization of an egg by inhibiting the movement of the sperm or the egg. If an egg becomes fertilized, then EC may disrupt transport of the fertilized egg to the uterus or, if the transport through the fallopian tube is complete, prevent the implantation of the fertilized egg in the woman's uterus. EC is most effective when used up to seventy-two hours after unprotected intercourse and becomes completely ineffective after implantation occurs, usually six or seven days after intercourse.

The Pharmacist's Role

During the past twenty years emergency contraception pills (ECPs) have been available to and used by American women. During this time frame non-emergency oral contraceptives (those taken as a daily pre-intercourse regimen) were used off-label as emergency contraception and were distributed as such "primarily in hospital emergency rooms, reproductive health clinics, and university health centers." These medical facilities would repackage oral contraceptives for use as emergency contraception; pharmacies associated with certain clinics would repackage oral contraceptives into EC regimens and label them as such; and private physicians would instruct patients to take a larger dosage of their regular birth control pills as EC.

In 1998 the FDA approved the Preven Emergency Contraceptive Kit, an EC based on the Yuzpe regimen. In 1999, the FDA also approved Plan B, another EC regimen. While different regimens of oral contraceptives had been distributed and used before 1998 as emergency contraceptives, Preven and Plan B are the first regimens specifically approved by the FDA as safe and effective emergency contraceptives, to be packaged and marketed as such. Additionally, modified doses of oral contraceptives, not specifically packaged for use as an EC, can still be prescribed in doses that would effect emergency contraception if doctor and patient desire such a method.

Emergency contraception pills are classified as prescription drugs, and "states are delegated the power and responsibility of determining which health care professionals . . . have prescriptive authority." Currently, many states have authorized collaborative practices that have expanded the role of pharmacists. These collaborative practices generally authorize greater independence of the pharmacist to initiate drug therapies not specifically prescribed by a patient's physician or other authorized health care professional. In other words, some patients may not require a prescription from their doctor before being distributed certain medications or drugs from a pharmacist. However, with the exception of Washington, California, and Alaska, states do not authorize this expanded pharmacist role in the distribution of ECPs. Pharmacists are generally limited to dispensing ECPs specifically prescribed by some other authorized health care professional. Other general duties of a pharmacist in the distribution of ECPs may include counseling and educating women on EC use at the time the prescription is filled.

In Washington, California, and Alaska, pharmacists have the dual authority to prescribe *and* dispense ECPs under each state's respective collaborative practices. Generally speaking, the pharmacist may dispense ECPs in accordance with "standardized procedures or protocols developed by the pharmacist and an authorized prescriber[.]" Thus, a woman need not receive authorization from her doctor prior to buying ECPs; the pharmacist acts not as a third party or indirect provider of ECPs, but as a direct provider in accordance with a general collaborative protocol.

If pro-choice groups and the American Medical Association have their way, pharmacists will have no future role in ECPs. This is because these groups support an FDA reclassification of ECPs as over-the-counter (OTC) drugs, rather than prescription. Many pro-choice groups claim as a top goal the persuasion of the FDA to reclassify ECPs as OTC. If OTC status were granted, then "women would be able to get ECPs without encountering any type of health care provider."

OTC status for ECPs is not generally supported by pharmacists however, and is not likely in today's political climate. Advocates on both sides of the issue believe the Bush administration, with its influence on the FDA, will delay or negate a switch in classification from prescription to OTC. The behavioral and social policy concerns raised by ECPs "may make switching ECPs to OTC status a politically unpopular move." In any event, ECPs are currently available only by prescription.

Many restrictions have been imposed by the FDA in the use and distribution of mifepristone. First, the drug can only be used during the first forty-nine days after a woman's last menstrual cycle. Also, the drug is distributed to women directly from doctors and certain health clinics. Mifepristone "is not and will not be available in pharmacies[.]" Thus, under the current FDA restrictions, pharmacists have no role in mifepristone-induced abortions.

While current mifepristone use is much lower than expected since its FDA approval and subsequent availability to the public, some signals suggest that future use or access may become more widespread. A survey of doctors by the Kaiser Family Foundation discovered that twenty-three percent of doctors said they were "likely" to offer mifepristone in 2002; up from the seven percent that actually provided the drug since its approval. Also, health centers offering mifepristone have reported a ninety-nine percent rate of abortion in women who have taken the drug. An expected increase in availability, a near perfect rate of achieving the desired ends of abortion, together with continued efforts by pro-choice groups, such as Planned Parenthood, to increase accessibility to abortion, could be the impetus to pharmaceutical distribution of mifepristone in the future.

FDA approval of mifepristone and ECPs, such as Preven and Plan B, has made drug related reproductive therapy a real and potentially widespread option for women. Marketing campaigns by women's and abortion-rights groups and the drug manufacturers themselves will further introduce these drug options to women. This drug therapy revolution of sorts has expanded the pharmacist's role in the provision of emergency contraception, and perhaps, in the future, the provision of mifepristone.

The more women that are aware of and desire EC, the more involved and important pharmacists will become in the contraception process. One can imagine that if more and more states adopt the liberal EC distribution procedures of Washington and California, then pharmacists would become the primary providers of ECPs. And if mifepristone distribution restrictions are relaxed, pharmacists could feasibly become key players in the furnishing of abortion drugs as well. Whether they like it or not, pharmacists are being thrust into the role of common, everyday providers of controversial reproductive medications, and this position may put some pharmacists in the predicament of having to choose between their moral convictions regarding EC and abortion and the patient's wishes. . . .

The Pharmacist's Professional Ethical Obligations

Pharmacy is a profession, and much like the professions of medicine and law, entails a duty to assure and promote the patient's best interests. As professionals, pharmacists are expected to give priority to the patient's interests over their own immediate interests. As key players in the implementation of drug therapies, pharmacists are expected to withhold drugs "from those who have no authority to use them" and not to withhold "medications from those who do have authority to use them."

The patient's best interests are the pharmacist's primary commitment and concern. Among other things, pharmacists are expected to "help individuals achieve optimum benefit from their medications, to be committed to their welfare, and to maintain their trust"; to place "concern for the well-being of the patient at the center of professional practice" taking into consideration the "needs stated by the patient"; and to hold "the patient's welfare paramount." Further, patient autonomy and "personal and cultural differences among patients" must be respected by the pharmacist. These professional duties, and others, encompass the "collective conscience" of the pharmaceutical profession, and their implementation by each pharmacist is considered a moral obligation.

When presented with a validly authorized prescription for a legal medication, by a patient aware of the risks involved in taking the medication, and for whom the medication would be reasonably safe, the aforementioned principles and expectations leave the pharmacist with an ethical duty to fill and dispense the prescription. The duty to dispense in these circumstances may give rise to a serious conflict between the pharmacist's personal conviction concerning abortion and her professional duty to the patient.

In 1998, the American Pharmaceutical Association (APhA), and subsequently various other pharmaceutical organizations, eased the conflict between personal and professional morals by adopting policies recognizing a pharmacist's right to refuse dispensing medications based on the pharmacist's personal beliefs. However, if the pharmacist exercises her right of conscience and refuses to fill the prescription, the duty to the patient is not extinguished, and could be fulfilled by referring the patient to another pharmacist or distributor. In any event, "the patient should not be required to abide by the pharmacist's personal, moral decision." For many pharmacists, a referral would be no more than passive participation in the activity they initially refused to actively assist. Thus the dilemma, while transformed into whether to refer or not, is equally troublesome to the pharmacist.

Section II: The Potential Ramifications of Choosing Conscience

The pharmacist who ultimately decides that her moral convictions regarding abortion outweigh her professional obligation to the patient may refuse to fill the prescription and refer the patient to another pharmacist; or, the pharmacist with conscientious objection may refuse to dispense and refuse to refer. While the former decision will, in practical terms, shield the pharmacist from most negative consequences, the latter decision could have serious implications for the pharmacist, including employment termination or demotion, civil tort liability, or disciplinary action from the state pharmacy board. . . .

⋘◉⋙

Legal protection must serve two purposes in order to appropriately ensure a pharmacist's right of conscientious refusal: 1) prevent and deter detrimental recriminatory action against the pharmacist; and 2) provide adequate remedies in the case that the pharmacist is sued or disciplined. The most efficient and effective means to these ends is the enactment of state and federal legislation.

The first step to successful enactment of pharmacist conscience legislation in each state and the United States is the cooperation of local, regional, and national pharmaceutical associations. The American Pharmaceutical Association took a large positive step when it adopted its pharmacist conscience clause.

However, in the same pronouncement it rejected adoption of a policy encouraging enactment of state and national legal protection of the right of conscience. If pharmacists themselves, as represented by their professional associations and organizations, do not call for state and national legislative action, the road to adequate protection will be more difficult.

In any event, an effective conscience statute should take into consideration many complex issues including broad protection against recriminatory action, efficient administration of pharmacies, and accommodation of patients. First and foremost the conscience clause should serve its purpose stating clearly that no pharmacist shall be required to dispense abortion or EC drugs, nor shall any pharmacist be required to refer to another pharmacist who will dispense abortion or EC drugs. Although pharmacists currently have no role in the distribution of mifepristone, the abortion language should nonetheless be included as the potential for future pharmaceutical access exists. Next, the conscience statute should prohibit discrimination, civil liability, and professional disciplinary action that result from exercising the aforementioned rights of refusal. The statute should also encompass provisions prohibiting discrimination in the hiring process so as to preclude pharmacy-employers from screening applicants to avoid hiring pro-life pharmacists in the first place. Finally, the statute should provide adequate methods of deterrence. Employment discrimination could be deterred through its criminalization or by providing an express cause of action in tort as a remedy to the discriminatory hiring, firing, demotion, or promotion of pharmacists.

Employer and patient considerations should also exist in a pharmacist conscience clause. Prior notification of a pharmacist's beliefs regarding abortion and EC should be disclosed to the employer so as to enable efficient administration of the pharmacy. Further, patients should be put on notice in advance regarding when pharmacists with moral objections to abortion and EC will be on duty. For example, schedules could be posted conspicuously within a pharmacy as to when abortion and EC drugs will and will not be available to customer-patients. This will enable patients to avoid the hassle of going to a pharmacy and having their prescription refused. In any event, matters such as the aforementioned should be considered when drafting a pharmacist conscience clause.

Conclusion

Pharmacists, like other professionals such as physicians and attorneys, have a general duty to ensure their client's best interests, and thus must put the health of patients above all other considerations. Thus, it would seem to follow, when a pharmacist is presented with a valid prescription of what is safe for the patient to consume, the drugs should be distributed without dispute. However, to require that a pharmacist, or any professional, participate in what she would equate to the taking of a human life should never be a principle of professional ethics.

Certain issues, because of their inherent complexity and ambiguity, must be resolved, with guidance from religion, philosophy, and science, in the heart and mind of each individual. The commencement of human life and the relative sanctity of unborn life are issues that fall within this category of subjective individual determination. The thoughtful decision should be respected and free from vilifying recrimination. If a pharmacist, in her heart of hearts, concludes that accommodating prescriptions for abortive and EC medications is akin to directly facilitating the destruction of a precious human life, a refusal to accommodate such prescriptions should be protected under the law and within the profession. A safeguard of the right to refuse is imminently necessary as abortive drugs and EC become more widespread and risk of liability and loss of employment may compel many pharmacists to disregard their sacred beliefs or reap the consequences of their objections. Proactive acceptance of a pharmacist's conscientious objection to abortion and EC within the pharmaceutical community would pave the way to legislative protection already afforded doctors and nurses.

Julie Cantor and
Ken Baum

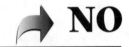 **NO**

The Limits of Conscientious Objection—May Pharmacists Refuse to Fill Prescriptions for Emergency Contraception?

Health policy decisions are often controversial, and the recent determination by the Food and Drug Administration (FDA) not to grant over-the-counter status to the emergency contraceptive Plan B was no exception. Some physicians decried the decision as a troubling clash of science, politics, and morality.[1] Other practitioners, citing safety, heralded the agency's prudence.[2] Public sentiment mirrored both views. Regardless, the decision preserved a major barrier to the acquisition of emergency contraception—the need to obtain and fill a prescription within a narrow window of efficacy. Six states have lowered that hurdle by allowing pharmacists to dispense emergency contraception without a prescription.[3-8] In those states, patients can simply bypass physicians. But the FDA's decision means that patients cannot avoid pharmacists. Because emergency contraception remains behind the counter, pharmacists can block access to it. And some have done just that.

Across the country, some pharmacists have refused to honor valid prescriptions for emergency contraception. In Texas, a pharmacist, citing personal moral grounds, rejected a rape survivor's prescription for emergency contraception.[9] A pharmacist in rural Missouri also refused to sell such a drug,[10] and in Ohio, Kmart fired a pharmacist for obstructing access to emergency and other birth control.[11] This fall, a New Hampshire pharmacist refused to fill a prescription for emergency contraception or to direct the patron elsewhere for help. Instead, he berated the 21-year-old single mother, who then, in her words, "pulled the car over in the parking lot and just cried."[12] Although the total number of incidents is unknown, reports of pharmacists who refused to dispense emergency contraception date back to 1991[13] and show no sign of abating.

Though nearly all states offer some level of legal protection for health care professionals who refuse to provide certain reproductive services, only Arkansas, Mississippi, and South Dakota explicitly protect pharmacists who refuse to

From *New England Journal of Medicine*, November 4, 2004, pp. 2008–2012. Copyright © 2004 by Massachusetts Medical Society. Reprinted by permission.

dispense emergency and other contraception.[14] But that list may grow. In past years, legislators from nearly two dozen states have taken "conscientious objection"—an idea that grew out of wartime tension between religious freedom and national obligation[15] and was co-opted into the reproductive-rights debate of the 1970s[16]—and applied it to pharmacists. One proposed law offers pharmacists immunity from civil lawsuits, criminal liability, professional sanctions, and employment repercussions.[17] Another bill, which was not passed, would have protected pharmacists who refused to transfer prescriptions.[18]

This issue raises important questions about individual rights and public health. Who prevails when the needs of patients and the morals of providers collide? Should pharmacists have a right to reject prescriptions for emergency contraception? The contours of conscientious objection remain unclear. This article elucidates those boundaries and offers a balanced solution to a complex problem. Because the future of over-the-counter emergency contraception is in flux, this issue remains salient for physicians and their patients.

Arguments in Favor of a Pharmacist's Right to Object

Pharmacists Can and Should Exercise Independent Judgment

Pharmacists, like physicians, are professionals. They complete a graduate program to gain expertise, obtain a state license to practice, and join a professional organization with its own code of ethics. Society relies on pharmacists to instruct patients on the appropriate use of medications and to ensure the safety of drugs prescribed in combination. Courts have held that pharmacists, like other professionals, owe their customers a duty of care.[19] In short, pharmacists are not automatons completing tasks; they are integral members of the health care team. Thus, it seems inappropriate and condescending to question a pharmacist's right to exercise personal judgment in refusing to fill certain prescriptions.

Professionals Should Not Forsake Their Morals as a Condition of Employment

Society does not require professionals to abandon their morals. Lawyers, for example, choose clients and issues to represent. Choice is also the norm in the health care setting. Except in emergency departments, physicians may select their patients and procedures. Ethics and law allow physicians, nurses, and physician assistants to refuse to participate in abortions and other reproductive services.[14,20] Although some observers argue that active participation in an abortion is distinct from passively dispensing emergency contraception, others believe that making such a distinction between active and passive participation is meaningless, because both forms link the provider to the final outcome in the chain of causation.

Conscientious Objection Is Integral to Democracy

More generally, the right to refuse to participate in acts that conflict with personal ethical, moral, or religious convictions is accepted as an essential element of a democratic society. Indeed, Oregon acknowledged this freedom in its Death with Dignity Act,[21] which allows health care providers, including pharmacists, who are disquieted by physician-assisted suicide to refuse involvement without fear of retribution. Also, like the draftee who conscientiously objects to perpetrating acts of death and violence, a pharmacist should have the right not to be complicit in what they believe to be a morally ambiguous endeavor, whether others agree with that position or not. The reproductive-rights movement was built on the ideal of personal choice; denying choice for pharmacists in matters of reproductive rights and abortion seems ironic.

Arguments Against a Pharmacist's Right to Object

Pharmacists Choose to Enter a Profession Bound by Fiduciary Duties

Although pharmacists are professionals, professional autonomy has its limits. As experts on the profession of pharmacy explain, "Professionals are expected to exercise special skill and care to place the interests of their clients above their own immediate interests."[22] When a pharmacist's objection directly and detrimentally affects a patient's health, it follows that the patient should come first. Similarly, principles in the pharmacists' code of ethics weigh against conscientious objection. Given the effect on the patient if a pharmacist refuses to fill a prescription, the code undermines the right to object with such broadly stated objectives as "a pharmacist promotes the good of every patient in a caring, compassionate, and confidential manner," "a pharmacist respects the autonomy and dignity of each patient," and "a pharmacist serves individual, community, and societal needs."[23] Finally, pharmacists understand these fiduciary obligations when they choose their profession. Unlike conscientious objectors to a military draft, for whom choice is limited by definition, pharmacists willingly enter their field and adopt its corresponding obligations.

Emergency Contraception Is Not an Abortifacient

Although the subject of emergency contraception is controversial, medical associations,[24] government agencies,[25] and many religious groups agree that it is not akin to abortion. Plan B and similar hormones have no effect on an established pregnancy, and they may operate by more than one physiological mechanism, such as by inhibiting ovulation or creating an unfavorable environment for implantation of a blastocyst.[26] This duality allowed the Catholic Health Association to reconcile its religious beliefs with a mandate adopted by Washington State that emergency contraception must be provided to rape survivors.[27] According to the association, a patient and a provider who aim only to prevent conception follow Catholic teachings and state law. Also, whether one believes that pregnancy begins with fertilization or implantation, emergency contraception cannot fit squarely within the concept of abortion because one cannot be sure that conception has occurred.

Pharmacists' Objections Significantly Affect Patients' Health

Although religious and moral freedom is considered sacrosanct, that right should yield when it hinders a patient's ability to obtain timely medical treatment. Courts have held that religious freedom does not give health care providers an unfettered right to object to anything involving birth control, an embryo, or a fetus.[28,29] Even though the Constitution protects people's beliefs, their actions may be regulated.[30] An objection must be balanced with the burden it imposes on others. In some cases, a pharmacist's objection imposes his or her religious beliefs on a patient. Pharmacists may decline to fill prescriptions for emergency contraception because they believe that the drug ends a life. Although the patient may disapprove of abortion, she may not share the pharmacist's beliefs about contraception. If she becomes pregnant, she may then face the question of abortion—a dilemma she might have avoided with the morning-after pill.

Furthermore, the refusal of a pharmacist to fill a prescription may place a disproportionately heavy burden on those with few options, such as a poor teenager living in a rural area that has a lone pharmacy. Whereas the savvy urbanite can drive to another pharmacy, a refusal to fill a prescription for a less advantaged patient may completely bar her access to medication. Finally, although Oregon does have an opt-out provision in its statute regulating assisted suicide, timing is much more important in emergency contraception than in assisted suicide. Plan B is most effective when used within 12 to 24 hours after unprotected intercourse.[31] An unconditional right to refuse is less compelling when the patient requests an intervention that is urgent.

Refusal Has Great Potential for Abuse and Discrimination

The limits to conscientious objection remain unclear. Pharmacists are privy to personal information through prescriptions. For instance, a customer who fills prescriptions for zidovudine, didanosine, and indinavir is logically assumed to be infected with the human immunodeficiency virus (HIV). If pharmacists can reject prescriptions that conflict with their morals, someone who believes that HIV-positive people must have engaged in immoral behavior could refuse to fill those prescriptions. Similarly, a pharmacist who does not condone extramarital sex might refuse to fill a sildenafil prescription for an unmarried man. Such objections go beyond "conscientious" to become invasive. Furthermore, because a pharmacist does not know a patient's history on the basis of a given prescription, judgments regarding the acceptability of a prescription may be medically inappropriate. To a woman with Eisenmenger's syndrome, for example, pregnancy may mean death. The potential for abuse by pharmacists underscores the need for policies ensuring that patients receive unbiased care.

Toward Balance

Compelling arguments can be made both for and against a pharmacist's right to refuse to fill prescriptions for emergency contraception. But even cogent ideas falter when confronted by a dissident moral code. Such is the nature of belief. Even so, most people can agree that we must find a workable and respectful balance between the needs of patients and the morals of pharmacists.

Three possible solutions exist: an absolute right to object, no right to object, or a limited right to object. On balance, the first two options are untenable. An absolute right to conscientious objection respects the autonomy of pharmacists but diminishes their professional obligation to serve patients. It may also greatly affect the health of patients, especially vulnerable ones, and inappropriately brings politics into the pharmacy. Even pharmacists who believe that emergency contraception represents murder and feel compelled to obstruct patients' access to it must recognize that contraception and abortion before fetal viability remain legal nationwide. In our view, state efforts to provide blanket immunity to objecting pharmacists are misguided. Pharmacies should follow the prevailing employment-law standard to make reasonable attempts to accommodate their employees' personal beliefs.[32] Although neutral policies to dispense medications to all customers may conflict with pharmacists' morals, such policies are not necessarily discriminatory, and pharmacies need not shoulder a heightened obligation of absolute accommodation.

Complete restriction of a right to conscientious objection is also problematic. Though pharmacists voluntarily enter their profession and have an obligation to serve patients without judgment, forcing them to abandon their morals imposes a heavy toll. Ethics and law demand that a professional's morality not interfere with the provision of care in life-or-death situations, such as a ruptured ectopic pregnancy.[29] Whereas the hours that elapse between intercourse and the intervention of emergency contraception are crucial, they do not meet that strict test. Also, patients who face an objecting pharmacist do have options, even if they are less preferable than having the prescription immediately filled. Because of these caveats, it is difficult to demand by law that pharmacists relinquish individual morality to stock and fill prescriptions for emergency contraception.

We are left, then, with the vast middle ground. Although we believe that the most ethical course is to treat patients compassionately—that is, to stock emergency contraception and fill prescriptions for it—the totality of the arguments makes us stop short of advocating a legal duty to do so as a first resort. We stop short for three reasons: because emergency contraception is not an absolute emergency, because other options exist, and because, when possible, the moral beliefs of those delivering care should be considered. However, in a profession that is bound by fiduciary obligations and strives to respect and care for patients, it is unacceptable to leave patients to fend for themselves. As a general rule, pharmacists who cannot or will not dispense a drug have an obligation to meet the needs of their customers by referring them elsewhere. This idea is uncontroversial when it is applied to common medications such as antibiotics and statins; it becomes contentious, but is equally valid, when it is applied to emergency contraception. Therefore, pharmacists who object should, as a matter of ethics and law, provide alternatives for patients.

Pharmacists who object to filling prescriptions for emergency contraception should arrange for another pharmacist to provide this service to customers promptly. Pharmacies that stock emergency contraception should ensure, to the extent possible, that at least one nonobjecting pharmacist is on duty at all times. Pharmacies that do not stock emergency contraception should give clear notice and refer patients elsewhere. At the very least, there should be a prominently displayed sign that says, "We do not provide emergency contraception. Please call Planned Parenthood at 800-230-PLAN (7526) . . . for assistance." However, a direct referral to a local pharmacy or pharmacist who is willing to fill the prescription is preferable. Objecting pharmacists should also redirect prescriptions for emergency contraception that are received by telephone to another pharmacy known to fill such prescriptions. In rural areas, objecting pharmacists should provide referrals within a reasonable radius.

Notably, the American Pharmacists Association has endorsed referrals, explaining that "providing alternative mechanisms for patients . . . ensures patient access to drug products, without requiring the pharmacist or the patient to abide by personal decisions other than their own."[33] A referral may also represent a break in causation between the pharmacist and distributing emergency contraception, a separation that the objecting pharmacist presumably seeks. And, in deference to the law's normative value, the rule of referral also conveys the importance of professional responsibility to patients. In areas of the country where referrals are logistically impractical, professional obligation may dictate providing emergency contraception, and a legal mandate may be appropriate if ethical obligations are unpersuasive.

Inevitably, some pharmacists will disregard our guidelines, and physicians—all physicians—should be prepared to fill gaps in care. They should identify pharmacies that will fill patients' prescriptions and encourage patients to keep emergency contraception at home. They should be prepared to dispense emergency contraception or instruct patients to mimic it with other birth-control pills. In Wisconsin, family-planning clinics recently began dispensing emergency contraception, and the state set up a toll-free hotline to help patients find physicians who will prescribe it.[34] Emergency departments should stock emergency contraception and make it available to rape survivors, if not all patients.

In the final analysis, education remains critical. Pharmacists may have misconceptions about emergency contraception. In one survey, a majority of pharmacists mistakenly agreed with the statement that repeated use of emergency contraception is medically risky.[35] Medical misunderstandings that lead pharmacists to refuse to fill prescriptions for emergency contraception are unacceptable. Patients, too, may misunderstand or be unaware of emergency contraception.[36] Physicians should teach patients about this option before the need arises, since patients may understand their choices better when they are not under stress. Physicians should discuss emergency contraception during office visits, offer prescriptions in advance of need, and provide education through pamphlets or the Internet. Web sites . . . allow users to search for physicians who prescribe emergency contraception by ZIP Code, area code, or address, and Planned Parenthood offers extensive educational information . . . , including details about off-label use of many birth-control pills for emergency contraception.

Our principle of a compassionate duty of care should apply to all health care professionals. In a secular society, they must be prepared to limit the reach of their personal objection. Objecting pharmacists may choose to find employment opportunities that comport with their morals—in a religious community, for example—but when they pledge to serve the public, it is unreasonable to expect those in need of health care to acquiesce to their personal convictions. Similarly, physicians who refuse to write prescriptions for emergency contraception should follow the rules of notice and referral for the reason previously articulated: the beliefs of health care providers should not trump patient care. It is difficult enough to be faced with the consequences of rape or of an unplanned pregnancy; health care providers should not make the situation measurably worse.

Former Supreme Court Chief Justice Charles Evans Hughes called the quintessentially American custom of respect for conscience a "happy tradition"[37]—happier, perhaps, when left in the setting of a draft objection than when pitting one person's beliefs against another's reproductive health. Ideally, conflicts about emergency contraception will be rare, but they will occur. In July, 11 nurses in Alabama resigned rather than provide emergency contraception in state clinics.[38] As patients understand their birth-control options, conflicts at the pharmacy counter and in the clinic may become more common. When professionals' definitions of liberty infringe on those they choose to serve, a respectful balance must be struck. We offer one solution. Even those who challenge this division of burdens and benefits should agree with our touchstone—although health professionals may have a right to object, they should not have a right to obstruct.

References

1. Drazen JM, Greene MF, Wood AJJ. The FDA, politics, and Plan B. N Engl J Med 2004;350:1561–2.

2. Stanford JB, Hager WD, Crockett SA. The FDA, politics, and Plan B. N Engl J Med 2004;350:2413–4.

3. Alaska Admin. Code tit. 12, § 52.240 (2004).

4. Cal. Bus. & Prof. Code § 4052 (8) (2004).

5. Hawaii Rev. Stat. § 461-1 (2003).

6. N.M. Admin. Code § 16.19.26.9 (2003).

7. Wash. Rev. Code § 246-863-100 (2004).

8. Me. Rev. Stat. Ann. tit.32, §§ 13821-13825 (2004).

9. Pharmacist refuses pill for victim. Chicago Tribune. February 11, 2004:C7.

10. Simon S. Pharmacists new players in abortion debate. Los Angeles Times. March 20, 2004:A18.

11. Sweeney JF. May a pharmacist refuse to fill a prescription? Plain Dealer. May 5, 2004:E1.

12. Associated Press. Pharmacist refuses to fill morning after prescription. (Accessed October 14, 2004. . . .)

13. Sauer M. Pharmacist to be fired in abortion controversy. St. Petersburg Times. December 19, 1991:1B.

14. State policies in brief: refusing to provide health services. New York: Alan Guttmacher Institute, September 1, 2004. (Accessed October 14, 2004. . . .)

15. Seeley RA. Advice for conscientious objectors in the armed forces. 5th ed. Philadelphia: Central Committee for Conscientious Objectors, 1998:1–2. (Accessed October 14, 2004. . . .)

16. 42 U.S.C. § 300a-7 (2004).

17. Mich. House Bill No. 5006 (As amended April 21, 2004).

18. Oregon House Bill No. 2010 (As amended May 11, 1999).

19. Hooks Super X, Inc. v. McLaughlin, 642 N.E. 2d 514 (Ind. 1994).

20. Section 2.01. In: Council on Ethical and Judicial Affairs. Code of medical ethics: current opinions with annotations. 2002–2003 ed. Chicago: American Medical Association, 2002.

21. Oregon Revised Statute § 127.885 § 4.01 (4) (2003).

22. Fassett WE, Wicks AC. Is pharmacy a profession? In: Weinstein BD, ed. Ethical issues in pharmacy. Vancouver, Wash.: Applied Therapeutics,1996:1–28.

23. American Pharmacists Association. Code of ethics for pharmacists: preamble. (Accessed October 14, 2004. . . .)

24. Hughes EC, ed. Obstetric-gynecologic terminology, with section on neonatology and glossary of congenital anomalies. Philadelphia: F.A. Davis, 1972.

25. Commodity Supplemental Food Program, 7 C.F.R. § 247.2 (2004).

26. Glasier A. Emergency postcoital contraception. N Engl J Med 1997;337:1058–64.

27. Daily reproductive health report: state politics & policy: Washington governor signs law requiring hospitals to offer emergency contraception to rape survivors. Menlo Park, Calif.: Kaisernetwork, April 2, 2002. (Accessed October 14, 2004. . . .)

28. Brownfield v. Daniel Freeman Marina Hospital, 208 Cal. App. 3d 405 (Cal. Ct. App. 1989).

29. Shelton v. Univ. of Medicine & Dentistry, 223 F.3d 220 (3d Cir. 2000).

30. Tribe LH. American constitutional law. 2nd ed. Mineola, N.Y.: Foundation Press, 1988:1183.

31. Brody JE. The politics of emergency contraception. New York Times. August 24, 2004:F7.

32. Trans World Airlines v. Hardison, 432 U.S. 63 (1977).

33. 1997–98 APhA Policy Committee report: pharmacist conscience clause. Washington, D.C.: American Pharmacists Association, 1997.

34. Politics wins over science. Capital Times. May 13, 2004:16A.

35. Alford S, Davis L, Brown L. Pharmacists' attitudes and awareness of emergency contraception for adolescents. Transitions 2001; 12(4):1–17.

36. Foster DG, Harper CC, Bley JJ, et al. Knowledge of emergency contraception among women aged 18 to 44 in California. Am J Obstet Gynecol 2004;191:150-6.

37. United States v. Macintosh, 283 U.S. 605, 634 (1931) (Hughes, C.J., dissenting).

38. Elliott D. Alabama nurses quit over morning-after pill. Presented on All Things Considered. Washington, D.C.: National Public Radio, July 28, 2004 (transcript). *Copyright © 2004 Massachusetts Medical Society.*

POSTSCRIPT

Should Pharmacists Be Allowed to Deny Prescriptions on Grounds of Conscience?

In November 2004, the FDA announced a labeling change for mifepristone. Because the FDA and the manufacturer Danco Laboratories had received reports of serious side effects, the warning label was changed to reflect this new information.

As of 2005, the federal government and 47 state governments had laws protecting conscientious objectors in health care. The Illinois Health Care Right of Conscience Act is the most detailed and protects physicians, health care personnel, health care facilities, and health care payers who refuse to participate in services that are contrary to their conscience. In April 2005, however, Gov. Rod Blagojevich issued an emergency rule requiring pharmacies to fill prescriptions for birth control and mifepristone "without delay." Bills have been introduced that specifically include pharmacists in the Health Care Right of Conscience Act.

Four states (South Dakota, Mississippi, Arkansas, and Georgia) have laws specifically recognizing a pharmacist's right of conscientious objection, while in 2005 California enacted a law requiring pharmacists to dispense these drugs. Considerable activity on both sides of the issue is going on in the states. The National Conference of State Legislatures monitors these bills. See http://www. ncsl.org/programs/health/conscienceclauses.htm.

In "Pharmacies, Pharmacists, and Conscientious Objection," Mark R. Wicclair argues that the health needs of patients and the professional obligations of pharmacists limit the extent to which they may refuse to assist patients who have lawful prescriptions for medically indicated drugs (*Kennedy Institute of Ethics Journal*, vol. 16, no. 3, 2006). On the other hand, Brian P. Knestout asserts that "conscience clauses" protect medical professionals who do not wish to perform or assist in procedures related to abortion, sterilization, or euthanasia ("An Essential Prescription: Why Pharmacist-Inclusive Clauses Are Necessary," *Journal of Contemporary Health Law and Policy*, Spring 2006).

ISSUE 21

Should Public Health Override Powers over Individual Liberty in Combatting Bioterrorism?

YES: Lawrence O. Gostin, from "Law and Ethics in a Public Health Emergency," *Hastings Center Report* (March–April 2002)

NO: George J. Annas, from "Bioterrorism, Public Health, and Human Rights," *Health Affairs* (November/December 2002)

ISSUE SUMMARY

YES: Law and public health professor Lawrence O. Gostin states that the threat of bioterrorism makes it imperative to reframe the balance between individual interests and society's need to protect itself so that the common good prevails.

NO: Law professor George J. Annas contends that taking human rights seriously is our best defense against terrorism and fosters public health on both a federal and global scale.

Most bioethical controversies develop over time, often with a single event crystallizing the debate. It would be hard to imagine a more dramatic and threatening series of events than those that occurred in the fall of 2001. First, there were the terrorist attacks on the World Trade Center in New York City and the Pentagon in Virginia on September 11. Second, beginning in October, there was the series of anthrax-related illnesses and deaths in Florida, New York, Washington, and other locations which, although unsolved, are presumed to be terror-related.

Suddenly Americans, accustomed to a level of personal security that is rare in the world, understood that they, too, are at risk. The possibility that more attacks using devastating biological, chemical, or nuclear agents could occur brought into high relief a debate that has gone on over the past few decades, primarily in the context of the HIV/AIDS epidemic. In circumstances where the public's health is endangered, how should the need to control the outbreak—whatever its source—be balanced against the fundamental rights of liberty and individual autonomy that are so basic to American values?

In the early- and mid-twentieth century, the U.S. public health system commanded a prominent role in identifying, tracking, and controlling epidemics. But in the antibiotic era, as infectious diseases waned in prevalence and severity, and as the more technological and groundbreaking aspects of medicine gained public attention and resources, the nation's public health infrastructure became outmoded. This was the conclusion of the 1988 Institute of Medicine (IOM) report, *The Future of Public Health;* the follow-up report in 2002, *The Future of the Public's Health in the Twenty-First Century*, concluded that the IOM's earlier recommendations had not been implemented. Simply put, the nation's public health system was not prepared for the anthrax attacks nor is it prepared for future possible attacks.

Against this background the federal Centers for Disease Control and Prevention (CDC), the nation's chief public health agency, asked the Center for Law and the Public's Health at Georgetown University to draft a Model State Emergency Health Powers Act. Although the CDC is a federally funded agency and provides support and technical assistance, public health activities are largely carried out by states under the "police powers" reserved for them by the Constitution.

Lawrence O. Goston is well known for his human rights advocacy, particularly in the HIV/AIDS epidemic. Therefore many bioethicists were surprised that the first draft of the Model Act (October 23, 2001), prepared with the cooperation of many individuals and groups, gave overwhelming powers to state governments. The first draft was withdrawn for revision, and a succeeding draft issued on December 21 answered some, but by no means all, of the objections.

In the following selections, Gostin and George J. Annas debate the provisions of the model law and the ethical principles that should undergird government's response in an age of bioterrorism. Gostin believes that the communitarian tradition of American thought, rather than the individualistic strain, must govern the appropriate balance between public health and individual liberty. Annas counters that it is unnecessary and counterproductive to sacrifice basic human rights to respond to terrorism.

YES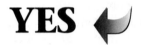

Lawrence O. Gostin

Law and Ethics in a Public Health Emergency

In 1974, the Surgeon General informed Congress that it was time to "close the book on infectious diseases." So sure was the United States that modern biomedicine would solve the problem of infectious diseases that government was already cutting funding from state and local public health agencies and beginning a massive build-up of biotechnology research and development. Having declared victory over infectious diseases, the new war would be waged against diseases of modern western civilization, principally cardiovascular disease and neoplasms.

The United States was also unconcerned about bioterrorism. To be sure, America had experienced bioterrorism in 1984 when the Rajneeshee cult contaminated salad bars in rural Oregon, causing over 750 cases of Salmonella poisoning. But the government and citizenry felt that America's geographic isolation meant it would be relatively immune from upheavals abroad.

Of course, the perception of safety and security evaporated on 11 September 2001. And then on 4 October, authorities confirmed the first case of inhalational anthrax in Florida, beginning a period in which five people died, hundreds were tested, and thousands treated. Although the method of delivery through the postal service was inefficient, the anthrax outbreak exposed the nation's vulnerability.

A sustained debate ensued about the public health system's preparedness to detect and respond quickly and effectively to bioterrorism and naturally occurring infectious diseases. Do public health agencies have sufficient laboratory capacity, information systems, and work force? Are there sufficient stockpiles of safe and effective vaccines and treatments? Do health and safety agencies efficiently share information and coordinate activities? Is communication to the public clear and authoritative? Unfortunately, the answer to these questions, and many others, is that the United States is ill prepared.[1]

Crumbling Foundations

The lack of preparedness for bioterrorism and naturally occurring infectious diseases is due primarily to insufficient financing. Before the recent influx of funding for homeland security,[2] traditional population-based public health

From *Hastings Center Report*, March–April 2002, pp. 9–11. Copyright © 2002 by Hastings Center Report. Reprinted by permission.

services received approximately 1 percent of all health dollars, with the rest going to health care and biotechnology.[3] At the federal level, over 95 percent of the health budget went to nondiscretionary spending, principally Medicaid and Medicare. Congress allocated half of the remaining 5 percent to the National Institutes of Health, whose budget has been approximately doubling in each of the last several years. The Public Health Service agencies together shared the remainder.[4] Even in the president's new bioterrorism budget for homeland security, biotechnology and health care take the lion's share, leaving relatively little for prevention.[5]

What is wrong with this picture? Expenditures on biotechnology and health care are not improper, but they are now out of proportion to the benefit derived. Biotechnology and health care contribute to only a small percentage of the population's health (estimated at less than 5 percent), but receive an inordinately high percentage of health funding (more than 95 percent). On the other hand, population-based services (such as sanitation, pure food and water, safe products and roads) contribute much more to health and longevity, but have been starved of resources.[6]

Individual health care services dominate federal and state budgets because of the values dominant in America. Both ends of the political spectrum celebrate personal freedom and choice—the political left emphasizes civil liberties while the political right focuses on markets and free enterprise. In this political climate, the public sees government as inefficient and burdensome. People would rather see ever-increasing advances in clinical medicine and freedom of choice in health care than stable and well-funded agencies regulating for the public welfare. The nation has lost the tradition of classical republicanism that valued the collective benefits of health, safety, and security.[7]

Public Health Law Reform

Another important reason for the lack of preparedness is that public health laws are antiquated. Many of these laws date back to the early twentieth century and predate modern science, medicine, and constitutional law.[8] Consequently, these laws do not provide a clear mission, essential services, or powers necessary for public health agencies to be effective.[9] These antiquated laws are often unconstitutional since they lack clear standards and procedural safeguards. Vague public health laws may be challenged in a crisis, adding to indecision and delay; more fundamentally, existing laws do not provide a hedge against arbitrary action and unfairness in the exercise of public health powers.

To rectify the problems of antiquity, inadequacy, and unfairness, the Robert Wood Johnson "Turning Point" program funded the development of a model public health law in collaboration with a consortium of states. The "Public Health Statute Modernization" Project, which began in 2001, had a three-year time horizon, with little public and political impetus for speedy reform. Following the events of 11 September and 4 October, however, the need for law reform captured the attention of political leaders. On 6 October, I received a call from Gene Matthews, general counsel of the Centers for Disease Control and Prevention (CDC), asking the Center for Law and the Public's Health to draft a Model State Emergency Health Powers Act (MSEHPA). Because the CDC feared that governors would introduce their own legislation in the absence of a model, Matthews asked for a draft within three to four weeks.

That began an intensive drafting process in collaboration with members of the National Governors Association, the National Conference of State Legislatures, the National Association of Attorneys General, the Association of State and Territorial Health Officials, and the National Conference of State and National Association of County and City Health Officials. The model law, or a version of it, has been introduced in nearly half of the states, with many more expected to consider it.

MSEHPA has been developed using an open and deliberative process. Federal agencies such as the CDC and Department of Justice provided intellectual support during its development, as did high-level staff of state governors, legislators, attorney generals, and health commissioners. The Center for Law and the Public's Health received thousands of comments about the model law from national organizations, academic institutions, practitioners, corporations, and the general public, and it has been widely discussed in the media.[10] Despite this rigorous and inclusive process, it has provoked criticism from a civil liberties and property rights perspective. As one governor's chief of staff said in a private meeting commenting on the model law: "The far left has met the far right, leaving the vast majority of Americans in the middle unprotected."

The Model Law

MSEHPA . . . is intended to support the vital functions of public health agencies while safeguarding personal and proprietary interests: planning, surveillance, management of property, and protection of persons. The planning and surveillance functions would be implemented immediately, but the measures affecting property and persons would be triggered only after a state's governor declares a public health emergency.

Declaration of a public health emergency.   A public health emergency is narrowly defined in the model law as involving an imminent threat caused by bioterrorism or a new or re-emerging infectious agent or biological toxin that poses a high probability of a large number of deaths or serious disabilities. Civil libertarians objected to a previous draft of the definition on two grounds: that it would permit compulsory powers against persons living with HIV/AIDS, and that state governors would have too much discretion. In response, the definition of a public health emergency was modified to exclude endemic diseases such as HIV/AIDS and to place checks on the governor. The legislature may, by majority vote, discontinue the state of emergency at any time. Similarly, the judiciary may overturn an emergency declaration if the governor has not complied with the standards and procedures in the model law. This reflects a preference for constitutional checks and balances, providing a role for each branch of government.

Emergency planning.   The governor must appoint a Public Health Emergency Planning Commission to design a plan for coordination of services; procurement of necessary materials and supplies; housing, feeding, and caring for affected populations; and vaccination and treatment. The planning requirement is important because most states do not have a systematic design for handling a public health emergency. Planning raises significant ethical issues, notably the proper criteria allocating vaccines, medicines, and health care services. On what basis should scarce resources be allocated: need, benefit, age, or utility? The model law does not resolve the numerous ethical or policy issues but insists that a rational plan be devised through a deliberative process.

Surveillance.   MSEHPA addresses measures necessary to detect and monitor infectious disease outbreaks. It requires prompt disease reporting, interviewing, and contact tracing. Existing law often does not facilitate, and may even hinder, surveillance. For example, most states do not require reporting of many of the critical agents of bioterrorism.[11] Consequently, if a case of smallpox or hemorrhagic fever is known or suspected, there is no assurance that public health authorities will be promptly notified. MSEHPA also facilitates exchange of health information if necessary to prevent, identify, or investigate a public health emergency. Existing state laws, due to privacy concerns, often prohibit the sharing of health information between public health and law enforcement agencies, between public health agencies and health care organizations, and among public health agencies in different states. While individuals have the right to expect a certain amount of privacy to prevent harms and embarrassment, a balance needs to be struck to ensure public health and safety. Consider the potential impact of a case of bioterrorism in New York City, if a health officer could not exchange data with the public safety officer, monitor hospitals and pharmacies for unusual clusters of symptoms, or obtain health records from New Jersey or Connecticut.

Management of property.   MSEHPA authorizes the public health authority to close, decontaminate, or procure facilities and materials to respond to a public health emergency; dispose of infectious waste safely; perform appropriate burials; and obtain and deploy health care supplies. These powers are necessary to ensure sufficient availability of vaccines, medicines, and hospital beds, and sufficient power to regulate, close, or destroy dangerous facilities. The political right has engaged in a sustained attack on these provisions, claiming that they interfere with the freedom to own and control personal property. Indeed, the drafters have been lobbied by virtually every major corporate sector, including the food, transportation, hospital, and pharmaceutical industries, some of which have hired large law firms to help press their case.

Although the right to possess and enjoy private property is important, owners have always been subject to the restriction that property not be used in a way that poses a health hazard.[12] MSEHPA provides a right of compensation to owners only if the government "takes" private property for public purposes—if, for example, it confiscates private stocks of drugs to treat patients or takes over a private hospital to quarantine persons exposed to infection. No compensation would be provided for a "nuisance abatement"—closing a facility that poses a public health threat or destroying property contaminated with smallpox or anthrax. Although entrepreneurs may complain that such private losses are unfair, MSEHPA fully comports with modern constitutional law and enlightened public policy.[13] If government were forced to compensate for all nuisance abatements, it would significantly chill public health regulation.

Protection of persons. MSEHPA permits public health authorities to physically examine, test, vaccinate, or treat individuals to prevent or ameliorate an infectious condition, and to isolate or quarantine individuals to prevent or limit the transmission of an infectious disease. Civil libertarians have argued that individuals should be neither confined nor compelled to receive vaccines or treatment. But this view has never been accepted even in the most liberal societies. It is generally accepted that persons who pose a significant risk to the public may be subject to restraint. MSEHPA's powers of vaccination, treatment, and civil confinement are not new, but have been part of public health law since the founding of the republic. The exercise of these powers has also been upheld by the courts on grounds of community health and security: "There are manifold restraints to which every person is necessarily subject for the common good. On any other basis organized society could not exist with safety to its members."[14]

To ensure an appropriate sphere of liberty and justice, MSEHPA contains many safeguards that do not exist in most statutes: vaccines and treatments cannot be imposed on persons who would suffer harm; cultural and religious beliefs must be respected; and the needs of persons isolated or quarantined must be met, including food, clothing, shelter, and health care. Orders for isolation or quarantine are subject to judicial review, with full procedural due process.

The Future of Public Health

In many ways, America has the public health system it deserves—underfunded, ill prepared, and dispirited. The government has starved public health agencies of resources, allowing the public health infrastructure to deteriorate. The public has valued high-glamour genetics and high-technology biomedicine over basic prevention and population-based services. And the legislature has neglected the legal foundations of public health. The law lacks a coherent vision of an appropriate mission, essential services, powers, and safeguards for public health agencies.

The *Institute of Medicine Report on Public Health Preparedness,* due to be published this year, will set out the intellectual critique of the public health system. The events of 11 September and 4 October will provide the impetus for change. Now it is time to change the nation's values, priorities, and funding to recognize the overwhelming importance of assuring the conditions in which the people can be healthy, safe, and secure.

Notes

1. Institute of Medicine, *The Future of Public Health* (Washington, D.C.: National Academy Press, 1988); Centers for Disease Control and Prevention, *Public Health's Infrastructure: A Status Report,* submitted to the Appropriations Committee of the United States Senate in 2001.

2. Protecting the Homeland: The President's Budget for 2003 (4 February 2002), . . . at p. 5.

3. K. W. Eilbert et al., *Measuring Expenditures for Essential Public Health Services* 17 (Washington, D.C.: Public Health Foundation, 1996). See also Centers for Disease Control, "Estimated National Spending on Prevention: United States, 1988," *Morbidity & Mortality Weekly Report* 41 (1992): 529, 531.

4. See J. I. Boufford and P. R. Lee, *Health Policies for the 21st Century: Challenges and Recommendations for the U.S. Department of Health and Human Services* (New York: Milbank Memorial Fund, 2001).

5. S. Gorman, "Shortchanging Prevention?" *National Journal,* 9 February 2002, 391.

6. L.O. Gostin, J. P. Koplan, and F. Grad, "The Law and the Public's Health: The Foundations," in *Law in Public Health Practice,* ed. R. A. Goodman et al., (New York: Oxford University Press, forthcoming).

7. D. E. Beauchamp, "Community: The Neglected Tradition of Public Health," *Hastings Center Report* 15 (1985): 28–36.

8. L.O. Gostin, S. Burris, and Z. Lazzarini, "The Law and the Public's Health: A Study of Infectious Disease Law in the United States," *Columbia Law Review* 99 (1999): 59–128.

9. L.O. Gostin, "Public Health Law Reform," *American Journal of Public Health* 91 (2001): 1365–68.

10. J. Gillis, "States Weighing Laws to Fight Bioterrorism," *The Washington Post,* 19 November 2001.

11. H. Horton et al., "Disease Reporting as a Tool for Bioterrorism Preparedness," *Journal of Law, Medicine and Ethics,* forthcoming.

12. Commonwealth v. Alger, 7 Cush.53, 84–85 (1851).

13. Lucas v. South Carolina Coastal Council, 505 U.S. 1992 (1992).

14. Jacobson v. Massachusetts, 197 U.S. 11, 26 (1905).

George J. Annas 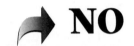 **NO**

Bioterrorism, Public Health, and Human Rights

A central lesson from 9/11 is that threats to public health are national and global. Unfortunately, public health as a field has an unappealing tendency to look backward when planning for the future. Even the influential 1988 report of the Institute of Medicine, *The Future of Public Health,* ignored the need for federal public health leadership and financing.[1] Rather than "moving public health into the 21st century [the report tried to] return it to the 19th century," leaving us poorly prepared for bioterrorism.[2] As Lawrence Gostin's paper outlines, the Centers for Disease Control and Prevention's (CDC's) request to develop a state emergency powers act in the wake of the anthrax attacks reflects this regressive tendency. Its exclusive concentration on the state level misses an important opportunity to exercise national public health leadership and instead promotes a return to the paternalistic pre-human rights days of nineteenth-century public health practices such as forced examination and quarantine.

In this brief commentary I make three arguments: (1) Bioterrorism should move us toward a more federalized and globalized public health system, (2) protecting basic human and constitutional rights is essential to effective coordination of medicine and public health, and (3) 9/11 and the suggested act should prompt thoughtful reflection, debate, and action to modernize public health practice.

Federal (and global) public health State public health laws are often antiquated, but their most antiquated feature is their underlying premise that public health is exclusively a state-level concern. A bioterrorist attack on the United States, for example, is inherently a matter of national security, making it a federal matter. That is why the FBI, not state or local police, took almost immediate control in the wake of the anthrax attacks. State laws regarding bioterrorism should be primarily aimed at preparing state and local authorities for their important job of assisting federal agencies, such as the new U.S. Department of Homeland Security, in the response. Biological attacks are different in kind from nuclear and chemical attacks, and they require specially tailored defenses.[3]

Public health policy should be national, and the addition of national security to federal financing and interstate commerce provides sufficient constitutional authority for Congress to enact legislation giving the federal government the leadership role in public health in the twenty-first century. In response to bioterrorism, in particular, it is imperative that the federal government develop a national plan that individual states can help implement, and that the federal government supply the states with badly needed financial and other resources to improve their public health infrastructure, training, and coordination.

At the outset of the twenty-first century, bioterrorism, although only one threat to public health, can be the catalyst to effectively "federalize" and integrate much of what are now uncoordinated and piecemeal state and local public health programs. This should include a renewed effort for national health insurance; national licensure for physicians, nurses, and allied health professionals; and national patient-safety standards. Federal public health leadership will also help us look outward and recognize that prevention of future bioterrorist attacks and even ordinary epidemics will require international cooperation.[4] In this regard, the threat of bioterrorism joins HIV/AIDS and other epidemics to demonstrate the need to globalize public health.

Public health and medicine   A major planning question in responding to a bioterrorist attack is the relationship between medicine and public health. It is almost certain that any attack will first be recognized by physicians working in a hospital emergency room.[5] Therefore, proposals to train emergency room personnel to recognize patients exposed to the most likely bioterrorist agents make perfect sense, as do up-to-date communication systems that can track relevant disease occurrences quickly and accurately (although there is no necessity to report data that identify patients). But who should be in charge after an outbreak has been confirmed?

The suggested act assumes that a state's governor will designate "public health officials" to be in charge and that these officials—who will be issued badges—will be empowered to take over hospitals and order physicians to examine and treat (and quarantine) individuals against their will, even when there is no evidence at all that the individual is either sick or contagious. The act's first draft was even more extreme, making it a crime for any individual to refuse to be examined or treated and a crime for a physician to refuse an order by a public health official to examine or treat a patient.[6] Moreover, should any patient be injured, or even killed, by the treatment (as, for example, immunocompromised individuals could be by smallpox vaccine), the public health officials and state would be immune from lawsuit.

This approach is likely to be counterproductive. Despite its talk about balancing human rights with disease prevention, the suggested act unnecessarily ignores basic human rights. Physicians, on the other hand, have effectively incorporated the doctrine of informed consent into their core medical ethics precepts. Public health still favors legal mandates and government-backed paternalism. Public health should be abandoning paternalism, rather than attempting to use 9/11 to increase it. Public health officials are likely to be much more effective in responding to emergencies if they work with both physicians and the public, rather than trying to exercise arbitrary and unaccountable power over them.

As evidenced by both 9/11 and the anthrax attacks, U.S. hospitals and physicians stand ready to help in any way they can in a mass emergency. The public is also eager—often too eager—to accept medications and line up to seek screening and care at hospitals. The real problem in a bioterrorist event will be supplying medical care, drugs, and vaccines to those who demand them. Nonetheless, the prospect of arbitrary forced treatment and quarantine would rightly engender distrust in government and public health officials and could actually discourage those who might have been exposed from seeking treatment at all—even encourage them to escape to another state. As 9/11 demonstrated, most people want to protect their families first and are likely to avoid public health officials who they believe might arbitrarily separate them from their families. As long as the public trusts its physicians and public health professionals, the problem will not be getting Americans to accept treatment, it will be persuading the worried well that they don't need treatment.

Democracy and public health   The suggested act has been criticized by both civil liberties and libertarian groups. But they are hardly alone. As the act's authors note on the cover page of their second (21 December 2001) and apparently final draft, not one of the groups involved in any way with the original draft and the revision, including the authors themselves, have endorsed the proposal as written.[7] The original "model" act has been relabeled as simply a "draft for discussion," prepared "to facilitate and encourage communication," and does "not represent the official policy, endorsement, or views" of the Center for Law and the Public's Health, the CDC, the National Governors Association (NGA), the National Conference of State Legislatures (NCSL), the Association of State and Territorial Health Officials (ASTHO), the National Association of County and City Health Officials (NACCHO), or the National Association of Attorneys General (NAAG), or anyone else.[8]

There is no chance that every state, or even many states, will adopt the suggested act, so if uniformity is seen as necessary, only a federal statute can provide it. So far, only Delaware and South Carolina have embraced the suggested act. More typically, states have ignored it, or like California, have considered it and rejected it outright. Other states, like Minnesota, have adopted some of its provisions but have rewritten them to be consistent with contemporary medical ethics and constitutional rights.

Under the new Minnesota law, for example, even in a public health emergency, "individuals have a fundamental right to refuse medical treatment, testing, physical or mental examination, vaccination, participation in experimental procedures and protocols, collection of specimens and preventive treatment programs."[9] Of course there are extreme circumstances under which isolation or quarantine can be employed. But the Minnesota legislature permits such measures only under much more limited conditions; the right to refuse all interventions continues in isolation and quarantine; and family members are permitted to visit. Most of the other provisions of the suggested act, including the immunity provisions, were referred to the Minnesota commissioner of health, who was instructed to study them and report back to the legislature, after having solicited public comment on any recommendations.[10] The Minnesota legislature properly recognized that human rights and health are not inherently conflicting goals that must be traded off against each other; they are, as Jonathan Mann and colleagues first articulated in the context of the international HIV/AIDS epidemic, "inextricably linked."[11]

The suggested act was drafted under extreme, albeit self-imposed, time constraints in the immediate aftermath of 9/11 and the anthrax attacks, when fear ruled reason. This is a predictable prescription for disaster. Sensible public health and bioterrorism legislation must be drafted in a calm atmosphere, in a transparent, public process.[12] Most importantly, as Ken Wing has noted, "statute drafting is a technical and instrumental job—one that should follow, not precede the more fundamental task of deciding what the statute ought to say."[13]

Ultimately, public health must rely not on force but on persuasion, and not on blind trust but on trust based on transparency, accountability, democracy, and human rights. There is plenty of time to draft and debate a twenty-first-century federal public health law that takes constitutional rights seriously, unites the public with its medical caretakers, treats medicine and public health as true partners, and moves us in the direction of global cooperation.

Notes

1. Institute of Medicine, *The Future of Public Health* (Washington: National Academy Press, 1988). But see more recently, IOM, *America's Vital Interest in Global Health: Protecting Our People, Enhancing Our Economy, and Advancing Our International Interests* (Washington: National Academy Press, 1997).

2. G. J. Annas, L. Glantz, and N. A. Scotch, "Back to the Future: The IOM Report Reconsidered," *American Journal of Public Health* (July 1991): 835–837.

3. M. Hamburg, "Homeland Security Research and Critical infrastructure," Testimony before the House Energy and Commerce Subcommittee on Oversight and Investigations, 9 July 2002. See also M. T. Osterholm, "Emerging Infections—Another Warning," *New England Journal of Medicine* (27 April 2000): 1280–1281.

4. J. Frenk and O. Gómez-Dantés, "Globalization and the Challenges to Health Systems," *Health Affairs* (May/June 2002): 160–165; D. P. Fidler, "A Globalized Theory of Public Health Law," *Journal of Law, Medicine, and Ethics* (Summer 2002): 150–161; and W. Mariner, "Bioterrorism Act: The Wrong Response," *National Law Journal* (17 December 2001): 18.

5. D. A. Henderson, "Public Health Preparedness," in *Science and Technology in a Vulnerable World,* ed. A. H. Teich, S. D. Nelson, and S. J. Lita (Washington: American Association for the Advancement of Science, 2002), 33–40.

6. G. J. Annas, "Bioterrorism, Public Health, and Civil Liberties," *New England Journal of Medicine* (25 April 2002): 1337–1342.

7. "The Model State Emergency Health Powers Act, as of December 21, 2001," . . . (28 August 2002). Text of the suggested act is also available in the *Journal of Law, Medicine, and Ethics* (Summer 2002): 322–348, although the disclaimer has been moved to the end in this publication.

8. "The Model State Emergency Health Powers Act, as of December 21, 2001."

9. *2002 Minnesota Chapter Law 402* (signed by the governor 22 May 2002).

10. Ibid.

11. J. Mann et al., "Health and Human Rights," *Health and Human Rights* 1, no. 1 (1994): 6–23. And see generally, J. Mann et al., eds., *Health and Human Rights: A Reader* (New York: Routledge, 1999); and G. J. Annas, "Is Privacy the Enemy of Public Health?" (Review of *The Limits of Privacy,* by Amitai Etzioni), *Health Affairs* (July/Aug 1999): 197–198.

12. M. T. Osterholm and J. Schwartz, *Living Terrors: What America Needs to Know to Survive the Coming Bioterrorist Catastrophe* (New York: Dell, 2000), 154–155.

13. K. Wing, "The Model Act: Is It the Best Way to Prepare for the Next Public Health Emergency?" *Northwest Public Health* (Spring/Summer 2002): 10–11.

POSTSCRIPT

Should Public Health Override Powers over Individual Liberty in Combatting Bioterrorism?

As of July 2006, 171 bills or resolutions based on the Model State Emergency Health Power Act had been introduced in 44 states and the District of Columbia; 38 states have passed some version of the Act. The most recent version, dated December 12, 2001, can be found at: http://www.publichealthlaw.net/Resources/Modellaws.htm#MSEHPA.

Many of the same issues that arise in the context of a bioterrorist threat also apply to natural disasters such as pandemic influenza, most recently the potential threat of a global avian flu epidemic. Although planning for such an event is ongoing, including stockpiling doses of Tamiflu, the only effective medication, the results are not encouraging. The main problems are the lack of an effective vaccine, a health care system that cannot accommodate an epidemic, and erratic regional planning, according to Dr. John G. Bartlett ("Planning for Avian Influenza," *Annals of Internal Medicine,* July 18, 2006). Larry Gostin analyzes public health strategies in terms of public benefits and private rights in "Public Health Strategies for Pandemic Influenza: Ethics and the Law" (*Journal of the American Medical Association,* April 12, 2006).

For other views on public health in an emergency, see Ronald Bayer and James Colgrove, "Bioterrorism, Public Health, and the Law," *Health Affairs* (November–December 2002). They argue that although the debates over the Model Act were triggered by the threat of bioterrorism, they illustrate broader philosophical differences between guarding the common welfare and respecting individual liberty. In the same issue of *Health Affairs*, Amitai Etzioni argues in "Public Health Law: A Communitarian Perspective" that the attacks on America's homeland clearly demonstrate the need to trim the individualistic excesses of the previous generation and make more room for the public interest. Also in this issue, George M. Gray and David P. Repeik describe how fear affects public health in "Dealing With the Dangers of Fear: The Role of Risk Communication." Griffin Trotter sees the threat of terrorism as a challenge to revise bioethicists' long-standing deference to individual autonomy in "Of Terrorism and Healthcare: Jolting the Old Habits," *Cambridge Quarterly of Healthcare Ethics* (vol. 11, 2002), pp. 411-414. See also Jonathan Moreno, ed., *In the Wake of Terror: Medicine and Morality in a Time of Crisis* (MIT Press, 2003). Karine Morin, Daniel Higginson, and Michael Goldrich, writing for the American Medical Association's Council on Ethical and Judicial Affairs, present the AMA's position on the responsibilities of physicians in terrorist attacks or disasters in "Physician Obligation in Disaster Preparedness and Response" (*Cambridge Quarterly of Healthcare Ethics,* vol. 15, 2006). Several commentaries follow this article.

Contributors to This Volume

EDITOR

CAROL LEVINE joined the United Hospital Fund in New York City in October 1996 where she directs the Families and Health Care Project. This project focuses on developing partnerships between health care professionals and family caregivers, who provide most of the long-term and chronic care to elderly, seriously ill, or disabled relatives. She founded the Orphan Project: Families and Children in the HIV Epidemic in 1991. She was director of the Citizens Commission on AIDS in New York City from 1987 to 1991. As a senior staff associate of The Hastings Center, she edited the *Hastings Center Report*. In 1993 she was awarded a MacArthur Foundation Fellowship for her work in AIDS policy and ethics. She has written several articles and books, most recently *Always On Call: When Illness Turns Families Into Caregivers* (Vanderbilt University Press, 2004); with Thomas H. Murray, *The Cultures of Caregiving: Conflict and Common Ground among Families, Health Professionals, and Policy Makers* (Johns Hopkin's University Press, 2004); and with Geoff Foster and John Williamson, *A Generation at Risk: The Global Impact of HIV/AIDS on Orphan and Vulnerable Children* (Cambridge University Press, 2005).

STAFF

Larry Loeppke	Managing Editor
Jill Peter	Senior Developmental Editor
Susan Brusch	Senior Developmental Editor
Beth Kundert	Production Manager
Jane Mohr	Project Manager
Tara McDermott	Design Coordinator
Nancy Meissner	Editorial Assistant
Julie Keck	Senior Marketing Manager
Mary Klein	Marketing Communications Specialist
Alice Link	Marketing Coordinator
Lori Church	Pemissions Coordinator

AUTHORS

FELICIA ACKERMAN is a professor of philosophy at Brown University in Providence, Rhode Island. Her articles have appeared in various philosophy journals and anthologies, including *Philosophical Perspectives* and the *Midwest Studies in Philosophy* book series. She is also a writer of short stories, some of which deal with issues in medical ethics. She received her Ph.D. from the University of Michigan.

MARCIA ANGELL is a senior lecturer in the department of social medicine at Harvard Medical School and the former editor-in-chief of *The New England Journal of Medicine*. Angell writes frequently in professional journals and the popular media on a wide range of topics, particularly medical ethics, health policy, the nature of medical evidence, the interface of medicine and the law, and care at the end of life. Her book, *Science on Trial: The Clash of Medical Evidence and the Law in the Breast Implant Case*, was published by W. W. Norton in 1996.

GEORGE J. ANNAS is the Edward R. Utley Professor of Health Law and chairman of the Health Law Department at the Boston University School of Public Health in Boston, Massachusetts. He is also the cofounder of Global Lawyers & Physicians and the Patients Rights Project. For five years, he was the director of the Boston University School of Law's Center for Law and Health Sciences. He is a widely published national expert in the field of law and medicine, whose books include *Some Choice: Law, Medicine, and the Market* (Oxford University Press, 1998) and *The Rights of Patients: The Basic ACLU Guide to Patient Rights* (Humana Press, 1992).

ROBERT M. ARNOLD is director of the Palliative Care Service at the University of Pittsburgh's Medical Center. He is coauthor, with Charles W. Lidz and Lynn Fisher, of *The Erosion of Autonomy in Long-Term Care* (Oxford University Press, 1992) and coeditor of *Procuring Organs for Transplant: The Debate Over Non-Heart-Beating Cadaver Protocols* (Johns Hopkins University Press, 1995).

KEN BAUM is a physician and attorney at the firm of Wiggin and Dana, New Haven, Connecticut.

GENE BISHOP, MD, is an internist at Pennsylvania Hospital and a consultant with the Pennsylvania Health Law Project in Philadelphia.

LESLIE J. BLACKHALL recently joined the faculty at the University of Virginia as an associate professor of medicine and an associate professor of medical education. She is a medical director at the Center for Geriatric and Palliative Care and coordinator for research at the Center for Biomedical Ethics.

M. GREGG BLOCHE is professor of law at Georgetown University and adjunct professor at the Bloomberg School of Public Health, Johns Hopkins University.

AMY C. BRODKEY, MD, is a clinical associate professor of psychiatry at the University of Pennsylvania School of Medicine and medical director of the behavioral health service of the Family Practice and Counseling Network, Philadelphia.

JULIE CANTOR is an attorney at Yale University School of Medicine.

MEGAN CLAYTON is a research associate at the Oxford Centre for Applied Ethics, Oxford University, England.

ROBERT W. DONNELL, MD, is a staff physician, Department of Medicine, St. Mary's Hospital, Rogers, Arkansas.

BENNETT FODDY is a research associate at the Oxford Centre for Applied Ethics, Oxford University, England.

KATHLEEN M. FOLEY holds The Society of Memorial Sloan-Kettering Cancer Center chair in pain research and is director of the Project on Death in America of the Open Society Institute. She is a professor of neurology and pharmacology at the Weill Medical College of Cornell University and attending neurologist in the Pain and Palliative Care Service at Memorial Sloan-Kettering.

GELYA FRANK is a professor of occupational science and occupational therapy and anthropology in the department of occupational science and occupational therapy at the University of Southern California, in Los Angeles, California.

ROBERT P. GEORGE is McCormick Professor of Jurisprudence at Princeton University and director of the James Madison Program in American Ideals and Institutions. A lawyer and constitutional scholar, George is the author of *Making Men Moral: Civil Liberties and Public Morality* (Oxford University Press, 1993) and *In Defense of Natural Law* (Oxford University Press, 1999).

LAWRENCE O. GOSTIN is a professor of law at Georgetown University, a professor of public health at the Johns Hopkins University, and the director of the Center for Law and the Public's Health at Johns Hopkins and Georgetown Universities. He is also the codirector of the Georgetown/Johns Hopkins Program on Law and Public Health. Gostin is the health law and ethics editor of the *Journal of the American Medical Association* (*JAMA*).

JEROME GROOPMAN is a professor of medicine at Harvard, the chief of experimental medicine at Beth-Israel Deaconess Medical Center, and the author, most recently, of *The Anatomy of Hope* (Random House).

MICHAEL L. GROSS is co-director of the Graduate Program in Applied and Professional Ethics, Division of International Relations, School of Political Science, University of Haifa, Israel.

DONALD W. HERBE is a law student at Cleveland State University.

MATTHEW F. HOLLON is an attending physician at the University of Washington Medical Center, Roosevelt, General Internal Medical Center. He is also acting instructor of medicine at the University of Washington.

ALAN F. HOLMER is president of the Pharmaceutical Research and Manufacturers of America. In 1981 President Reagan appointed him deputy assistant to the president for intergovernmental affairs, with responsibility for liaison with state and local officials. Holmer has served as an adjunct professor at Georgetown University Law Center and as a guest lecturer at various law schools and universities.

THE INSTITUTE OF MEDICINE serves as adviser to the nation on matters of health. Established in 1970 under the charter of the National Academy of Sciences, the Institute provides objective, independent, evidence-based advice to policymakers, health professionals, the private sector, and the public.

MARK KUCZEWSKI is a philosopher and director of the Neiswanger Institute for Bioethics and Health Policy at the Stritch School of Medicine, Loyola University, in Chicago.

PATRICK LEE is associate professor of philosophy at the Franciscan University in Steubenville, Ohio. He is the author of *Abortion and Unborn Life* (1996).

CHARLES W. LIDZ is a professor of psychiatry at the University of Pittsburgh. Currently, he is on leave from the University of Pittsburgh and works at the University of Massachusetts Medical School, where he is director of the Center for Mental Health Services Research.

MARGARET OLIVIA LITTLE is a philosopher at the Kennedy Institute of Ethics, Georgetown University. Her research interests focus on the intersection of ethics, feminist theory, and public policy.

JEROD M. LOEB is vice president for research and performance measurement, Division of Research at the Joint Commission on Accreditation of Healthcare Organizations. Prior to joining the Joint Commission, Loeb was assistant vice president for science, technology, and public health at the American Medical Association (AMA) in Chicago where he also served as secretary of the AMA's Council on Scientific Affairs.

STEVEN LUTTRELL is senior registrar in the department of health care for older people at Whittington Hospital, London, England.

JONATHAN H. MARKS is a barrister at Matrix Chambers, London, and Greenwall Fellow in Bioethics at Georgetown University Law Center and Bloomberg School of Public Health, Johns Hopkins University.

MARY FAITH MARSHALL, Ph.D., is a professor of bioethics and associate dean for Social Medicine and Medical Humanities, College of Medicine, University of Minnesota.

MASSACHUSETTS CITIZENS FOR CHILDREN (MCC) is a nonprofit statewide child advocacy organization whose mission is to improve the lives of the state's most vulnerable children. It is a national leader in child abuse prevention. To effect change, MCC works to improve state services for children, pushes for needed legislation and, when necessary, takes legal action.

PATRICK J. McCRUDEN is vice president of mission and ethics at St. Joseph's Mercy Health Center in Hot Springs, Arkansas.

VICKI MICHEL is an adjunct professor at Loyola Law School in Los Angeles, California.

STEVEN H. MILES is an associate professor of medicine in the division of geriatric medicine at the Hennepin County Medical Center and in the Center for Biomedical Ethics at the University of Minnesota in Minneapolis, Minnesota.

SHEILA MURPHY is an associate professor at the Annenberg School for Communication and in the department of psychology at the University of Southern California, in Los Angeles.

THOMAS H. MURRAY is president of The Hastings Center in Garrison, New York. He was formerly a professor of biomedical ethics and director of the Center for Biomedical Ethics in the School of Medicine at Case Western Reserve University in Cleveland, Ohio. He is a founding editor of the journal *Medical Humanities Review* and the author or editor of over 100 publications, including *The Worth of a Child* (University of California Press, 1996), *Feeling Good, Doing Better* (Humana Press, 1984), and *Which Babies Shall Live?* (Humana Press, 1985), coauthored with Arthur L. Caplan.

ONORA O'NEILL is principal of Newnham College, Cambridge University, England. She has chaired the Nuffield Council on Bioethics and is currently chair of the Nuffield Foundation. She has written widely on political philosophy and ethics, international justice, and the philosophy of Immanuel Kant.

LYNN M. PALTROW is an attorney and executive director of National Advocates for Pregnant Women.

CHARLES PETERS is an associate professor of clinical pediatrics in the division of hematology-oncology and blood and marrow transplantation at the University of Minnesota Medical School in Minneapolis, Minnesota.

THE PRESIDENT'S COUNCIL ON BIOETHICS was created by President George W. Bush in November 2001 to advise the president on bioethical issues that may arise in connection with advances in biomedical science and technology.

JANET RADCLIFFE-RICHARDS is a member of the Centre for Bioethics and Philosophy of Medicine, department of medicine, University College London.

TOM REGAN is a professor of philosophy and a department chair at North Carolina State University in Raleigh, North Carolina, where he has been teaching since 1967. He has published many books and articles on animal rights and environmental ethics, including *The Struggle for Animal Rights* (ISAR, 1987). In addition to his scholarly activities, his work as a video author and director has earned him major international awards.

LAINIE FRIEDMAN ROSS is an assistant professor of pediatrics in the McLean Center for Clinical Medical Ethics, Department of Medicine, at the University of Chicago in Chicago, Illinois. She is also director of the Ethics Case Consultation Service and codirector of the Multidisciplinary Ethics Lecture Series at the university. Her many articles have appeared in such journals as *The New England Journal of Medicine, Bioethics,* and *The Hastings Center Report,* and she is the author of *Children, Families, and Health Care Decision Making* (Clarendon Press, 1998).

CHRISTOPHER JAMES RYAN is a consultant-liaison psychiatrist in the Department of Psychiatry at Westmead Hospital in Westmead, New South Wales, Australia.

MICHAEL J. SANDEL teaches political philosophy at Harvard University, where he is the Anne T. and Robert M. Bass Professor of Government. He serves on the President's Council on Bioethics.

MARK SHELDON is a lecturer in philosophy and also in the medical ethics and humanities program at the Feinberg School of Medicine. He has served as adjunct senior scholar at the MacLean Center for Clinical Medical Ethics at the University of Chicago and senior policy analyst at the American Medical Association. Formerly professor of philosophy and adjunct professor of medicine at Indiana University and the Indiana University School of Medicine, he currently serves as adjunct faculty at the Neiswanger Institute for Bioethics and Health Policy at the Loyola University Stritch School of Medicine and as adjunct faculty and ethicist at Rush-Presbyterian-St. Luke's Medical Center in Chicago.

SILJA J. A. TALVI is a senior editor at *These Times*, an investigative journalist and essayist with credits in many newspapers and magazines, including *The Nation*, *Salon*, and the *Christian Science Monitor.*

ANN SOMMERVILLE is head of the ethics department of the British Medical Association in London, England.

JEAN TOAL is a justice of the South Carolina supreme court.

HOWARD TRACHTMAN, MD, is a physician at Schneider Children's Hospital, New Hyde Park, New York.

ROBERT F. WEIR is director of the Program in Biomedical Ethics and Medical Humanities in the College of Medicine at the University of Iowa. A professor of pediatrics, he is also on the faculty of the university's School of Religion. His major research interests include ethical issues at the beginning of life, at the end of life, and in genetics. He is the editor of *Physician-Assisted Suicide* (Indiana University Press, 1997) and *Stored Tissue Samples: Ethical, Legal, and Public Policy Implications* (University of Iowa Press, 1998).

WEST VIRGINIA DEPARTMENT OF HEALTH AND HUMAN RESOURCES administers the Medicaid program in the state.

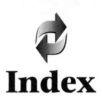

Index